Diabetes Mellitus: Associated Conditions

Editors

LEONID PORETSKY
EMILIA PAULINE LIAO

ENDOCRINOLOGY AND METABOLISM CLINICS OF NORTH AMERICA

www.endo.theclinics.com

Consulting Editor
DEREK LeROITH

March 2014 • Volume 43 • Number 1

ELSEVIER

1600 John F. Kennedy Boulevard • Suite 1800 • Philadelphia, Pennsylvania, 19103-2899

http://www.theclinics.com

ENDOCRINOLOGY AND METABOLISM CLINICS OF NORTH AMERICA Volume 43, Number 1
March 2014 ISSN 0889-8529, ISBN 13: 978-0-323-28704-3

Editor: Jessica McCool
Developmental Editor: Susan Showalter

Endocrinology and Metabolism Clinics of North America (ISSN 0889-8529) is published quarterly by Elsevier Inc., 360 Park Avenue South, New York, NY 10010-1710. Months of issue are March, June, September, and December. Periodicals postage paid at New York, NY and additional mailing offices. Subscription prices are USD 330.00 per year for US individuals, USD 581.00 per year for US institutions, USD 165.00 per year for US students and residents, USD 415.00 per year for Canadian individuals, USD 718.00 per year for Canadian institutions, USD 480.00 per year for international individuals, USD 718.00 per year for international institutions, and USD 245.00 per year for international and Canadian and foreign students/residents. To receive student/resident rate, orders must be accompanied by name of affiliated institution, date of term, and the signature of program/residency coordinator on institution letterhead. Orders will be billed at individual rate until proof of status is received. Foreign air speed delivery is included in all *Clinics* subscription prices. All prices are subject to change without notice. **POSTMASTER:** Send address changes to *Endocrinology and Metabolism Clinics of North America*, Elsevier Health Sciences Division, Subscription Customer Service, 3251 Riverport Lane, Maryland Heights, MO 63043. **Customer Service: Telephone: 1-800-654-2452** (U.S. and Canada); **1-314-447-8871** (outside U.S. and Canada). **Fax: 1-314-447-8029. E-mail: journalscustomerservice-usa@elsevier.com** (for print support); **journalsonlinesupport-usa@elsevier.com** (for online support).

Reprints. For copies of 100 or more, of articles in this publication, please contact the Commercial Rights Department, Elsevier Inc., 360 Park Avenue South, New York, NY 10010-1710; phone: +1-212-633-3874; fax: +1-212-633-3820; E-mail: reprints@elsevier.com.

Endocrinology and Metabolism Clinics of North America is covered in *MEDLINE/PubMed (Index Medicus)*, *EMBASE/Excerpta Medica, Current Contents/Clinical Medicine, Current Contents/Life Sciences, Science Citation Index, ISI/BIOMED, BIOSIS,* and *Chemical Abstracts.*

Printed and bound by CPI Group (UK) Ltd, Croydon, CR0 4YY

Contributors

CONSULTING EDITOR

DEREK LeROITH, MD, PhD
Director of Research, Division of Endocrinology, Metabolism, and Bone Diseases,
Department of Medicine, Mount Sinai School of Medicine, New York, New York

EDITORS

LEONID PORETSKY, MD
Chief, Division of Endocrinology and Metabolism; Vice-Chairman for Research,
Department of Medicine; Director, Gerald J. Friedman Diabetes Institute,
Gerald J. Friedman Chair for Endocrinology, Beth Israel Medical Center; Professor of
Medicine, Albert Einstein College of Medicine, New York, New York

EMILIA PAULINE LIAO, MD
Assistant Professor, Department of Medicine, Albert Einstein College of Medicine,
Bronx; Associate Program Director, Endocrinology, Beth Israel Medical Center, New York,
New York

AUTHORS

MOSTAFA A. ALBAYATI, BSc, MBBS
Research Fellow, Department of Vascular Surgery, Southampton General Hospital,
University Hospital Southampton NHS Foundation Trust, Southampton, United Kingdom

TOM BATEMARCO, BS
Division of Pulmonary, Critical Care and Sleep Medicine, Department of Medicine,
Hofstra-North Shore Long Island Jewish School of Medicine, New Hyde Park, New York

NORMAN BEATTY, BS
Division of Pulmonary, Critical Care and Sleep Medicine, Department of Medicine,
Hofstra-North Shore Long Island Jewish School of Medicine, New Hyde Park, New York

CHRISTOPH BUETTNER, MD, PhD
Associate Professor of Medicine and Neuroscience, Division of Endocrinology, Mount
Sinai Medical Center, New York, New York

ALEXANDER BYSTRITSKY, MD, PhD
Department of Psychiatry and Biobehavioral Sciences, Semel Institute for Neuroscience
and Human Behavior, David Geffen School of Medicine, University of California,
Los Angeles, Los Angeles, California

JOSE M. CASTELLANO, MD, PhD
Zena and Michael A. Wiener Cardiovascular Institute and Marie-Josée and Henry R. Kravis
Cardiovascular Health Center, Mount Sinai School of Medicine, New York, New York

ZIJIAN CHEN, MD
Fellow, Division of Endocrinology and Metabolism, Beth Israel Medical Center, Albert Einstein College of Medicine, New York, New York

JESSICA DANIAL, MA
California School of Professional Psychology, Alliant International University, Los Angeles, California

JAIME A. DAVIDSON, MD, FACP, MACE
Clinical Professor of Medicine, Division of Endocrinology, Diabetes and Metabolism, Touchstone Diabetes Center, University of Texas Southwestern Medical Center, Dallas, Texas

SUZANNE M. DE LA MONTE, MD, MPH
Departments of Medicine, Pathology (Neuropathology), Neurology and Neurosurgery, Rhode Island Hospital, The Warren Alpert Medical School of Brown University, Providence, Rhode Island

MICHAEL E. FARKOUH, MD
Zena and Michael A. Wiener Cardiovascular Institute and Marie-Josée and Henry R. Kravis Cardiovascular Health Center, Mount Sinai School of Medicine, New York, New York; Peter Munk Cardiac Centre and Heart and Stroke Richard Lewar Centre of Excellence in Cardiovascular Research, University of Toronto, Toronto, Ontario, Canada

DOROTHY A. FINK, MD
Fellow, Division of Endocrinology, Department of Medicine, Columbia University Medical Center, New York, New York

VALENTIN FUSTER, MD, PhD
Zena and Michael A. Wiener Cardiovascular Institute and Marie-Josée and Henry R. Kravis Cardiovascular Health Center, Mount Sinai School of Medicine, New York, New York; The Centro Nacional de Investigaciones Cardiovasculares (CNIC), Madrid, Spain

EMILY JANE GALLAGHER, MD
Assistant Professor of Medicine, Division of Endocrinology, Diabetes and Bone Diseases, Icahn School of Medicine at Mount Sinai, New York, New York

ALAN J. GARBER, MD, PhD, FACE
Professor, Departments of Medicine, Molecular and Cellular Biology, and Biochemistry and Molecular Biology, Baylor College of Medicine, Houston, Texas

ELIZA B. GEER, MD
Assistant Professor of Medicine, Division of Endocrinology; Assistant Professor of Neurosurgery, Mount Sinai Medical Center, New York, New York

HARLY GREENBERG, MD, FAASM, FCCP
Division of Pulmonary, Critical Care and Sleep Medicine, Department of Medicine, Hofstra-North Shore Long Island Jewish School of Medicine, New Hyde Park, New York

DARRYL M. HOFFMAN, MD, FRCS
Division of Cardiothoracic Surgery, Beth Israel Medical Center, New York, New York

JULIE ISLAM, MD
Friedman Research Fellow, Division of Endocrinology and Metabolism, Beth Israel Medical Center, New York, New York

EDWARD B. JUDE, MD, MRCP
Consultant Diabetologist and Endocrinologist, Reader in Medicine, Department of Endocrinology, Tameside Hospital NHS Foundation Trust, Ashton-Under-Lyne, Lancashire; University of Manchester, Manchester, United Kingdom

JASON C. KOVACIC, MD, PhD
Zena and Michael A. Wiener Cardiovascular Institute and Marie-Josée and Henry R. Kravis Cardiovascular Health Center, Mount Sinai School of Medicine, New York, New York

DAVID KRONEMYER, MA
Department of Psychiatry and Biobehavioral Sciences, Semel Institute for Neuroscience and Human Behavior, David Geffen School of Medicine, University of California, Los Angeles, Los Angeles, California

SALILA KURRA, MD
Assistant Professor of Medicine, Columbia University Medical Center; Department of Medicine, Metabolic Bone Diseases Unit, Toni Stabile Osteoporosis Center, Columbia University Medical Center, New York, New York

L. ROMAYNE KURUKULASURIYA, MD
Associate Professor of Medicine, Division of Endocrinology, Diabetes and Metabolism, Department of Internal Medicine, University of Missouri Columbia School of Medicine, Columbia, Missouri

GUIDO LASTRA, MD
Assistant Professor of Medicine, Division of Endocrinology, Diabetes and Metabolism, Department of Internal Medicine, University of Missouri Columbia School of Medicine; Diabetes and Cardiovascular Research Center, University of Missouri; Harry S Truman Memorial Veterans Hospital, Columbia, Missouri

CAMILA MANRIQUE, MD
Assistant Professor of Medicine, Division of Endocrinology, Diabetes and Metabolism, Department of Internal Medicine, University of Missouri Columbia School of Medicine; Diabetes and Cardiovascular Research Center, University of Missouri; Harry S Truman Memorial Veterans Hospital, Columbia, Missouri

JANICE V. MASCARENHAS, MBBS
Clinical Research Fellow, Department of Endocrinology, Tameside General Hospital, Tameside Hospital NHS Foundation Trust, Ashton-Under-Lyne, Lancashire; University of Manchester, Manchester, United Kingdom

JOANNA MITRI, MD, MS
Division of Endocrinology, Diabetes and Metabolism, Prima CARE Medical Center, Fall River, Massachusetts

MICHAEL MORGENSTERN, MD
Division of Pulmonary, Critical Care and Sleep Medicine, Department of Medicine, Hofstra-North Shore Long Island Jewish School of Medicine, New Hyde Park, New York

ANINDITA NANDI, MD
Attending Physician, Division of Endocrinology and Metabolism, Beth Israel Medical Center, Albert Einstein College of Medicine, New York, New York

RONAK PATEL, MD
Fellow, Division of Endocrinology and Metabolism, Beth Israel Medical Center, Albert Einstein College of Medicine, New York, New York

ANASTASSIOS G. PITTAS, MD, MS
Associate Professor of Medicine, Tufts University School of Medicine; Division of
Endocrinology, Diabetes and Metabolism, Tufts Medical Center, Boston, Massachusetts

LEONID PORETSKY, MD
Chief, Division of Endocrinology and Metabolism; Vice-Chairman for Research,
Department of Medicine; Director, Gerald J. Friedman Diabetes Institute,
Gerald J. Friedman Chair for Endocrinology, Beth Israel Medical Center; Professor
of Medicine, Albert Einstein College of Medicine, New York, New York

SUSAN L. SAMSON, MD, PhD, FRCPC, FACE
Assistant Professor, Department of Medicine, Baylor College of Medicine, Houston,
Texas

CLIFFORD P. SHEARMAN, BSc, MBBS, MS, FRCS
Professor of Surgery, Department of Vascular Surgery, Southampton General Hospital,
University Hospital Southampton NHS Foundation Trust, Southampton, United Kingdom

ANTHONY L. SICA, PhD, FAASM
Division of Pulmonary, Critical Care and Sleep Medicine, Department of Medicine,
Hofstra-North Shore Long Island Jewish School of Medicine, New Hyde Park, New York

ETHEL S. SIRIS, MD
Madeline C. Stabile Professor of Medicine, Columbia University Medical Center; Director,
Toni Stabile Osteoporosis Center, Metabolic Bone Diseases Unit, Columbia University
Medical Center, New York-Presbyterian Hospital, New York, New York

JAMES R. SOWERS, MD
Professor of Medicine, and Medical Pharmacology and Physiology, Division of
Endocrinology, Diabetes and Metabolism, Department of Internal Medicine, University of
Missouri Columbia School of Medicine; Diabetes and Cardiovascular Research Center,
University of Missouri; Harry S Truman Memorial Veterans Hospital; Department of
Medical Physiology and Pharmacology, University of Missouri, Columbia, Missouri

SOFIA SYED, MD
Endocrine Fellow, Division of Endocrinology, Diabetes and Metabolism, Department of
Internal Medicine, University of Missouri Columbia School of Medicine; Diabetes and
Cardiovascular Research Center, University of Missouri, Columbia, Missouri

MAGDALENE M. SZUSZKIEWICZ-GARCIA, MD
Assistant Professor, Division of Endocrinology and Metabolism, Department of Medicine,
Center for Human Nutrition, University of Texas Southwestern Medical Center, Dallas,
Texas

ROBERT F. TRANBAUGH, MD
Division of Cardiothoracic Surgery, Beth Israel Medical Center, New York, New York

JANICE WANG, MD
Division of Pulmonary, Critical Care and Sleep Medicine, Department of Medicine,
Hofstra-North Shore Long Island Jewish School of Medicine, New Hyde Park, New York

ZARA ZELENKO, BA, PhD(c)
Division of Endocrinology, Diabetes and Bone Diseases, Icahn School of Medicine at
Mount Sinai, New York, New York

Contents

Foreword   xiii

Derek LeRoith

Preface: Why Are Associated Conditions Important?   xvii

Leonid Poretsky and Emilia Pauline Liao

Metabolic Syndrome   1

Susan L. Samson and Alan J. Garber

> Metabolic syndrome is not a disease per se, but is a term that highlights
> traits that may have an increased risk of disease, approximately 2-fold
> for cardiovascular disease and 5-fold or more for type 2 diabetes mellitus.
> Obesity and insulin resistance are believed to be at the core of most cases
> of metabolic syndrome, although further research is required to truly under-
> stand the pathophysiology behind the syndrome and the gene-environ-
> ment interactions that increase susceptibility. The mainstay of treatment
> remains lifestyle changes with exercise and diet to induce weight loss
> and pharmacologic intervention to treat atherogenic dyslipidemia, hyper-
> tension, and hyperglycemia.

Cardiovascular Disease in Diabetes Mellitus: Risk Factors and Medical Therapy   25

Magdalene M. Szuszkiewicz-Garcia and Jaime A. Davidson

> Cardiovascular disease is a serious complication of diabetes mellitus. In
> the last 2 decades, great strides have been made in reducing microvascu-
> lar complications in patients with diabetes through improving glycemic
> control. Decreasing rates of cardiovascular events have proved to be
> more difficult than simply intensifying the management of hyperglycemia.
> A tremendous effort has been made to deepen understanding of cardio-
> vascular disease in diabetes and to formulate the best treatment approach.
> This review summarizes the current state of knowledge and discusses
> areas of uncertainty in the care of patients with diabetes who are at risk
> for cardiovascular disease.

**The Relationships Between Cardiovascular Disease and Diabetes: Focus on
Pathogenesis**   41

Jason C. Kovacic, Jose M. Castellano, Michael E. Farkouh, and Valentin Fuster

> There is a looming global epidemic of obesity and diabetes. Of all the end-
> organ effects caused by diabetes, the cardiovascular system is particularly
> susceptible to the biologic perturbations caused by this disease, and many
> patients may die from diabetes-related cardiovascular complications.
> Substantial progress has been made in understanding the pathobiology
> of the diabetic vasculature and heart. Clinical studies have illuminated
> the optimal way to treat patients with cardiovascular manifestations of
> this disease. This article reviews these aspects of diabetes and the cardio-
> vascular system, broadly classified into diabetic vascular disease, diabetic

cardiomyopathy, and the clinical management of the diabetic cardiovascular disease patient.

Interventions for Coronary Artery Disease (Surgery vs Angioplasty) in Diabetic Patients   59

Darryl M. Hoffman and Robert F. Tranbaugh

Patients with diabetes develop more widespread and more severe atherosclerotic coronary artery disease than patients without diabetes. Medical management of this coronary disease is inferior to revascularization for more complex or more widespread disease. Revascularization by percutaneous intervention (PCI) for patients with diabetes is associated with high mortality and complication rates. Surgical revascularization by coronary artery bypass grafting, yields superior results to PCI for patients with diabetes and coronary artery disease. Patients with diabetes benefit from the same medical management of their coronary artery disease and secondary risk modification as patients without diabetes.

Mechanisms of Glucocorticoid-Induced Insulin Resistance: Focus on Adipose Tissue Function and Lipid Metabolism   75

Eliza B. Geer, Julie Islam, and Christoph Buettner

Glucocorticoids (GCs) are critical in the regulation of the stress response, inflammation and energy homeostasis. Excessive GC exposure results in whole-body insulin resistance, obesity, cardiovascular disease, and ultimately decreased survival, despite their potent anti-inflammatory effects. This apparent paradox may be explained by the complex actions of GCs on adipose tissue functionality. The wide prevalence of oral GC therapy makes their adverse systemic effects an important yet incompletely understood clinical problem. This article reviews the mechanisms by which supraphysiologic GC exposure promotes insulin resistance, focusing in particular on the effects on adipose tissue function and lipid metabolism.

Type 2 Diabetes Mellitus and Hypertension: An Update   103

Guido Lastra, Sofia Syed, L. Romayne Kurukulasuriya, Camila Manrique, and James R. Sowers

Patients with hypertension and type 2 diabetes are at increased risk of cardiovascular and chronic renal disease. Factors involved in the pathogenesis of both hypertension and type 2 diabetes include inappropriate activation of the renin-angiotensin-aldosterone system, oxidative stress, inflammation, impaired insulin-mediated vasodilatation, augmented sympathetic nervous system activation, altered innate and adaptive immunity, and abnormal sodium processing by the kidney. The renin-angiotensin-aldosterone system blockade is a key therapeutic strategy in the treatment of hypertension in type 2 diabetes. Emerging therapies for resistant hypertension as often exists in patients with diabetes, include renal denervation and carotid body denervation.

Polycystic Ovary Syndrome   123

Anindita Nandi, Zijian Chen, Ronak Patel, and Leonid Poretsky

Polycystic ovary syndrome (PCOS), a heterogeneous and chronic condition, today affects about 5% of women of reproductive age. PCOS is strongly associated with states of insulin resistance and hyperinsulinemia. Risk factors include genetics, metabolic profiles, and the in utero environment. Long-term consequences of PCOS include metabolic complications such as diabetes, obesity, and cardiovascular disease. Dysregulation of insulin action is closely linked to the pathogenesis of PCOS. However, whether insulin resistance is the causative factor in the development of PCOS remains to be ascertained. Moreover, the mechanism by which insulin resistance may lead to reproductive dysfunction requires further elucidation.

Peripheral Arterial Disease   149

Janice V. Mascarenhas, Mostafa A. Albayati, Clifford P. Shearman, and Edward B. Jude

Peripheral arterial disease (PAD) is an atherosclerotic-driven condition that remains underdiagnosed and undertreated. In diabetic patients, PAD begins early, progresses rapidly, and is frequently asymptomatic, making it difficult to diagnose. Strict management of the metabolic instigators and use of screening techniques for PAD in diabetes can facilitate early diagnosis and reduce progression. Exercise is an equally effective treatment option in improving walking distance. Early revascularization must be offered early in suitable patients. Surgical bypass and endovascular revascularization are complementary and the choice of intervention should be applied appropriately by a multidisciplinary vascular team on a selective, patient-specific basis.

Diabetes and Cancer   167

Zara Zelenko and Emily Jane Gallagher

Diabetes is a worldwide health problem that has been increasingly associated with various types of cancers. Epidemiologic studies have shown an increased risk of cancer as well as a higher mortality rate in patients with type 2 diabetes (T2D). The biologic mechanisms driving the link between T2D and cancer are not well understood. In this review, various proposed mechanisms are addressed to explain the relationship between T2D and cancer. Understanding the precise mechanisms that link T2D, obesity, and the metabolic syndrome with cancer will aid in developing treatments that will reduce mortality in individuals with T2D and cancer.

Obstructive Sleep Apnea: An Unexpected Cause of Insulin Resistance and Diabetes   187

Michael Morgenstern, Janice Wang, Norman Beatty, Tom Batemarco, Anthony L. Sica, and Harly Greenberg

Obstructive sleep apnea (OSA) is prevalent with type 2 diabetes. Conversely, nondiabetic patients with OSA are at increased risk of developing insulin resistance and diabetes. These disorders independently contribute to increased cardiovascular and cerebrovascular morbidity and mortality. The pathophysiology of OSA may help explain these associations. Evidence demonstrates that treatment of OSA with continuous positive airway pressure may lead to improvement in insulin sensitivity, hemoglobin A1c, systemic hypertension, and other components of the metabolic syndrome. Recognizing and treating OSA in patients with insulin resistance or diabetes ameliorates OSA-related symptoms and improves cardiometabolic risk.

Vitamin D and Diabetes   205

Joanna Mitri and Anastassios G. Pittas

There has been increasing evidence that vitamin D may have a role in modifying risk of diabetes. Vitamin D has both direct and indirect effects on various mechanisms related to the pathophysiology of type 2 diabetes, including pancreatic beta cell dysfunction, impaired insulin action and systemic inflammation. This article describes the biologic plausibility behind the potential association between vitamin D and type 2 diabetes and summarizes the current evidence from human studies that suggests but does not prove a relation between vitamin D and type 2 diabetes, and briefly reports on the potential association between vitamin D and type 1 diabetes.

Osteoporosis-associated Fracture and Diabetes   233

Salila Kurra, Dorothy A. Fink, and Ethel S. Siris

Osteoporosis and diabetes mellitus are chronic diseases with significant associated morbidity and mortality. Recent evidence suggests that both type 1 and type 2 diabetes are associated with an increased fracture risk. Fracture as a complication of diabetes must be considered when evaluating and treating patients with diabetes.

Relationships Between Diabetes and Cognitive Impairment   245

Suzanne M. de la Monte

Epidemics of obesity, diabetes, nonalcoholic fatty liver disease, and cognitive impairment/Alzheimer disease have emerged over the past 3 to 4 decades. These diseases share in common target-organ insulin resistance with a constellation of molecular and biochemical abnormalities that lead to organ/tissue degeneration over time. This article discusses the fundamental links among these diseases and how peripheral organ insulin resistance diseases contribute to cognitive impairment and neurodegeneration. A future role of endocrinologists and diabetologists could be to provide integrative diagnostic and treatment approaches for this collection of diseases that seem to share pathophysiological and pathogenetic bases.

Interactions Between Diabetes and Anxiety and Depression: Implications for Treatment   269

Alexander Bystritsky, Jessica Danial, and David Kronemyer

Anxiety or depression may be a risk factor for the development of diabetes. This relationship may occur through a combination of genetic predispositions; epigenetic contingencies; exacerbating conditions such as metabolic syndrome (a precursor to diabetes); and other serious medical conditions. Medications used to treat anxiety and depression have significant side effects, such as weight gain, further increasing the possibility of developing diabetes. These components combine, interact, and reassemble to create a precarious system for persons with, or predisposed to, diabetes. Clinicians must be aware of these interrelationships to adequately treat the disease.

Index   285

ENDOCRINOLOGY AND METABOLISM CLINICS OF NORTH AMERICA

FORTHCOMING ISSUES

June 2014
Thyroid Cancer and Other Thyroid Disorders
Kenneth D. Burman and
Jacqueline Jonklaas, *Editors*

September 2014
HIV and Endocrine Disorders
Paul Hruz, *Editor*

December 2014
Lipids
Donald A. Smith, *Editor*

RECENT ISSUES

December 2013
Acute and Chronic Complications of Diabetes
Leonid Poretsky and Emilia Pauline Liao, *Editors*

September 2013
Endocrine and Neuropsychiatric Disorders
Eliza B. Geer, *Editor*

June 2013
Aging and Endocrinology
Anne R. Cappola, *Editor*

RELATED INTEREST

Medical Clinics of North America, Volume 97, Issue 1 (January 2013)
Diabetic Chronic Kidney Disease
Mark E. Williams, *Editor*
Available at: http://www.medical.theclinics.com/

THE CLINICS ARE NOW AVAILABLE ONLINE!
Access your subscription at:
www.theclinics.com

Foreword

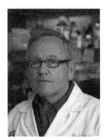

Derek LeRoith, MD, PhD
Consulting Editor

In this second issue on diabetic complications and associated conditions, Drs Liao and Poretsky have assembled articles that further describe the problems that physicians and their patients face. As with the first issue, the articles cover both basic mechanisms and clinical approaches, making these issues very topical and of value to endocrinologists and health care professionals.

Metabolic syndrome remains a description of a number of risk factors that independently increase the risk of cardiovascular complications in both obese individuals and those with type 2 diabetes. The definition includes waist circumference as a measure of visceral adiposity, hypertension, hypertriglyceridemia with low HDL, and glucose intolerance. The underlying cause remains the overweight-associated insulin resistance and hyperinsulinemia. As Drs Samson and Garber discuss, there is some debate as to the utility of the syndrome because the group of risk factors does not influence the outcomes more than the sum of the individual risk factors and the appropriate management is to address each risk factor individually.

Drs Szuszkiewicz-Garcia and Davidson describe the increased cardiovascular complications of diabetes, interestingly more in women than in men. The cardiometabolic risk factors are well known and need to be controlled fairly aggressively. Although the evidence for tight glucose control has not been demonstrated to reduce the impact on macrovascular complications, health care professionals and patients should be aware that prevention of microvascular complications is still dependent on glucose control.

Drs Kovacic, Castellano, Farkouh, and Fuster discuss the epidemic of type 2 diabetes and one of its most important complications, namely, cardiovascular disease. As they discuss, prevention is critical and the judicious use of medications for the cardiometabolic risk factors needs emphasizing both to health-care professionals and to patients. Recent outcome trials have demonstrated that bypass surgery surpasses angioplasties and stents of various kinds in diabetic patients and this needs to be seriously considered when advising patients on therapy following diagnostic catheterization.

In the subsequent article, Drs Hoffman and Tranbaugh develop the theme further and describe the evidence that diabetic patients often have more extensive coronary

Endocrinol Metab Clin N Am 43 (2014) xiii–xvi
http://dx.doi.org/10.1016/j.ecl.2013.10.004
0889-8529/14/$ – see front matter © 2014 Elsevier Inc. All rights reserved.

disease. Furthermore, percutaneous coronary intervention is inferior to coronary artery bypass and the technique of using the radial artery instead of saphenous vein for the bypass is superior. They also conclude that medical therapy after bypass is critical for secondary prevention.

Glucocorticoids have long been known to affect the metabolic status of patients. Whether due to pituitary or adrenal tumors, chronic administration for immune disorders, or even stress with overactivity of the hypothalamic-pituitary-adrenal axis, these effects are seen. The effects include central obesity and excessive hepatic lipogenesis that are mediated, in part, by 11β-hydroxysteroid dehydrogenase 1. Drs Geer, Islam, and Buettner go on to discuss the effects of glucocorticoids on adipocyte lipolysis and how overall chronic glucocorticoid excess causes increased insulin resistance and worsening of the metabolic status, including type 2 diabetes.

Hypertension is commonly seen in obese individuals, those with metabolic syndrome, and most diabetic patients, especially those with type 2 diabetes, although eventually those with type 1 diabetes as well. Traditionally, the cause of hypertension has been considered to be secondary to the insulin resistance and hyperinsulinemia. Concomitant secondary effects are the oxidative stress, activation of the renin-angiotensin system, impaired insulin-mediated vasodilatation, augmented sympathetic nervous system activity, and excessive sodium reabsorption in the kidney. Drs Lastra, Syed, Kurukulasuriya, Manrique, and Sowers also stress that antihypertensive therapy in diabetic patients should include blockers of the renin-angiotensin axis.

Drs Nandi, Jian, Chen, Patel, and Poretsky discuss the polycystic ovarian syndrome (PCOS), one of the most common causes of infertility in women. There is strong evidence of the presence and role of insulin resistance in the cause of PCOS. The evidence is from both laboratory and animal studies, as well as from human studies that include the existence of hyperandrogenism. Because insulin resistance and hyperinsulinemia are the underlying pathophysiological mechanisms in obesity, metabolic syndrome, and type 2 diabetes, it is not surprising that PCOS is common in these conditions. Furthermore, therapies like metformin and thiazolidinediones that reduce insulin resistance have been successful in treating PCOS.

Because the incidence of peripheral vascular disease in patients with diabetes is four-fold greater than in the general population, it presents many problems to both patients and health care providers. Clearly the cause is related to the general atherosclerotic process that is accelerated in diabetic individuals, especially those that are poorly controlled in regard to hypertension, hyperlipidemia, and hyperglycemia. Drs Mascarenhas, Albayati, Shearman, and Jude discuss how, in addition to general physical examination, the use of ankle brachial pressure index has become an excellent screening tool. They also stress, of course, that prevention is critical because the poor outcomes, including amputation in diabetic patients, can be devastating.

In the article by Drs Zelenko and Gallagher there is a description of the impact of obesity and diabetes on cancer risk and cancer-related mortality. Many different common cancers are involved and, as described, the mechanisms probably involve many of the factors that present in these syndromes, namely, insulin resistance, hyperinsulinemia, inflammatory cytokines, hyperglycemia, insulin-like growth factors, and leptin, to name a few important examples. The connection between obesity, metabolic syndrome, and type 2 diabetes is exemplified by the response to bariatric surgery, where the risk of cancer-related mortality is reduced. In their article, the authors cover the epidemiology and the potential mechanisms involved in the association between these metabolic syndromes and cancer risk.

Obesity (and therefore type 2 diabetes) has always been known to be associated with obstructive sleep apnea. What Drs Morgenstein, Wang, Beatty, Batemarco, Sica, and Greenberg discuss is the opposite sequence of events, namely, that sleep apnea may actually be causative in insulin resistance, obesity, and diabetes. Sleep apnea causes hypoxia that in turn induces an inflammatory process with resultant insulin resistance. Further studies have shown that lack of sleep is associated with overeating and obesity. Most interestingly, type 2 diabetic individuals who are not overweight have an increased incidence of sleep apnea, suggesting a central effect of the diabetic abnormality; as yet, the cause is unknown.

Over the past decade there have been multiple reports of the value of measuring serum vitamin D levels and supplementation of vitamin D for numerous conditions other than for bone health. There have even been reports of its value in type 1 and type 2 diabetes. As Drs Mitri and Pittas discuss in their article, most of the evidence on the effect of vitamin D on β-cell function, insulin action, and immunological function arises from laboratory and animal studies. Unfortunately clinical trials have shown mixed results and have been generally disappointing. Of interest is the recent announcement by the NIH that a controlled clinical trial is to be funded. Given the very few side effects seen with vitamin D, it would be very advantageous if a clinical successful trial could be seen.

A largely less well-recognized complication of diabetes is osteoporosis in patients with type 1 and type 2 diabetes. Although these types of diabetes have different origins and pathophysiology, there are often similarities in the effects on bone. One of the more perplexing effects of diabetes on bone has been the increase in bone fragility that often results in nonclassic fractures of peripheral bones. Although further research is warranted and on-going, Drs Kurra, Fink, and Siris discuss the importance of evaluating all patients with diabetes for osteoporosis and that standard therapies for osteoporosis are equally effective in patients with diabetes as they are in nondiabetic individuals. Finally, the use of medications, such as thiazolidinediones that may increase the bone fragility and/or osteoporosis in type 2 diabetes, needs to be carefully evaluated.

It is now well-recognized that in diabetic patients the incidence of cognitive dysfunction and even neurodegenerative diseases such as Alzheimers is increased. The causes for this association are discussed in the article by Dr de la Monte. Evidence suggests that genetics may play a role as well as central nervous system insulin and insulin-like growth factor-1 resistance as well as insulin deficiency. Another suggestion is that the diabetes including the abnormalities in glycemic control may be exacerbating the underlying cognitive dysfunction that has a separate cause. This would suggest that tight glycemic control and delivering insulin locally, for example, by nasal insulin administration, should be capable of reducing the cognitive decline seen in diabetic patients and others with Alzheimers.

Health care professionals have been aware for a long time that in dealing with patients with diabetes, both type 1 and type 2, anxiety and depression are common and often complicate many aspects of the therapeutic armamentarium, leading to poor compliance. Drs Bystritsky, Danial, and Kronemyer remind us that there is a further component that should be considered and that is the effects of antianxiety and antidepressant medications on metabolic syndrome. For example, antipsychotics are well known to cause increased weight and frank obesity in some patients. Furthermore, anxiety and changes in the hormonal axes can enhance the clinical presentations of type 2 diabetes, if not actually precipitating the appearance of the disorder.

As the reader will find, the articles in this issue are written by experts and should be extremely important for understanding of the pathophysiology and management of diabetic patients with the various complications. I personally would like to thank both the issue editors and the authors for an amazing compilation of articles.

Derek LeRoith, MD, PhD
Division of Endocrinology, Metabolism, and Bone Diseases
Department of Medicine
Mount Sinai School of Medicine
One Gustave L. Levy Place
Box 1055, Altran 4-36
New York, NY 10029, USA

E-mail address:
derek.leroith@mssm.edu

Preface

Why Are Associated Conditions Important?

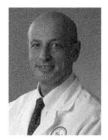 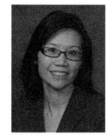

Leonid Poretsky, MD   Emilia Pauline Liao, MD
Editors

This issue of *Endocrinology and Metabolism Clinics of North America* focuses on the conditions closely associated with diabetes mellitus. Unlike microvascular complications of diabetes, which are seen exclusively in the setting of diabetes, conditions closely associated with diabetes might be seen independently or in association with this disease, but their prevalence in patients with diabetes exceeds that in the general population. The associated conditions are diverse and include such apparently unrelated syndromes as, for example, coronary artery disease and sleep apnea. However, on closer inspection, many of these have common background characterized by insulin resistance and increased oxidative stress.

What is the importance of these conditions? Although not as closely linked to hyperglycemia as the specific complication of diabetes (diabetic retinopathy, diabetic nephropathy, diabetic neuropathy), the associated conditions contribute greatly to morbidity and mortality in patients with diabetes. In fact, heart disease, one such associated condition, continues to be responsible for most of the diabetes-related mortality. Therefore, treating these conditions, as well as understanding their pathophysiology and their relationship to diabetes, remains a major challenge.

We hope that the current issue summarizes and clarifies the relationship between diabetes and conditions that are closely associated with it. We thank Dr Derek LeRoith, the Consulting Editor, for the opportunity to edit both this issue and the previous issue, "Acute and Chronic Complications of Diabetes." We also thank all the authors, as well as the editorial staff of *Endocrinology and Metabolism Clinics of North America*, for their invaluable contributions.

Endocrinol Metab Clin N Am 43 (2014) xvii–xviii
http://dx.doi.org/10.1016/j.ecl.2013.10.002
0889-8529/14/$ – see front matter © 2014 Elsevier Inc. All rights reserved.

endo.theclinics.com

We learned a lot while editing these two issues. We hope that the readers will have a similarly enlightening experience.

Leonid Poretsky, MD
Department of Medicine
Albert Einstein College of Medicine
1300 Morris Park Avenue
Bronx, NY 10461, USA

Endocrinology
Gerald J. Friedman Diabetes Institute
Beth Israel Medical Center
16th Street, First Avenue
New York, NY 10003, USA

Emilia Pauline Liao, MD
Department of Medicine
Albert Einstein College of Medicine
1300 Morris Park Avenue
Bronx, NY 10461, USA

Endocrinology
Beth Israel Medical Center
16th Street, First Avenue
New York, NY 10003, USA

E-mail addresses:
LPoretsk@chpnet.org (L. Poretsky)
eliao@chpnet.org (E.P. Liao)

Metabolic Syndrome

Susan L. Samson, MD, PhD[a], Alan J. Garber, MD, PhD[b,c,d],*

KEYWORDS

- Metabolic syndrome • Obesity • Dyslipidemia • Hypertension • Cardiovascular risk
- Diabetes risk • National Cholesterol Education Program Adult Treatment Panel III

KEY POINTS

- Metabolic syndrome is a clustering of clinical findings made up of abdominal obesity, high glucose, high triglyceride, and low high-density lipoprotein cholesterol levels, and hypertension.
- Several definitions of metabolic syndrome have been proposed, with varied requirements, including those by the International Diabetes Federation and the National Cholesterol Education Program Adult Treatment Panel III.
- There is a proposed harmonized international definition that incorporates the criteria for the National Cholesterol Education Program definition and suggests that population-specific waist circumference thresholds should be used for obesity.
- Diagnosis of metabolic syndrome has a relative risk of approximately 2-fold for cardiovascular disease over 5 to 10 years and at least 5-fold for type 2 diabetes.
- Treatment involves diet and exercise to promote weight loss and pharmacologic treatment of atherogenic dyslipidemia, hypertension, and hyperglycemia.

INTRODUCTION

A medical syndrome is a clustering of clinical findings that occur together more often than would be expected by chance. The constellation of components that make up the metabolic syndrome (MetS) has had several labels over the years including the eponymous Reaven syndrome, syndrome X, dysmetabolic syndrome X (ICD-9 code 277.7), CHAOS, plurimetabolic syndrome, the deadly quartet, and insulin resistance syndrome. Although increased attention and research have been focused on MetS in the last 2 to 3 decades, syndromes analogous to MetS have been described in the

[a] Department of Medicine, Baylor College of Medicine, One Baylor Plaza, ABBR R615, Houston, TX 77030, USA; [b] Department of Medicine, Baylor College of Medicine, One Baylor Plaza, BCM 620, Houston, TX 77030, USA; [c] Department of Molecular and Cellular Biology, Baylor College of Medicine, One Baylor Plaza, BCM 620, Houston, TX 77030, USA; [d] Department of Biochemistry and Molecular Biology, Baylor College of Medicine, One Baylor Plaza, BCM 620, Houston, TX 77030, USA
* Corresponding author. Department of Medicine, Baylor College of Medicine, One Baylor Plaza, BCM 620, Houston, TX 77030.
E-mail address: agarber@bcm.edu

Endocrinol Metab Clin N Am 43 (2014) 1–23
http://dx.doi.org/10.1016/j.ecl.2013.09.009
0889-8529/14/$ – see front matter © 2014 Elsevier Inc. All rights reserved.

medical literature for nearly a century. The descriptions of these syndromes may differ by components or criteria, but all point toward a similar dysmetabolic phenotype. Swedish physician Eskil Kylin, with a keen interest in hypertension, described its relationship with hyperglycemia and gout in 1923.[1] In 1956, Dr Jean Vague of Marseilles, France published the association of atherosclerosis, diabetes, gout, and renal calculi with central obesity.[2,3] Both Haller and Singer used the term "metabolic syndrome" in German language publications that reported on their observations from studies of patients with dyslipidemia. Haller[4] included obesity, diabetes, hyperlipoproteinemia, gout, and fatty liver in the syndrome, whereas Singer[5] included the first 4 components but added hypertension. Professor Phillips (Columbia University) recognized the coexistence of impaired glucose metabolism with hyperinsulinemia, hyperlipidemia, and hypertension, leading to increased risk for myocardial infarction (MI); in also observing the increased prevalence of this MetS with aging, he focused on changes in sex hormone levels as important to the underlying disease.[6] However, it was Dr Gerald Reaven, in his 1988 Banting medal lecture for the American Diabetes Association (ADA), who discussed the constellation of metabolic findings of syndrome X, proposing a central role for insulin resistance in the pathophysiology of the syndrome and the risk of diabetes and cardiovascular disease (CVD), with the goal to foster new hypotheses and research in the field.[7] According to the World Health Organization (WHO), worldwide prevalence of obesity has doubled in the last 3 decades and at least one-third of adults older than 20 years are overweight or obese.[8] As the prevalence of obesity increases, it follows that the prevalence of MetS also will increase in parallel. Alarmingly, nearly one-half of the diabetes burden and one-quarter of the heart disease burden are attributable to being overweight or obese.[9]

DEFINITIONS

Despite multiple labels in the past, the term MetS is now used universally. It was first formalized by use in a working definition proposed by a diabetes consultation panel for WHO in 1998 and finalized in 1999.[10] The section on MetS is a small portion of a document primarily focused on the diagnosis and classification of type 2 diabetes mellitus (T2DM),[10] but it provoked discussion and position statements such as from the European Group for the Study of Insulin Resistance (EGIR)[11] and the American Association of Clinical Endocrinologists (AACE) in 2003.[12] In the United States, the National Cholesterol Education Program (NCEP) Adult Treatment Panel III (ATPIII) was published in 2001 to guide therapy for low-density lipoprotein (LDL) cholesterol (LDL-C) to reduce coronary heart disease (CHD).[13] MetS was seen as an additional target beyond LDL decreasing that could result in reduction of CHD risk. The NCEP/ATPIII was followed by a similar definition from the International Diabetes Federation (IDF) in 2005.[14] The commonality among the different definitions is that each recognizes the components of: (1) obesity, abdominal adiposity or indicators of insulin resistance, (2) impaired glucose metabolism, (3) hypertension, and (4) atherogenic dyslipidemia. The dissimilarities are in how the components are detected clinically and, in some cases, there is an emphasis on a particular trait that is obligate to meet the definition (**Table 1**).

NCEP/ATPIII MetS criteria were proposed requiring 3 of 5 factors: abdominal obesity measured as sex-specific waist circumference (WC), triglyceride levels, low high-density lipoprotein (HDL) cholesterol (HDL-C), hypertension, and increased fasting glucose (IFG), without exclusion of diabetes.[13] A 2004 update was provided by the American Heart Association (AHA) and National Heart Lung and Blood Institute (NHLBI) to decrease the threshold for IFG from 110 mg/dL (6.1 mmol/L) to 100 mg/dL

(5.6 mmol/L) as recommended by the ADA, and to clarify that it could include patients already on treatment of dyslipidemia or hypertension.[15] Although the later IDF criteria were in agreement with the NCEP definition, abdominal obesity was made a requirement, as measured by WC, or it was assumed if body mass index (BMI, calculated as weight in kilograms divided by the square of height in meters) was 30 kg/m^2 or higher.[16] The IDF WC threshold for Europoids was lower than that used by NCEP, and the document also discussed the need for thresholds for WC dependent on ethnic background (**Table 2**).[16]

The clinical usefulness of a MetS diagnosis partially has been hampered by the multiple definitions. Efforts have been made to unify the definition of MetS. In 2009, 5 groups released a joint interim statement regarding the harmonization of the criteria: IDF, AHA, NHLBI, World Heart Federation, International Atherosclerosis Society, and International Association for the Study of Obesity (see **Table 1**).[17] Obesity was removed as an obligate component and HDL-C, triglyceride, blood pressure, and fasting glucose criteria were identical to the modified NCEP definition. The higher NCEP threshold for Europoid WC was kept for North American patients, but it was acknowledged that lower values used by the IDF could be important for those at higher risk.[17] This document also noted that the criteria used for abdominal obesity, as WC, required refinement with regard to country-specific and population-specific definitions, as originally discussed by the IDF, with more study and evidence needed to determine the WC cutoffs in different populations that are associated with higher risk.[17] The WC thresholds suggested for the harmonized definition of the joint interim statement are shown in **Table 2**,[17] and the physician is left to clinical judgment regarding patients with mixed ethnicity.

Adult MetS criteria have been modified for pediatric and adolescent age groups, and there have also been multiple MetS definitions used in this population.[18] The earliest definition was proposed by Cook and colleagues[19] and was a modification of the original NCEP criteria with WC and blood pressure equal to or greater than the 90th percentile for age, sex, and height with triglyceride levels greater than 110 mg/dL (1.23 mmol/L) and HDL levels less than 40 mg/dL (1.03 mmol/L). Additional definitions followed with varied age-specific and sex-specific triglyceride and HDL-C cutoffs, and differing approaches to measuring abdominal obesity with WC or BMI.[20] In 2007, an IDF consensus panel proposed unified criteria.[20] For children aged 10 to 16 years, obesity was diagnosed if WC was equal to or greater than the 90th percentile for age. Over 16 years, the criteria were the same as adult IDF WC criteria, with cutoffs of 94 cm or higher in males and 80 cm or higher in females.[20] A MetS diagnosis required an additional 2 of increased triglyceride levels (≥1.7 mmol/L or 150 mg/dL), low HDL-C levels (≤1.03 mmol/L or 40 mg/dL), increased blood pressure (≥130 bpm systolic, ≥85 bpm diastolic), and impaired fasting glucose level (≥5.6 mmol/L or 100 mg/dL) or overt diabetes. For children younger than 10 years, obesity was defined as WC equal to or greater than the 90th percentile, but the panel did not support that a MetS diagnosis could be made in this age group, although testing for additional components could be undertaken in high-risk children.

EPIDEMIOLOGY

The reported prevalence of MetS varies depending on the definition used, age, sex, socioeconomic status, and the ethnic background of study cohorts. However, from studies published in the last decade, an estimated one-quarter to one-third of adults meet MetS criteria in multiple ethnic backgrounds. Cross-sectional data from 1999 to 2010 from the National Health and Nutrition Examination Survey (NHANES) in the

Table 1
Comparison of definitions of MetS

	WHO	EGIR	NCEP/ATPIII	AACE	AHA/NHLBI/ADA Updated NCEP/ATPIII	IDF	Harmonized Definition[a]
Year	1999	1999	2001	2003	2004	2005	2009
Number of risk factors	IFG/IGT/T2DM or insulin resistance[b] and 2 of...	Insulin resistance[c] and 3 or more of...	Three or more of....	IGT/IFG with any of the following...	Three or more of...	Obesity and 2 of...	Three or more of...
Obesity	Waist/hip ratio >0.9 M, >0.85 F or BMI >30 kg/m²	Waist circumference ≥94 cm M ≥80 cm F	Waist circumference ≥102 cm M ≥88 cm F	BMI ≥25 kg/m²	Waist circumference ≥102 cm M ≥88 cm F	Waist circumference ≥94 cm M ≥90 (Asian M) ≥80 cm F	Waist circumference[d] Geographic and ethnic specific
Dyslipidemia	HDL-C <0.91 mmol/L M (35 mg/dL) <1.0 mmol/L F (<39 mg/dL) TG ≥1.7 mmol/L (150 mg/dL)	HDL-C <1.0 mmol/L (39 mg/dL) TG ≥2.0 mmol/L (177 mg/dL) or treated	HDL-C <1.0 mmol/L M (40 mg/dL) <1.3 mmol/L F (50 mg/dL) TG ≥1.69 mmol/L (150 mg/dL)	HDL-C <1.0 mmol/L M (40 mg/dL) <1.3 mmol/L F (50 mg/dL) TG ≥1.69 mmol/L (150 mg/dL)	HDL-C <1.0 mmol/L M (40 mg/dL) <1.3 mmol/L F (50 mg/dL) TG ≥1.69 mmol/L (150 mg/dL) or treated	HDL-C <1.0 mmol/L M (40 mg/dL) <1.3 mmol/L F (50 mg/dL) TG ≥1.7 mmol/L (150 mg/dL) or treated	HDL-C <1.0 mmol/L M (40 mg/dL) <1.3 mmol/L F (50 mg/dL) TG ≥1.7 mmol/L (150 mg/dL) or treated

	(Definition 1)	(Definition 2)	(Definition 3)	(Definition 4)	(Definition 5)	(Definition 6)	(Definition 7)
Hyperglycemia	T2DM FPG >6.1 mmol/L (110 mg/dL) 2 h OGT >7.7 mmol/L (140 mg/dL)	Not T2DM FPG >6.1 mmol/L (110 mg/dL)	T2DM FPG ≥110 mg/dL (6.1 mmol/L)	Not T2DM FPG ≥110 mg/dL (6.1 mmol/L) 2 h OGT >7.7 mmol/L (140 mg/dL)	T2DM FPG ≥5.6 mmol/L (100 mg/dL)	T2DM FPG ≥5.6 mmol/L (100 mg/dL)	T2DM FPG ≥5.6 mmol/L (100 mg/dL) or treated
Hypertension	SBP ≥140 DBP ≥90	SBP ≥140 DBP ≥90 or treated	SBP ≥130 DBP ≥85	SBP ≥130 DBP ≥85	SBP ≥130 DBP ≥85 or treated	SBP ≥130 DBP ≥85 or treated	SBP ≥130 DBP ≥85 or treated
Additional components	Microalbuminuria ≥20 µg/min Albumin/creatinine ≥30 mg/g	—	—	Insulin resistance (family history T2DM, age, ethnicity, sedentary, lifestyle, PCOS)	—	—	—

Abbreviations: AHA, American Heart Association; BMI, body mass index; DBP, diastolic blood pressure in mm Hg; F, female; FPG, fasting plasma glucose; HDL-C, high-density lipoprotein cholesterol; IFG, impaired fasting glucose; IGT, impaired glucose tolerance; M, male; NHLBI, National Heart, Lung and Blood Institute; OGT, oral glucose tolerance test; PCOS, polycystic ovarian syndrome; SBP, systolic blood pressure in mm Hg; TG, triglyceride.

[a] Joint statement from the IDF, AHA/NHLBI, the World Heart Federation, the International Atherosclerosis Society, and the International Association for the Study of Obesity.

[b] If fasting glucose <110 mg/dL (6.1 mmol/L), insulin resistance measured by hyperinsulinemic-euglycemic clamp with lowest quartile for glucose uptake.

[c] Modification to WHO definition to use upper quartile of fasting insulin levels.

[d] See **Table 2** for suggested population-specific values.

Data from Refs.[11–13,15–17]

Table 2
Suggested cutoffs for WC to determine abdominal obesity from the harmonized definition (2009) and national organizations

Population/Ethnicity	WC (cm)	
	Male	Female
United States (NCEP/ATPIII)	≥102	≥88
Health Canada	≥102	≥88
Europoid	≥94	≥80
European Cardiovascular Societies	≥102	≥88
South Asian	≥90	≥80
Chinese	≥90	≥80
China Cooperative Task Force	≥85	≥80
Japanese	≥85	≥90
Ethnic South and Central Americans	≥90	≥80
Eastern Mediterranean and Middle East	≥94	≥80
Sub-Saharan African	≥94	≥80

Adapted from Alberti KG, Eckel RH, Grundy SM, et al. Harmonizing the metabolic syndrome: a joint interim statement of the International Diabetes Federation Task Force on Epidemiology and Prevention; National Heart, Lung, and Blood Institute; American Heart Association; World Heart Federation; International Atherosclerosis Society; and International Association for the Study of Obesity. Circulation 2009;120(16):1642; with permission.

United States show that, in adults older than 20 years, the age-adjusted overall prevalence of MetS was 25.5% in 1999 to 2000, declining slightly to 22.9% in 2009 to 2010.[21] However, this finding was tempered by the fact that the prevalence of hyperglycemia increased from 12.9% to 19.9% and that of abdominal obesity, because WC had increased from 45.4% to 56.1%.[21] From Europe, the DECODE (Diabetes Epidemiology: Collaborative Analysis of Diagnostic Criteria in Europe) study included data from 9 population studies performed in Finland, the Netherlands, the United Kingdom, Sweden, Poland, and Italy.[22] Using the lower IDF WC cutoffs, 41% of the men and 38% of women met MetS criteria at baseline at ages 47 to 71 years.[22]

The high prevalence of MetS is not unique to the United States and Europe. In Asian Indians, the prevalence of MetS is 5% in rural populations but increases to greater than one-third of the population in urban settings.[23] The prevalence of MetS in the States of the Gulf Cooperative Council (Kuwait, Oman, Qatar, Bahrain, Saudi Arabia, and United Arab Emirates) is higher than for US population data, at 21% to 37% in men and 32% to 43% in women.[24] From the Korean NHANES (KNHANES) held from 1998 to 2008, MetS was present in 25% of the population older than 20 years using NCEP criteria but with a lower Asian WC threshold.[25] Japanese participants of KOPS (Kyushu and Okinawa Population Study) (ages 30–69 years) had a prevalence of 36% in men, but only 10% in women using BMI 25 kg/m^2 or greater or Japanese WC cutoffs.[26] In China, a cross-sectional survey of subjects aged 30 to 74 years revealed a prevalence of 10% in men and 18% in women, but the prevalence was higher in urban settings.[27]

The prevalence of MetS also increases with aging. Analysis of US data from the cohort of the Framingham Offspring Study showed that the prevalence of MetS increased by approximately 50% from baseline at 50 years old from 21% to 34% in men and from 12.5% to 24% in women at 8 years of follow-up.[28] From CHS (Cardiovascular Health Study) in the United States, in adults older than 65 years, there was an overall prevalence of MetS of 35%.[29] The US prevalence of MetS in older individuals is echoed by studies using the NCEP definition from the United Kingdom and Europe. The cohort of PROSPER (Prospective Study of Pravastatin in the Elderly at Risk) included nondiabetic participants 70 to 82 years old from the United Kingdom, Ireland, and the Netherlands, using BMI of 30 kg/m^2 or higher as the criterion for obesity. The prevalence of MetS was 28%, similar to the BRHS (British Regional Heart Study) of 27% in men 60 to 79 years old.[30] In China, the estimated prevalence of MetS in the elderly ages 60 to 95 years is higher than in younger cohorts, at nearly 60% using the harmonized definition.[31]

In the pediatric population, MetS prevalence in the United States is estimated to be low overall but is highly prevalent when studied in overweight and obese children.[18,19] From NHANES III data (1988–1994), the overall prevalence was 6% in males and 2% in females aged 12 to 19 years using Cook and colleagues'[19] modified NCEP definition. Differences were apparent when the data were analyzed for ethnic background, with higher prevalence in White and Mexican-American adolescents compared with African Americans.[19] Analysis of data from individuals who were in the 95th percentile or higher for weight revealed a prevalence of 28%.[19] Follow-up analysis of NHANES data from 1999 to 2002 by the same investigators showed an increased prevalence of 9% overall (13% male and 5% female) and 44% in overweight adolescents.[32] The presence of MetS in children and adolescents is closely associated with parental history of obesity.[33]

The MetS phenotype is also associated with other primary diseases. Abdominal obesity is present in 40% to 85% of women with polycystic ovary syndrome (PCOS), and other MetS components (insulin resistance, dyslipidemia, and hypertension) are also concentrated in this population.[34] The prevalence of MetS in US studies of women with PCOS is twice that of age-matched individuals.[35–37] A study of Italian women with PCOS found a lower prevalence of MetS than in the United States, at 8% compared with age-matched and weight-matched individuals, but the prevalence of MetS in the controls was only 2.4%.[38] The 2003 Rotterdam consensus on PCOS recommended screening for MetS in this population using the NCEP criteria, except that the addition of oral glucose testing criteria was advocated for in this population for patients with BMI of 27 kg/m^2 or higher.[39]

Living with human immunodeficiency virus (HIV) infection long-term has been facilitated by the use of combination antiretroviral therapy (cART). However, HIV-positive patients can develop dysmetabolic features, including hyperlipidemia, central adipose deposits, peripheral lipoatrophy, glucose intolerance, and insulin resistance.[40] They are also at risk for CVD.[40] The lipodystrophic syndrome is often, although not always, attributable to the use of cART.[40] The reported prevalence of MetS in this population varies widely across different cohorts. Determining the prevalence of MetS attributable to HIV or cART is complicated by the background population and heterogeneity in the use of cART in a cohort. Also, the diagnosis of MetS in this population can be more challenging if there is lipodystrophy and fat partitioning, so that abdominal obesity is not the predominant phenotype and WC thresholds are not met. Some MetS prevalence estimates in HIV-positive patients are lower than for population studies, despite the propensity for dyslipidemia. From ALLRT (AIDS Clinical Trials Group Longitudinal Linked Randomized Trials), treatment-naive patients had a MetS prevalence of 20% by NCEP criteria overall but this increased to more than one-third of patients who were older than 50 years.[41] The risk was increased for high HIV-1 RNA levels or the use of protease inhibitors.[41] Other international studies report prevalence of MetS just lower than 20%, but associated with cART use.[42,43] In a more homogeneous cohort of patients, all of whom were on cART, the prevalence of MetS was higher, at 54.5% in male and 47.2% in female patients with HIV in their 40s.[44] The prevalence of MetS was the same with or without lipodystrophy, diagnosed clinically by the presence of lipoatrophy or abdominal prominence. Only 4% of participants in this cohort were free of all MetS components.

Hypopituitarism is also associated with metabolic abnormalities and increased cardiometabolic risk. Verhelst and colleagues[45] analyzed the prevalence of MetS criteria in patients with untreated adult-onset growth hormone (GH) deficiency (GHD) from an international database of patients from Europe and Argentina. MetS prevalence was more than 40% overall, but ranged from 38% to 60%, depending on the country. It was not influenced by the presence of additional pituitary deficiencies. In the Hypopituitary Control and Complications Study, the baseline prevalence of MetS in adult patients with GHD was 42% with age-adjusted prevalence of 52% in the United States and 29% in Europe.[46] After 3 years of GH therapy, there was a significant reduction in the number of patients meeting the threshold for central obesity. Overall, MetS prevalence did not change, because of the increase in the prevalence of hypertension and impaired fasting glucose.

CONSEQUENCES OF METS

MetS, by definition, is not a disease, but is a clustering of individual risk factors for disease, drawing the attention of the clinician to the probable coexistence of multiple cardiometabolic risk factors in patients when one of the components is found.[47] Therefore, a diagnosis of MetS could be expected to predict risk. The goal is to target the different components of MetS with lifestyle and pharmacologic therapies to prevent disease, particularly CVD and diabetes.

Among the differing MetS definitions, the NCEP criteria better concentrate cardiovascular risk in a population[48,49] with the best predictive accuracy at identifying individuals at risk for acute MI independently of age, sex, previous CVD, smoking, hypercholesterolemia, diabetes, and hypertension.[50] Other studies support that NCEP criteria are more accurate and sensitive for prediction of CVD.[51–53] The most recent harmonized definition of MetS proposed by the joint interim statement is essentially the AHA/NHLBI updated NCEP criteria.[17]

Overall, a MetS diagnosis portends an adjusted relative risk (RR) of CVD outcomes, which hovers around 2-fold. From the Framingham Heart Study Offspring Study, participants with MetS had an age-adjusted RR of CVD of 2.88 for men and 2.25 for women older than 8 years.[28,54] Using data from the Hypertension Heredity in Malmö Evaluation Study, the RR of a cardiovascular event was 2.04 after adjusting for age, sex, family history of MI, current smoking, and LDL cholesterol.[29] From the DECODE study, using a modified IDF definition because of the lack of information on lipid medication use, the analysis showed a hazard ratio (HR) of 2.24 for males and 2.32 for females with abdominal obesity and 2 or more other components.[22] For patients without abdominal obesity, the risk also was higher: the HR with 3 or more components was 2.44 for men, although it was not calculable for women because of the low event rate. Nonetheless, the results emphasized that patients with MetS who do not meet obesity thresholds are also at risk for CVD. In contrast to these reports, analysis of data from PROSPER and the male BRHS cohorts did not find a significant increase in risk for CVD using NCEP criteria with BMI of 30 kg/m^2 or higher instead of WC at a mean follow-up of 3 and 7 years, respectively.[30]

The absence of MetS diagnosis does not imply safety from CVD. From NHANES data, the chance of a future MI was 23% to 42% without a MetS diagnosis.[49] In CHS, CVD events occurred in 18% of those without a MetS diagnosis.[29] These findings emphasize the importance of additional cardiovascular risk factors not accounted for in the definition of MetS.

The presence of MetS does signify higher risk than is predicted by its components when analyzed individually. From MRFIT (Multiple Risk Factor Intervention Trial),[55] the presence of a MetS diagnosis by NCEP criteria, but using BMI of 30 kg/m² or higher, increased total mortality (HR = 1.21) and CVD mortality (HR = 1.49). Separating the components, the HR became significant only when more than 2 components were present and was further increased with the addition of more MetS components.[55] For example, the HR for CVD mortality was 2.98 if all 5 components were present compared with 1.51 with 3 components.[55] Using the US NHANES data, Eddy and colleagues[49] examined the importance of each MetS component for CVD risk. Fasting glucose level greater than 110 mg/dL concentrated CVD risk and predicted a future MI better than any MetS definition used.[49]

With hyperglycemia as a component of MetS, does the diagnosis of MetS added to a known diagnosis of T2DM predict a worsened cardiovascular outcome? Cull and colleagues[56] examined data from UKPDS 78 (UK Prospective Diabetes Study 78). Newly diagnosed patients with T2DM had a MetS prevalence of 61%, and this subgroup did have significantly increased risk of MI or stroke over 10 years of follow-up.[56] However, there was significant overlap of 10-year risk estimates with or without MetS. The investigators concluded that there is little clinical value in an added diagnosis of MetS for risk stratification in patients already diagnosed with T2DM.[56] This finding is in agreement with other published data that show that a MetS diagnosis does not provide further predictive power for CVD events and mortality,[57] because T2DM is already a CVD risk equivalent.[58,59]

Although the original intent for defining MetS was to identify those at risk for CVD, there has been investigation of its ability to predict T2DM. Analysis of data from the Framingham Heart Study Offspring participants revealed an age-adjusted RR of diabetes of 7-fold in males and females.[28,54] Investigators from EPIC (European Prospective Investigation into Cancer) and the Nutrition-Potsdam study examined the incidence of self-reported diabetes from 2796 male and female participants. The HR for patients fitting NCEP criteria was 3.7 in men and 6.1 in women, with abdominal obesity and hyperglycemia as the 2 strongest individual predictors.[60] When the data were analyzed using a reference group with no cardiometabolic risk factors, the adjusted HR for those meeting 3 or more criteria was 22.5.[60] The elderly cohorts from PROSPER and the BRHS had an increased risk for diabetes if diagnosed with MetS, with HRs of 4.4 and 7.5, respectively.[30] All 5 components of the MetS definition caused significantly increased risk of new-onset diabetes when analyzed independently.[30] From a meta-analysis of prospective cohort studies, the RR of incident diabetes was 5.1 and, despite the heterogeneity of the studies, the investigators concluded that MetS predicts incident diabetes in individuals from numerous backgrounds.[61]

The more MetS components you have, the higher the risk of T2DM. For example, in WOSCOPS (West of Scotland Coronary Prevention Study), the HR for diabetes using NCEP criteria was 7.3 with 3 components and 24.4 with 4 or more.[62] In the BRHS, the RR of T2DM in men with 3 NCEP abnormalities was 4.6 but higher at 10.9 with 4 abnormalities.[63]

Of all MetS criteria, IFG and impaired glucose tolerance (IGT) are most strongly associated with diabetes.[60,61] The AusDiab study showed that fasting glucose was a superior predictor of incident diabetes than a diagnosis of MetS.[64] Similarly, fasting glucose levels of 6.1 mmol/L (110 mg/dL) or higher had the highest risk of all MetS components, with HR = 18.42 for the PROSPER cohort and HR = 5.97 for the

BRHS cohort.[30] In the Framingham cohort, fasting plasma glucose level greater than 100 mg/dL alone best predicted the risk for diabetes (RR = 12.1), whereas other components singled out had RRs in the range of 2.4 to 4.1.[28] Even with various combinations of 2 or 3 of the remaining MetS components without glucose, the RRs (range 3.1–5.4) were still lower than for IFG alone.[28]

MetS also is associated with nonalcoholic fatty liver disease (NAFLD). The prevalence of NAFLD has paralleled the increase in obesity, and it is the most common cause of chronic liver disease.[65] NAFLD encompasses a continuum of pathologic changes to the liver from steatosis to steatohepatitis, which can further develop into cirrhosis and increased risk of hepatocellular carcinoma.[65,66] NAFLD has sometimes been referred to as MetS of the liver, and there has been some discussion as to whether this could be included as a MetS component. NAFLD is significantly associated with MetS components of increased WC, triglycerides, blood pressure, glucose, homeostatic model assessment insulin resistance, and lower HDL levels, and the prevalence of NAFLD increases with the number of MetS components present.[67] In a cross-sectional study from Mexico,[68] NAFLD was present in 87% of males and 76% of females with MetS. In a study from Spain,[69] the prevalence of NAFLD by ultrasonography was 53% in patients with MetS. The prevalence of ultrasonographic NAFLD from NHANES III (1988–1994) data is lower, with NAFLD present in only 30% of patients with MetS. There was also some discordance in that nearly 20% had NAFLD without MetS, whereas 10% with MetS did not have NAFLD.[67] Statistical modeling did not support that NAFLD is an independent manifestation that should be added as a component of MetS.[67] Nonetheless, a diagnosis of MetS could mean that NAFLD is present, with all of its attendant risks.

Additional disease risk can be considered to be associated with MetS in relation to the component of obesity. Twenty percent of all cancer deaths in women and 14% in men can be attributed to obesity.[70] There are data to support that there is increased risk of colon, kidney, prostate, endometrial, and breast cancer with obesity.[71] Obesity also portends a worsened outcome with cancer treatment.[71] The underlying reason behind these observations remains to be elucidated, but possibilities are promotion of cancer growth by adipose tissue inflammation, hyperglycemia or hyperinsulinemia, or even increased insulin-like growth factor 1 levels.[3,71,72]

Overall, the diagnosis of MetS predicts an approximately 2-fold increase in CVD over 5 to 10 years, at least a 5-fold increase in development of diabetes, and there is an association with other health problems, including fatty liver and cancer. A finding of impaired glucose metabolism seems to be a better predictor for development of diabetes. However, in the clinical realm, a patient presenting with abdominal obesity or with other components of MetS should be tested for IFG or IGT. Also, there is much debate as to whether a MetS diagnosis has any value for predicting CVD risk, given the availability of risk engines that take into account the presence of additional well-known risk factors. Again, in a patient with a MetS phenotype, there should be the impetus for clinicians to look for and treat additional CVD risk factors aggressively.

PATHOPHYSIOLOGY

With extra caloric intake and a sedentary lifestyle, the excess energy balance is stored as fat. Adipose tissue depots are not metabolically equal. Visceral fat, compared with subcutaneous fat,[73–75] has distinct gene expression patterns and is associated with higher insulin resistance, smaller LDL-C and HDL-C particle size, and increased LDL-C and very low–density lipoprotein (VLDL) particle numbers.[76] In susceptible individuals, the inability for the β cell to compensate for insulin resistance results in relative hypoinsulinemia, promoting increased hormone-sensitive lipase activity and excess lipolysis of stored triglycerides from adipocytes, especially from abdominal fat depots, with excess release of free fatty acids (FFAs).[77] The portal theory of MetS envisages that the FFAs derived from visceral fat are released into the portal circulation and shuttled to the liver to be stored as triglyceride (**Fig. 1**).[78,79] The FFA flux stimulates hepatic output of VLDL, resulting in hypertriglyceridemia.[80] Exchange of triglycerides from VLDL for cholesterol esters from HDL-C by cholesterol ester transfer protein results in rapid clearance of HDL-C.[81] Excess triglycerides also are transferred to LDL, which then becomes a more attractive substrate for hepatic lipase, which brings about lipolysis of the triglycerides and results in small dense LDL particles.[79] Small dense LDL is more atherogenic than larger LDL subclasses and is more prone to oxidation and uptake into the arterial wall.[80] Clinically, the dyslipidemia of obesity is shown as hypertriglyceridemia, with low HDL-C and an increased small dense LDL/LDL-C ratio.

Increased FFA flux to peripheral tissues also inhibits insulin signaling (see **Fig. 1**). With hepatic insulin resistance and an abundance of FFA substrate, gluconeogenesis is increased, contributing to hyperglycemia. Myocellular insulin resistance also results in decreased glucose disposal peripherally. Over time, the pancreatic β cell continues to decompensate for the increased need for insulin to overcome resistance, and T2DM is the consequence (see **Fig. 1**).

The development of hypertension is likely multifactorial, partially mediated by endothelial dysfunction caused by FFA-mediated generation of reactive oxygen species (ROS), hyperinsulinemia-induced sympathetic nervous system activation and inhibition of nitric oxide synthase, and the effects of adipose tissue–derived cytokines.[78,82–84] There also is hyperactivity of the renin-angiotensin-aldosterone system (RAAS) in obesity.[85]

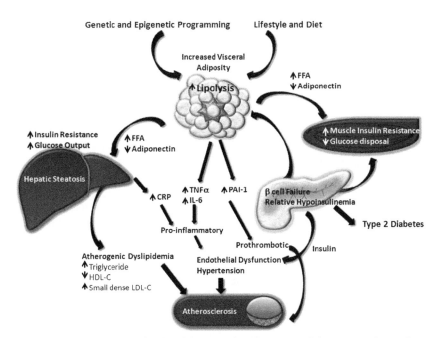

Fig. 1. Proposed mechanisms for the clustering of MetS traits and the increased risk of T2DM and CVD. CRP, C-reactive protein; IL-6, interleukin 6; PAI-1, plasminogen activator inhibitor 1; TNFα, tumor necrosis factor α.

Consideration also has to be given to the secretory products of adipose tissue. Fat is not an inert storage depot for triglycerides, but it is an active endocrine organ.[86] Adipokines are secreted by adipose tissue with far-reaching metabolic effects: these include leptin, resistin, visfatin, monocyte chemoattractant protein 1, retinol binding protein 4, adipocyte-type fatty acid binding protein, plasminogen activating factor 1, and adiponectin.[73,87] Among these adipokines, adiponectin is a positive player, and higher levels result in decreased systemic inflammation and promotion of insulin sensitivity.[87]

There also is a close relationship with bone marrow–derived cells, specifically macrophages, in the adipose tissue of obese individuals, which likely are responsible for increases in cytokines such as interleukin 6 (IL-6) and tumor necrosis factor α (TNF-α), which increase inflammation and postreceptor resistance to insulin and may also have a role in the increased CVD risk associated with obesity.[82] In rodent models of obesity, adipocytes can be seen to be surrounded by a syncytium of macrophages, histopathologically described as crownlike structures.[3,73,88] This finding has also been reported in adipose tissue of obese humans.[89] The adipocytes are undergoing necrosis, and these findings correlate with insulin resistance. What makes the adipocytes sick? One hypothesis is that the prevalence of excess fuel leads to cell stress at the level of the organelles with increased ROS production in the mitochondria caused by FFA oxidation and pathologic activation of the unfolded protein response in the endoplasmic reticulum caused by excess demands for protein synthesis for adipose tissue expansion.[90,91]

Although obesity features prominently in discussions of MetS, approximately one-third of obese individuals, as defined by their BMI, are considered to have metabolically healthy obesity[92] and do not manifest dyslipidemia, hypertension, or hyperglycemia. These healthy obese individuals have less macrophage infiltration in their adipose tissue[93,94] and decreased levels of C-reactive protein (CRP), IL-6, TNF-α, and plasminogen activator inhibitor 1, with increased adiponectin.[92] Those obese individuals who do develop MetS must be predisposed toward metabolic deterioration in their response to obesity, which may be caused by a pathologic combination of genetic and epigenetic factors, along with dietary and environmental influences.

Genome-wide association studies have provided a powerful tool to identify gene loci that could predispose individuals to MetS traits.[91,95] For example, an inability for the β cell to compensate for insulin resistance may be a key trait, and many of the genes that have been found to predict risk for T2DM are associated with β-cell function, rather than a propensity for obesity. For example, human genetic variation in transcription factor 7-like 2 (TCF7L2) a component of the Wnt signaling pathway, is highly associated with risk of developing T2DM among multiple ethnic backgrounds.[96,97] Individuals with the at-risk allele have impaired glucose-stimulated insulin secretion, which worsens over time, resulting in progression from IGT to T2DM, as has been observed in diabetes prevention cohorts.[98,99] It is possible that the genes influencing the development of the MetS phenotype may be the same as for individuals with prediabetes, because individuals with IFG, IGT, and MetS all have similar risk of developing T2DM, and there is additivity in individuals with both impaired glucose metabolism plus additional MetS components.[28] There is also an association of the at-risk TCF7L2 genetic variation with MetS traits, including atherogenic dyslipidemia.[100,101] Studies of TCF7L2 also show the importance of gene interactions with lifestyle and diet, because the association of TCF7L2 variations with risk of developing MetS is influenced by dietary fat intake.[100,101] Also, in the Diabetes Prevention Program (DPP) cohort, the at-risk TCF7L2 variation was associated with progression to T2DM in the control group but not for those with intensive lifestyle changes.[99]

Apart from impaired β-cell function, there are likely additional genetic or epigenetic factors that interact with the environment and diet to influence the development of MetS.[91,102] For example, the melanocortin 4 receptor, involved in brain satiety signaling, has been implicated in risk for increased fat mass and obesity in Europeans and Asian Indians.[103] The fat mass and obesity–associated gene (FTO) is also linked to increased BMI in Europeans, possibly because of effects on appetite or lipolysis.[104–106] Triglyceride levels are affected by variations in the gene for MLX interacting proteinlike.[107] However, the many genes identified account for only 10% of the variance of MetS traits and are likely responsible for only a little genetic susceptibility for MetS,[91] so there is still much research to be carried out in this area. Epigenetic contributions to MetS have also been discovered in studying fetal nutrition in animal models, specifically intrauterine growth retardation, which may result in a postnatal gene expression program that manifests as MetS.[91]

TREATMENT

The treatment of patients with MetS aims to decrease the risk for CVD and T2DM. Overall management involves (1) implementation of lifestyle and dietary changes for weight loss, (2) treatment of atherogenic dyslipidemia, and (3) treatment of hypertension. Many patients with MetS are overweight or obese, and weight reduction through lifestyle changes with caloric restriction and increased physical activity is an important part of the strategy.[108] In a systematic review of 11 randomized controlled studies of lifestyle interventions for a minimum of 6 months and a median length of 1 year,[109] the proportion of patients with resolution of MetS was approximately 2-fold over controls: there were reductions in systolic and diastolic blood pressure, triglycerides, WC, and fasting glucose levels but without a significant change in HDL-C. The DPP enrolled participants with IGT at baseline and randomized them to standard lifestyle counseling with placebo or metformin, or intensive lifestyle intervention in which individuals were encouraged to lose 7% of body weight with a low calorie diet and moderate physical activity (eg, brisk walking) a minimum of 150 minutes per week. Secondary analysis of DPP data showed that, for individuals without MetS at the outset, the risk of incident MetS was reduced 41% by intensive lifestyle changes for 3 years compared with controls.[110] In patients with MetS at baseline, 38% of patients in the lifestyle intervention no longer met MetS criteria at 3 years compared with 18% in the placebo group, mostly attributable to decreased WC and blood pressure.[110] Studies which incorporate intensive lifestyle changes frequently rely on close follow-up of patients, which can be challenging to achieve in real-life practice. The design of the DPP intensive lifestyle program has been adapted for use in a group setting as the Group Lifestyle Balance Program for community primary care practices, with success at promoting weight loss.[111] In patients struggling with weight loss with lifestyle changes, the use of approved pharmacologic agents or bariatric procedures in those meeting criteria could be considered.

It is important to temper the encouraging results of the DPP data regarding diabetes prevention, because they also showed that successful intensive lifestyle changes cannot delay or prevent T2DM in all individuals, and a portion of those with prediabetes continue to have glucose intolerance rather than revert to normoglycemia.[112] One interpretation is that once the process of β-cell failure has been initiated, it cannot be reversed in genetically susceptible individuals.

Dietary recommendations have been published in the AHA/NHLBI update on the NCEP criteria. Fat intake is recommended to be 25% or less of calories, with limitation of saturated and trans fats, cholesterol intake, and simple sugars (**Table 3**).[108]

Table 3	
Interventions for MetS as recommended by the AHA/NHLBI scientific statement (2005)	
Abdominal obesity	Reduce body weight by 7%–10% by 1 y
	Continue weight loss to achieve <25 kg/m^2 and achieve WC of <102 cm (40 inches) in men and <88 cm (35 inches) in women
	Encourage weight maintenance after weight loss
Physical activity	Moderate intensity aerobic activity (eg, brisk walking) of at least 30–60 min and at least 5 d per wk to daily
	Supplement with increased activities of daily living
	Resistance training 2 d per wk
Diet composition	Reduce total fat to 25% of calories
	Reduce saturated fat to <7% of calories
	Reduce trans fat
	Limit cholesterol
	Choose unsaturated fat
	Avoid simple sugars
Dyslipidemia	The primary target is to lower LDL-C as guided by NCEP/ATPIII using statins
	A secondary target is increased non-HDL-C
	If triglyceride level is ≥500 mg/dL, initiate fibrate or nicotinic acid
Increased blood pressure (BP)	Reduce BP to at least achieve BP of <140/90 mm Hg
	For BP ≥140/90 mm Hg, add BP medication as needed to achieve goal
	For BP ≥120/80 mm Hg, use lifestyle modification
Increased glucose level	For IFG, delay progression to T2DM with lifestyle changes

Adapted from Grundy SM, Cleeman JI, Daniels SR, et al. Diagnosis and Management of the Metabolic Syndrome: An American Heart Association/National Heart, Lung, and Blood Institute Scientific Statement. Circulation 2005;112:2741; with permission.

However, there are no clear indications on the type of diet that could be most successful in promoting weight loss as well as improvement in MetS components. The Mediterranean and DASH (Dietary Approaches to Stop Hypertension) diets have been used with success in patients with MetS.[113] Nonpharmacologic alternative or complementary substances such as omega-3 fatty acids, red wine, dark chocolate, cinnamon, ginseng, soy, green tea, and bitter melon lack a vigorous evidence base.[113]

Weight loss and lifestyle changes may improve individual MetS components, but reduction of cardiovascular risk through treatment of atherogenic dyslipidemia is a key focus. For patients with MetS, the increased triglyceride and lower HDL levels are associated with small dense LDL.[80] Statins (3-hydroxy-3-methylglutaryl coenzyme A reductase inhibitors) are the cornerstone as a monotherapy or in combination with a cholesterol absorption inhibitor (ezetimibe) or a bile acid sequestrant (colestipol, cholestyramine, or colesevelam) to decrease LDL-C levels. The ATPIII provides recommendations for LDL-C goals based on a patient's 10-year risk category as moderate (10%–20%), high (>20% as CHD or risk equivalent), or very high (CHD with additional risk factors).[108] For patients with MetS without a CHD risk equivalent, such as diabetes or a history of CVD, Framingham Risk tables facilitate estimation of 10-year risk. There has been evidence that statins can increase risk of developing T2DM, particularly relevant in the population with MetS. From the JUPITER (Justification for the Use of Statins in Primary Prevention) trial data, there was an HR = 1.28 for diabetes in those with 1 diabetes risk factor, including a MetS diagnosis, but there was nearly a 40% reduction in end points, and the investigators concluded that the CVD and mortality benefits of statin therapy outweighed the concern about T2DM risk.[114] There is residual risk for CVD even after maximal decrease of LDL levels,[115] and there has been speculation that this is caused by additional pathologic contributions by low HDL-C and increased triglycerides. HDL-C levels inversely correlate with CVD risk[116] and non-HDL-C is a secondary target after decreasing LDL-C levels as recommended by the ATPIII.[108] Can additional CVD prevention be derived from lipid therapies in addition to statins? Niacin increases HDL levels and decreases triglyceride levels, and, in the prestatin era, niacin monotherapy was shown to improve cardiovascular outcomes, such as secondary prevention with the Coronary Drug Project.[117] However, 2 recent trials have not shown benefit of treating low HDL-C with niacin in patients with known CVD already on statins with well-controlled LDL-C. The results of AIM-HIGH (Atherothrombosis Intervention in Metabolic Syndrome with Low HDL/ High Triglycerides)[118,119] and HPS2-THRIVE (Heart Protection Study 2)[120] were negative, and both studies were stopped early because of futility and concerns regarding adverse events. The CVD effects of addition of fenofibrate to a simvastatin was studied in patients with T2DM in the ACCORD (Action to Control Cardiovascular Risk in Diabetes) trial. Although there was no overall benefit for CVD outcomes, a subset of patients in the worst tertile for triglycerides and HDL-C may derive some benefit from this combination.[121,122] Gemfibrozil as monotherapy had a positive effect on secondary prevention of CHD in VA-HIT (Veterans Affairs High-Density Lipoprotein Intervention Trial), but it is not used in combination with a statin because of risk of myopathy.[123]

Hypertension should be treated to a goal of less than 140 bpm systolic and less than 80 bpm diastolic with guidance from the Seventh Report of the Joint National Committee on Prevention, Detection, Evaluation and Treatment of High Blood Pressure (JNC 7).[124] Lifestyle changes with increased exercise, decreased alcohol intake, and a low salt diet are recommended in obesity.[85] The choice of an angiotensin-converting enzyme inhibitor or angiotensin receptor blocker is supported by increased activity of the RAAS in obesity.[85] A role for diuretics because of the salt sensitivity of obese patients is acknowledged, but the use of thiazides should be judicious because of their effects on lipids and insulin resistance.[85] Spironolactone could be helpful by counteracting aldosterone activity. β-blockers increase insulin resistance, and use is limited to cardiac indications.[85]

From diabetes prevention trials, it is also apparent that lifestyle modifications have a large impact on the delay or prevention of T2DM, even beyond pharmacotherapy with metformin[125,126] which is not approved for this indication in the United States.

CONTROVERSIES

Multiple critiques have been leveled at the construct of the MetS over the last decade. A Joint Statement of the ADA and the European Association for the Study of Diabetes outlined several thoughtful and now famous concerns regarding MetS.[127] Because it is a vehicle first proposed to identify individuals at high risk for CVD, one criticism is that obvious risk factors are not accounted for in the definitions, including age, sex, smoking history, and LDL-C. These additional risk factors may partially explain why 20% to 40% of patients who have a cardiovascular event do not have an MetS diagnosis.[29,49] The ATPIII also discussed the importance of prothrombotic and proinflammatory factors for CVD, but there has not been movement to incorporate additional markers of CVD into mainstream clinical practice: apolipoprotein B, lipoprotein(a), small dense LDL particles, CRP, decreased adiponectin, and albuminuria all have been associated with risk for CVD.[47,87,128] Another criticism is that if the clinical focus is on the presence of MetS components, the presence of additional CVD risk factors could be ignored, and they could be left untreated. With regard to the usefulness of MetS for risk prediction, algorithms such as the Framingham score perform superiorly and provide an estimate of absolute risk, rather than the RR or HRs reported for population studies of MetS.[30,49,129,130] For diabetes, in the Framingham offspring cohort, fasting plasma glucose alone best predicted risk compared with varied permutations of the MetS with or without glucose.[28]

Reconciling the components of MetS to a single underlying cause, such as obesity or insulin resistance, has also been challenging. Kahn pointed out that not everyone who fits criteria for MetS has insulin resistance and oppositely, not all with insulin resistance have MetS.[47] Further, only half of obese individuals are insulin resistant,[47] indicating that there are additional yet unexplored factors and unique gene-environment and gene-diet interactions which require further research.

SUMMARY AND FUTURE CONSIDERATIONS

The definition of MetS has been harmonized to the NCEP definition and there are likely to be additional iterations and discussions of the syndrome in the future. The relationship of WC to cardiovascular risk in varied populations needs further research and refinement.[17] The basic research focus will be on further elucidation of pathophysiology and the gene interactions that underpin the clustering of MetS components.

There is no doubt that the clinical use of MetS has had its controversies. Perhaps the usefulness of MetS as a diagnosis is to be found in a sort of pattern recognition of a phenotype that allows clinicians to further explore the presence of all MetS components as well as additional cardiovascular risk factors not included in the definition, facilitating the use of established risk engines, which give a closer estimate of absolute risk to communicate to the patient. Once discovered, it is also essential that clinicians and patients take action to reduce these risk factors through lifestyle interventions and pharmacologic therapy.

REFERENCES

1. Rossner S. Eskil Kylin (1885–1974). Obes Rev 2009;10:362.
2. Vague J. The degree of masculine differentiation of obesities: a factor determining predisposition to diabetes, atherosclerosis, gout, and uric calculous disease. Am J Clin Nutr 1956;4(1):20–34.
3. Oda E. Metabolic syndrome: its history, mechanisms, and limitations. Acta Diabetol 2012;49(2):89–95.
4. Haller H. Epidemiology and associated risk factors of hyperlipoproteinemia. Z Gesamte Inn Med 1977;32(8):124–8 [in German].
5. Singer P. Diagnosis of primary hyperlipoproteinemias. Z Gesamte Inn Med 1977;32(9):129–33 [in German].
6. Phillips GB. Sex hormones, risk factors and cardiovascular disease. Am J Med 1978;65(1):7–11.
7. Reaven GM. Banting lecture 1988. Role of insulin resistance in human disease. Diabetes 1988;37(12):1595–607.
8. WHO obesity and overweight fact sheet no. 311. Available at: http://www.who.int/mediacentre/factsheets/fs311/en/. Accessed October 23, 2013.
9. Hossain P, Kawar B, El NM. Obesity and diabetes in the developing world–a growing challenge. N Engl J Med 2007;356(3):213–5.

10. Alberti KG, Zimmet PZ. Definition, diagnosis and classification of diabetes mellitus and its complications. Part 1: diagnosis and classification of diabetes mellitus provisional report of a WHO consultation. Diabet Med 1998;15(7):539–53.
11. Balkau B, Charles MA. Comment on the provisional report from the WHO consultation. European Group for the Study of Insulin Resistance (EGIR). Diabet Med 1999;16(5):442–3.
12. Einhorn D, Reaven GM, Cobin RH, et al. American College of Endocrinology position statement on the insulin resistance syndrome. Endocr Pract 2003;9(3): 237–52.
13. Expert Panel on Detection, Evaluation, and Treatment of High Blood Cholesterol in Adults. Executive summary of the third report of The National Cholesterol Education Program (NCEP) expert panel on detection, evaluation, and treatment of high blood cholesterol in adults (adult treatment panel III). JAMA 2001;285(19): 2486–97.
14. Available at: http://www.idf.org/webdata/docs/Metac_syndrome_def.pdf. Accessed October 23, 2013.
15. Grundy SM, Brewer HB Jr, Cleeman JI, et al. Definition of metabolic syndrome: report of the National Heart, Lung, and Blood Institute/American Heart Association conference on scientific issues related to definition. Arterioscler Thromb Vasc Biol 2004;24(2):e13–8.
16. Alberti KG, Zimmet P, Shaw J. Metabolic syndrome–a new world-wide definition. A Consensus Statement from the International Diabetes Federation. Diabet Med 2006;23(5):469–80.
17. Alberti KG, Eckel RH, Grundy SM, et al. Harmonizing the metabolic syndrome: a joint interim statement of the International Diabetes Federation Task Force on Epidemiology and Prevention; National Heart, Lung, and Blood Institute; American Heart Association; World Heart Federation; International Atherosclerosis Society; and International Association for the Study of Obesity. Circulation 2009;120(16):1640–5.
18. Marcovecchio ML, Chiarelli F. Metabolic syndrome in youth: chimera or useful concept? Curr Diab Rep 2013;13(1):56–62.
19. Cook S, Weitzman M, Auinger P, et al. Prevalence of a metabolic syndrome phenotype in adolescents: findings from the third National Health and Nutrition Examination Survey, 1988–1994. Arch Pediatr Adolesc Med 2003;157(8): 821–7.
20. Zimmet P, Alberti KG, Kaufman F, et al. The metabolic syndrome in children and adolescents–an IDF consensus report. Pediatr Diabetes 2007;8(5):299–306.
21. Beltran-Sanchez H, Harhay MO, Harhay MM, et al. Prevalence and trends of metabolic syndrome in the adult US population, 1999–2010. J Am Coll Cardiol 2013;62:697–703.
22. Gao W. Does the constellation of risk factors with and without abdominal adiposity associate with different cardiovascular mortality risk? Int J Obes (Lond) 2008;32(5):757–62.
23. Pandit K, Goswami S, Ghosh S, et al. Metabolic syndrome in South Asians. Indian J Endocrinol Metab 2012;16(1):44–55.
24. Mabry RM, Reeves MM, Eakin EG, et al. Gender differences in prevalence of the metabolic syndrome in Gulf Cooperation Council Countries: a systematic review. Diabet Med 2010;27(5):593–7.
25. Lee SR, Cha MJ, Kang DY, et al. Increased prevalence of metabolic syndrome among hypertensive population: ten years' trend of the Korean National Health and Nutrition Examination Survey. Int J Cardiol 2013;166(3):633–9.

26. Unno M, Furusyo N, Mukae H, et al. The utility of visceral fat level by bioelectrical impedance analysis in the screening of metabolic syndrome–the results of the Kyushu and Okinawa Population Study (KOPS). J Atheroscler Thromb 2012; 19(5):462–70.

27. Gu D, Reynolds K, Wu X, et al. Prevalence of the metabolic syndrome and overweight among adults in China. Lancet 2005;365(9468):1398–405.

28. Wilson PW, D'Agostino RB, Parise H, et al. Metabolic syndrome as a precursor of cardiovascular disease and type 2 diabetes mellitus. Circulation 2005; 112(20):3066–72.

29. Scuteri A, Najjar SS, Morrell CH, et al. The metabolic syndrome in older individuals: prevalence and prediction of cardiovascular events: the Cardiovascular Health Study. Diabetes Care 2005;28(4):882–7.

30. Sattar N, McConnachie A, Shaper AG, et al. Can metabolic syndrome usefully predict cardiovascular disease and diabetes? Outcome data from two prospective studies. Lancet 2008;371(9628):1927–35.

31. Liu M, Wang J, Jiang B, et al. Increasing prevalence of metabolic syndrome in a Chinese elderly population: 2001–2010. PLoS One 2013;8(6):e66233.

32. Cook S, Auinger P, Li C, et al. Metabolic syndrome rates in United States adolescents, from the National Health and Nutrition Examination Survey, 1999–2002. J Pediatr 2008;152(2):165–70.

33. Monzani A, Rapa A, Fuiano N, et al. Metabolic syndrome is strictly associated with parental obesity beginning from childhood. Clin Endocrinol (Oxf) 2013. [Epub ahead of print].

34. Randeva HS, Tan BK, Weickert MO, et al. Cardiometabolic aspects of the polycystic ovary syndrome. Endocr Rev 2012;33(5):812–41.

35. Apridonidze T, Essah PA, Iuorno MJ, et al. Prevalence and characteristics of the metabolic syndrome in women with polycystic ovary syndrome. J Clin Endocrinol Metab 2005;90(4):1929–35.

36. Glueck CJ, Papanna R, Wang P, et al. Incidence and treatment of metabolic syndrome in newly referred women with confirmed polycystic ovarian syndrome. Metabolism 2003;52(7):908–15.

37. Moran LJ, Misso ML, Wild RA, et al. Impaired glucose tolerance, type 2 diabetes and metabolic syndrome in polycystic ovary syndrome: a systematic review and meta-analysis. Hum Reprod Update 2010;16(4):347–63.

38. Carmina E, Napoli N, Longo RA, et al. Metabolic syndrome in polycystic ovary syndrome (PCOS): lower prevalence in southern Italy than in the USA and the influence of criteria for the diagnosis of PCOS. Eur J Endocrinol 2006;154(1):141–5.

39. Rotterdam ESHRE/ASRM-Sponsored PCOS Consensus Workshop Group. Revised 2003 consensus on diagnostic criteria and long-term health risks related to polycystic ovary syndrome (PCOS). Hum Reprod 2004;19(1):41–7.

40. Gutierrez AD, Balasubramanyam A. Dysregulation of glucose metabolism in HIV patients: epidemiology, mechanisms, and management. Endocrine 2012;41(1): 1–10.

41. Krishnan S, Schouten JT, Atkinson B, et al. Metabolic syndrome before and after initiation of antiretroviral therapy in treatment-naive HIV-infected individuals. J Acquir Immune Defic Syndr 2012;61(3):381–9.

42. Samaras K, Wand H, Law M, et al. Prevalence of metabolic syndrome in HIV-infected patients receiving highly active antiretroviral therapy using International Diabetes Foundation and Adult Treatment Panel III criteria: associations with insulin resistance, disturbed body fat compartmentalization, elevated C-reactive protein, and [corrected] hypoadiponectinemia. Diabetes Care 2007;30(1):113–9.

43. Alencastro PR, Wolff FH, Oliveira RR, et al. Metabolic syndrome and population attributable risk among HIV/AIDS patients: comparison between NCEP-ATPIII, IDF and AHA/NHLBI definitions. AIDS Res Ther 2012;9(1):29.
44. Freitas P, Carvalho D, Souto S, et al. Impact of lipodystrophy on the prevalence and components of metabolic syndrome in HIV-infected patients. BMC Infect Dis 2011;11:246.
45. Verhelst J, Mattsson AF, Luger A, et al. Prevalence and characteristics of the metabolic syndrome in 2479 hypopituitary patients with adult-onset GH deficiency before GH replacement: a KIMS analysis. Eur J Endocrinol 2011; 165(6):881–9.
46. Attanasio AF, Mo D, Erfurth EM, et al. Prevalence of metabolic syndrome in adult hypopituitary growth hormone (GH)-deficient patients before and after GH replacement. J Clin Endocrinol Metab 2010;95(1):74–81.
47. Kahn R. Metabolic syndrome: is it a syndrome? Does it matter? Circulation 2007; 115(13):1806–10.
48. Boronat M, Saavedra P, Varillas VF, et al. Differences in traditional and emerging cardiovascular risk factors of subjects discordantly classified by metabolic syndrome definitions of the International Diabetes Federation and the National Cholesterol Education Program. Nutr Metab Cardiovasc Dis 2009; 19(6):417–22.
49. Eddy DM, Schlessinger L, Heikes K. The metabolic syndrome and cardiovascular risk: implications for clinical practice. Int J Obes (Lond) 2008;32(Suppl 2): S5–10.
50. Fedorowski A, Burri P, Hulthen L, et al. The metabolic syndrome and risk of myocardial infarction in familial hypertension (hypertension heredity in Malmö evaluation study). J Hypertens 2009;27(1):109–17.
51. Milionis HJ, Kostapanos MS, Liberopoulos EN, et al. Different definitions of the metabolic syndrome and risk of first-ever acute ischaemic non-embolic stroke in elderly subjects. Int J Clin Pract 2007;61(4):545–51.
52. Nilsson PM, Engstrom G, Hedblad B. The metabolic syndrome and incidence of cardiovascular disease in non-diabetic subjects–a population-based study comparing three different definitions. Diabet Med 2007;24(5):464–72.
53. Jeppesen J, Hansen TW, Rasmussen S, et al. Insulin resistance, the metabolic syndrome, and risk of incident cardiovascular disease: a population-based study. J Am Coll Cardiol 2007;49(21):2112–9.
54. Wilson PW, Meigs JB. Cardiometabolic risk: a Framingham perspective. Int J Obes (Lond) 2008;32(Suppl 2):S17–20.
55. Eberly LE, Prineas R, Cohen JD, et al. Metabolic syndrome: risk factor distribution and 18-year mortality in the multiple risk factor intervention trial. Diabetes Care 2006;29(1):123–30.
56. Cull CA, Jensen CC, Retnakaran R, et al. Impact of the metabolic syndrome on macrovascular and microvascular outcomes in type 2 diabetes mellitus: United Kingdom Prospective Diabetes Study 78. Circulation 2007;116(19):2119–26.
57. Bruno G, Merletti F, Biggeri A, et al. Metabolic syndrome as a predictor of all-cause and cardiovascular mortality in type 2 diabetes: the Casale Monferrato Study. Diabetes Care 2004;27(11):2689–94.
58. Kahn R, Buse J, Ferrannini E, et al. The metabolic syndrome: time for a critical appraisal. Joint statement from the American Diabetes Association and the European Association for the Study of Diabetes. Diabetologia 2005;48(9):1684–99.
59. Laakso M. Hyperglycemia and cardiovascular disease in type 2 diabetes. Diabetes 1999;48(5):937–42.

60. Ford ES, Schulze MB, Pischon T, et al. Metabolic syndrome and risk of incident diabetes: findings from the European Prospective Investigation into Cancer and Nutrition-Potsdam Study. Cardiovasc Diabetol 2008;7:35.

61. Ford ES, Li C, Sattar N. Metabolic syndrome and incident diabetes: current state of the evidence. Diabetes Care 2008;31(9):1898–904.

62. Sattar N, Gaw A, Scherbakova O, et al. Metabolic syndrome with and without C-reactive protein as a predictor of coronary heart disease and diabetes in the West of Scotland Coronary Prevention Study. Circulation 2003;108(4):414–9.

63. Wannamethee SG, Shaper AG, Lennon L, et al. Metabolic syndrome vs Framingham risk score for prediction of coronary heart disease, stroke, and type 2 diabetes mellitus. Arch Intern Med 2005;165(22):2644–50.

64. Cameron AJ, Magliano DJ, Zimmet PZ, et al. The metabolic syndrome as a tool for predicting future diabetes: the AusDiab study. J Intern Med 2008;264(2): 177–86.

65. Krawczyk M, Bonfrate L, Portincasa P. Nonalcoholic fatty liver disease. Best Pract Res Clin Gastroenterol 2010;24(5):695–708.

66. Starley BQ, Calcagno CJ, Harrison SA. Nonalcoholic fatty liver disease and hepatocellular carcinoma: a weighty connection. Hepatology 2010;51(5): 1820–32.

67. Smits MM, Ioannou GN, Boyko EJ, et al. Non-alcoholic fatty liver disease as an independent manifestation of the metabolic syndrome: results of a US national survey in three ethnic groups. J Gastroenterol Hepatol 2013;28(4):664–70.

68. Castro-Martinez MG, Banderas-Lares DZ, Ramirez-Martinez JC, et al. Prevalence of nonalcoholic fatty liver disease in subjects with metabolic syndrome. Cir Cir 2012;80(2):128–33.

69. Caballeria L, Pera G, Rodriguez L, et al. Metabolic syndrome and nonalcoholic fatty liver disease in a Spanish population: influence of the diagnostic criteria used. Eur J Gastroenterol Hepatol 2012;24(9):1007–11.

70. Calle EE, Rodriguez C, Walker-Thurmond K, et al. Overweight, obesity, and mortality from cancer in a prospectively studied cohort of U.S. adults. N Engl J Med 2003;348(17):1625–38.

71. Gilbert CA, Slingerland JM. Cytokines, obesity, and cancer: new insights on mechanisms linking obesity to cancer risk and progression. Annu Rev Med 2013;64:45–57.

72. Giovannucci E, Harlan DM, Archer MC, et al. Diabetes and cancer: a consensus report. CA Cancer J Clin 2010;60(4):207–21.

73. Oda E. The metabolic syndrome as a concept of adipose tissue disease. Hypertens Res 2008;31(7):1283–91.

74. Bremer AA, Jialal I. Adipose tissue dysfunction in nascent metabolic syndrome. J Obes 2013;2013:393192.

75. Fox CS, Massaro JM, Hoffmann U, et al. Abdominal visceral and subcutaneous adipose tissue compartments: association with metabolic risk factors in the Framingham Heart Study. Circulation 2007;116(1):39–48.

76. Neeland IJ, Ayers CR, Rohatgi AK, et al. Associations of visceral and abdominal subcutaneous adipose tissue with markers of cardiac and metabolic risk in obese adults. Obesity (Silver Spring) 2012;21:E439–47.

77. Bergman RN, Kim SP, Catalano KJ, et al. Why visceral fat is bad: mechanisms of the metabolic syndrome. Obesity (Silver Spring) 2006;14(Suppl 1):16S–9S.

78. Bergman RN, Kim SP, Hsu IR, et al. Abdominal obesity: role in the pathophysiology of metabolic disease and cardiovascular risk. Am J Med 2007; 120(2 Suppl 1):S3–8.

79. Klop B, Elte JW, Cabezas MC. Dyslipidemia in obesity: mechanisms and potential targets. Nutrients 2013;5(4):1218–40.
80. Nikolic D, Katsiki N, Montalto G, et al. Lipoprotein subfractions in metabolic syndrome and obesity: clinical significance and therapeutic approaches. Nutrients 2013;5(3):928–48.
81. Subramanian S, Chait A. Hypertriglyceridemia secondary to obesity and diabetes. Biochim Biophys Acta 2012;1821(5):819–25.
82. Gupta A, Gupta V. Metabolic syndrome: what are the risks for humans? Biosci Trends 2010;4(5):204–12.
83. Reaven GM. Relationships among insulin resistance, type 2 diabetes, essential hypertension, and cardiovascular disease: similarities and differences. J Clin Hypertens (Greenwich) 2011;13(4):238–43.
84. Andreassi MG. Metabolic syndrome, diabetes and atherosclerosis: influence of gene-environment interaction. Mutat Res 2009;667(1–2):35–43.
85. Landsberg L, Aronne LJ, Beilin LJ, et al. Obesity-related hypertension: pathogenesis, cardiovascular risk, and treatment–a position paper of the Obesity Society and the American Society of Hypertension. Obesity (Silver Spring) 2013;21(1):8–24.
86. Kershaw EE, Flier JS. Adipose tissue as an endocrine organ. J Clin Endocrinol Metab 2004;89(6):2548–56.
87. Matsuzawa Y, Funahashi T, Nakamura T. The concept of metabolic syndrome: contribution of visceral fat accumulation and its molecular mechanism. J Atheroscler Thromb 2011;18(8):629–39.
88. West M. Dead adipocytes and metabolic dysfunction: recent progress. Curr Opin Endocrinol Diabetes Obes 2009;16(2):178–82.
89. Cinti S, Mitchell G, Barbatelli G, et al. Adipocyte death defines macrophage localization and function in adipose tissue of obese mice and humans. J Lipid Res 2005;46(11):2347–55.
90. Semenkovich CF. Insulin resistance and atherosclerosis. J Clin Invest 2006; 116(7):1813–22.
91. Lusis AJ, Attie AD, Reue K. Metabolic syndrome: from epidemiology to systems biology. Nat Rev Genet 2008;9(11):819–30.
92. Phillips CM. Metabolically healthy obesity: definitions, determinants and clinical implications. Rev Endocr Metab Disord 2013;14:219–27.
93. O'Connell J, Lynch L, Cawood TJ, et al. The relationship of omental and subcutaneous adipocyte size to metabolic disease in severe obesity. PLoS One 2010; 5(4):e9997.
94. O'Connell J, Lynch L, Hogan A, et al. Preadipocyte factor-1 is associated with metabolic profile in severe obesity. J Clin Endocrinol Metab 2011;96(4):E680–4.
95. Povel CM, Boer JM, Reiling E, et al. Genetic variants and the metabolic syndrome: a systematic review. Obes Rev 2011;12(11):952–67.
96. Jin T. The WNT signalling pathway and diabetes mellitus. Diabetologia 2008; 51(10):1771–80.
97. Ingelsson E, Langenberg C, Hivert MF, et al. Detailed physiologic characterization reveals diverse mechanisms for novel genetic loci regulating glucose and insulin metabolism in humans. Diabetes 2010;59:1266–75.
98. Lyssenko V, Lupi R, Marchetti P, et al. Mechanisms by which common variants in the TCF7L2 gene increase risk of type 2 diabetes. J Clin Invest 2007;117(8): 2155–63.
99. Florez JC, Jablonski KA, Bayley N, et al. TCF7L2 polymorphisms and progression to diabetes in the Diabetes Prevention Program. N Engl J Med 2006;355(3): 241–50.

100. Phillips CM, Goumidi L, Bertrais S, et al. Dietary saturated fat, gender and genetic variation at the TCF7L2 locus predict the development of metabolic syndrome. J Nutr Biochem 2012;23(3):239–44.
101. Warodomwichit D, Arnett DK, Kabagambe EK, et al. Polyunsaturated fatty acids modulate the effect of TCF7L2 gene variants on postprandial lipemia. J Nutr 2009;139(3):439–46.
102. Loos RJ, Rankinen T. Gene-diet interactions on body weight changes. J Am Diet Assoc 2005;105(5 Suppl 1):S29–34.
103. Loos RJ, Lindgren CM, Li S, et al. Common variants near MC4R are associated with fat mass, weight and risk of obesity. Nat Genet 2008;40(6):768–75.
104. Loos RJ, Bouchard C. FTO: the first gene contributing to common forms of human obesity. Obes Rev 2008;9(3):246–50.
105. Frayling TM, Timpson NJ, Weedon MN, et al. A common variant in the FTO gene is associated with body mass index and predisposes to childhood and adult obesity. Science 2007;316(5826):889–94.
106. Scuteri A, Sanna S, Chen WM, et al. Genome-wide association scan shows genetic variants in the FTO gene are associated with obesity-related traits. PLoS Genet 2007;3(7):e115.
107. Kooner JS, Chambers JC, Aguilar-Salinas CA, et al. Genome-wide scan identifies variation in MLXIPL associated with plasma triglycerides. Nat Genet 2008;40(2):149–51.
108. Grundy SM, Hansen B, Smith SC Jr, et al. Clinical management of metabolic syndrome: report of the American Heart Association/National Heart, Lung, and Blood Institute/American Diabetes Association conference on scientific issues related to management. Arterioscler Thromb Vasc Biol 2004;24(2):e19–24.
109. Yamaoka K, Tango T. Effects of lifestyle modification on metabolic syndrome: a systematic review and meta-analysis. BMC Med 2012;10:138.
110. Orchard TJ, Temprosa M, Barrett-Connor E, et al. Long-term effects of the Diabetes Prevention Program interventions on cardiovascular risk factors: a report from the DPP Outcomes Study. Diabet Med 2013;30(1):46–55.
111. Kramer MK, Kriska AM, Venditti EM, et al. Translating the Diabetes Prevention Program: a comprehensive model for prevention training and program delivery. Am J Prev Med 2009;37(6):505–11.
112. Perreault L, Pan Q, Mather KJ, et al. Effect of regression from prediabetes to normal glucose regulation on long-term reduction in diabetes risk: results from the Diabetes Prevention Program Outcomes Study. Lancet 2012;379(9833):2243–51.
113. Potenza MV, Mechanick JI. The metabolic syndrome: definition, global impact, and pathophysiology. Nutr Clin Pract 2009;24(5):560–77.
114. Ridker PM, Pradhan A, MacFadyen JG, et al. Cardiovascular benefits and diabetes risks of statin therapy in primary prevention: an analysis from the JUPITER trial. Lancet 2012;380(9841):565–71.
115. Gotto AM Jr, Moon JE. Pharmacotherapies for lipid modification: beyond the statins. Nat Rev Cardiol 2013;10:560–70.
116. Boekholdt SM, Arsenault BJ, Hovingh GK, et al. Levels and changes of HDL cholesterol and apolipoprotein A-I in relation to risk of cardiovascular events among statin-treated patients: a meta-analysis. Circulation 2013;128:1504–12.
117. Clofibrate and niacin in coronary heart disease. JAMA 1975;231(4):360–81.
118. AIM-HIGH Investigators. The role of niacin in raising high-density lipoprotein cholesterol to reduce cardiovascular events in patients with atherosclerotic

cardiovascular disease and optimally treated low-density lipoprotein cholesterol: baseline characteristics of study participants. The Atherothrombosis Intervention in Metabolic syndrome with low HDL/high triglycerides: impact on Global Health outcomes (AIM-HIGH) trial. Am Heart J 2011;161(3):538–43.

119. Guyton JR, Slee AE, Anderson T, et al. Relationship of lipoproteins to cardiovascular events in the Atherothrombosis Intervention in Metabolic Syndrome with Low HDL/High Triglycerides and Impact on Global Health Outcomes (AIM-HIGH) Trial. J Am Coll Cardiol 2013. [Epub ahead of print].

120. HPS2-THRIVE Collaborative Group. HPS2-THRIVE randomized placebo-controlled trial in 25 673 high-risk patients of ER niacin/laropiprant: trial design, pre-specified muscle and liver outcomes, and reasons for stopping study treatment. Eur Heart J 2013;34(17):1279–91.

121. Ginsberg HN, Bonds DE, Lovato LC, et al. Evolution of the lipid trial protocol of the Action to Control Cardiovascular Risk in Diabetes (ACCORD) trial. Am J Cardiol 2007;99(12A):56i–67i.

122. Ginsberg HN, Elam MB, Lovato LC, et al. Effects of combination lipid therapy in type 2 diabetes mellitus. N Engl J Med 2010;362(17):1563–74.

123. Rubins HB, Robins SJ, Collins D, et al. Gemfibrozil for the secondary prevention of coronary heart disease in men with low levels of high-density lipoprotein cholesterol. Veterans Affairs High-Density Lipoprotein Cholesterol Intervention Trial Study Group. N Engl J Med 1999;341(6):410–8.

124. Chobanian AV, Bakris GL, Black HR, et al. The Seventh Report of the Joint National Committee on Prevention, Detection, Evaluation, and Treatment of High Blood Pressure: the JNC 7 report. JAMA 2003;289(19):2560–72.

125. Knowler WC, Fowler SE, Hamman RF, et al. 10-year follow-up of diabetes incidence and weight loss in the Diabetes Prevention Program Outcomes Study. Lancet 2009;374(9702):1677–86.

126. Knowler WC, Barrett-Connor E, Fowler SE, et al. Reduction in the incidence of type 2 diabetes with lifestyle intervention or metformin. N Engl J Med 2002; 346(6):393–403.

127. Kahn R, Buse J, Ferrannini E, et al. The metabolic syndrome: time for a critical appraisal: joint statement from the American Diabetes Association and the European Association for the Study of Diabetes. Diabetes Care 2005;28(9): 2289–304.

128. Haffner SM. The metabolic syndrome: inflammation, diabetes mellitus, and cardiovascular disease. Am J Cardiol 2006;97(2A):3A–11A.

129. Simmons RK, Alberti KG, Gale EA, et al. The metabolic syndrome: useful concept or clinical tool? Report of a WHO Expert Consultation. Diabetologia 2010;53(4):600–5.

130. Kohli P, Greenland P. Role of the metabolic syndrome in risk assessment for coronary heart disease. JAMA 2006;295(7):819–21.

Cardiovascular Disease in Diabetes Mellitus
Risk Factors and Medical Therapy

Magdalene M. Szuszkiewicz-Garcia, MD[a],*,
Jaime A. Davidson, MD[b]

KEYWORDS

- Cardiovascular disease • Diabetes • Myocardial infarction • Coronary heart disease
- Hyperglycemia • Risk • Therapy

KEY POINTS

- Diabetes mellitus (DM) is a condition on the increase, carrying a high risk of cardiovascular (CV) complications.
- Diabetes carries a higher risk for cardiovascular events in women than in men.
- Clinicians still do not have the ability to precisely and reliably stratify risk among patients with diabetes.
- Treatment of known cardiovascular risks such as hypertension, hyperlipidemia, and smoking is key in decreasing the risk for cardiovascular events.
- Some glucose-lowering drugs may have a more positive impact on minimizing cardiovascular disease, but more research needs to be done to confirm this possibility.

INTRODUCTION

Diabetes mellitus (DM) is a disease on the rise. A 2011 report from the Centers for Disease Control and Prevention indicated that 25.8 million people, 8.3% of the United States population, have DM. Among adults age 65 years or older, 26.9% had diabetes in 2010.[1] Worldwide there are 240 million people with DM, and it is projected that by 2030 there will be 439 million affected by diabetes.[2] The most common cause of death among patients with diabetes is cardiovascular disease, with heart disease responsible for 70% of deaths.[3] The risk of increased cardiovascular morbidity and mortality has been recognized for years, dubbing diabetes "cardiovascular disease equivalent."

The authors have no conflict of interest.
[a] Division of Endocrinology and Metabolism, Center for Human Nutrition, Department of Medicine, University of Texas Southwestern Medical Center, 5323 Harry Hines Boulevard, Dallas, TX 75390-8857, USA; [b] Division of Endocrinology, Diabetes and Metabolism, Touchstone Diabetes Center, University of Texas Southwestern Medical Center, 5323 Harry Hines Boulevard K5.246, Dallas, TX 75390, USA
* Corresponding author.
E-mail address: Magda.Szuszkiewicz-Garcia@UTSouthwestern.edu

Endocrinol Metab Clin N Am 43 (2014) 25–40
http://dx.doi.org/10.1016/j.ecl.2013.09.001
0889-8529/14/$ – see front matter © 2014 Elsevier Inc. All rights reserved.

EPIDEMIOLOGY

There is no argument that individuals with diabetes have a significantly increased risk of macrovascular complications, but how accurate is this label of "cardiovascular disease equivalent?" Fifteen years ago a landmark Finnish study attempted to answer this question. A 7-year risk of myocardial infarction in middle-aged patients with diabetes was 20%, similar to that of patients with a previous myocardial infarction.[4] Following this study there have been a flurry of epidemiologic studies arguing for or against the risk equivalence. Results are as varied as the studies themselves. The risk seems to vary by severity of diabetes as well as definition of coronary heart disease (CHD) used. For example, in patients with diet-controlled diabetes, the risk of mortality and myocardial infarction was smaller than that in patients with a previous myocardial infarction.[5,6] On the other hand, diabetic patients treated with glucose-lowering agents had a risk of mortality similar to that of patients who had a previous myocardial infarction, and a much greater risk of death than patients with angina, evidence of ischemia or infarct on electrocardiogram, but no history of an infarct. This risk was disproportionately high in women.[6,7]

In long-standing diabetes, women carried almost twice as high a hazard ratio for all-cause mortality and for death from CHD when compared with men with diabetes and patients with CHD without diabetes. The highest risk of death occurred in patients with both CHD and diabetes: hazard ratio of 4.44 for men and 5.86 for women.[8]

It is clear, therefore, that patients with diabetes are not a homogeneous group. Women are at a higher risk than men. Younger patients and those with shorter, milder disease are at a lower risk of events. Patients with type 1 diabetes may also have a lower risk when young and early in the disease course.[9]

ASSESSING THE RISK OF CARDIOVASCULAR EVENTS

There is significant amount of dispute regarding which parameters allow for most accurate assessment of risk and prediction of cardiovascular event. There is no doubt that chronic hyperglycemia imparts increased risk for mortality and events in both type 1 and type 2 diabetes; however, the association is not linear and is not consistent in all types of vascular disease. In one study, elevated fasting glucose has been found to increase the risk for all types of vascular disease, including ischemic and hemorrhagic stroke.[10] This increased risk of mortality was noted already when fasting glucose was greater than 100 mg/dL, and it was linked to a 6-year shorter life span in a 50-year-old individual with DM. Sixty percent of this risk is attributable to vascular death.[11] On the other hand, other studies show less consistent results in some groups. Postmenopausal women with established CHD and impaired fasting glucose of 100 to 125 mg/dL had no increased risk of coronary events. However, when the old definition of impaired fasting glucose was applied (glucose >110 mg/dL), women had an increased risk of myocardial infarction and cardiac death. Strokes, transient ischemic attacks (TIAs) and congestive heart failure (CHF) were not predicted by impaired fasting glucose by either definition.[12]

Postprandial glucose has been studied extensively as a predictor of cardiovascular outcomes. Hyperglycemia at 1 hour and 2 hours after a standard 75-g oral glucose tolerance test, as well as after a meal challenge, has proved to be a good predictor of cardiovascular events and mortality.[13] This relationship is linear. In some groups such as older adults and women, postprandial glucose may have a better ability to predict mortality than a fasting value, although combination of both fasting and 2-hour glucose may allow for more accurate risk estimation.[13–15] Given that acute hyperglycemia may cause vasoconstriction, there is a sound physiologic base for concern, even in patients with normal fasting glucose.

Elevation of glycosylated hemoglobin (HbA1c) appears to correlate with mortality and cardiovascular events in a linear manner as well: a 1% increase of HbA1c carries a significant increase in risk (20%–30%) for cardiovascular events or death.[16] This risk exists for coronary artery disease, fatal and nonfatal myocardial infarction and stroke, and perhaps most strongly for peripheral artery disease, in patients with both type 1 and type 2 diabetes.[17] Even in the absence of diabetes a small increase in HbA1c (>5%) is associated with an increased risk of CHD.[18]

Here again, not all data are consistent. In one study of women with no diabetes, elevation of HbA1c did not predict the risk of cardiovascular events.[19] It is controversial whether HbA1c is a better or worse prognosticator of cardiovascular events. However, attempts to lower HbA1C do not consistently lower mortality in all patients, complicating this issue further.[20]

In addition to elevated glucose, patients with diabetes have several other risk factors. Comorbidities such as renal disease, hypertension, dyslipidemia, sleep apnea, obesity, and poor physical fitness all carry a significant increase in cardiovascular risk. Some of the risks, such as macroproteinuria, may be a better predictor of mortality than glucose or HbA1c.[21] This heterogeneity of risks makes event prediction difficult. Unfortunately, treatment of cardiovascular complications is costly and, therefore, precise identification of the most vulnerable patients would be important in early prevention.

Framingham, UKPDS Risk Engine, SCORE, and DECODE are among calculators that have attempted to better estimate risk for individual patients. The results, however, are inconsistent: the accuracy varies in men and women, and none of these risk engines have been validated against a pool of American patients.[22,23]

PATHOPHYSIOLOGY

There are several potential mechanisms through which diabetes causes acceleration of atherosclerosis. Persons with type 2 diabetes have hypertension as well as abnormalities of lipid metabolism and insulin resistance, all of which are linked to increasing cardiovascular risk. Hyperglycemia likely also plays a central role in pathogenesis of vascular diseases, evidenced by the increased prevalence of atherosclerosis in people with type 1 diabetes without dyslipidemia or hypertension.

Within the blood vessels, endothelial cells come into direct contact with high glucose levels and play several key regulatory functions. These cells mediate vasodilation through production of bradykinin and nitric oxide, which acts on smooth muscle, resulting in relaxation and vasodilation. Endothelial cells also regulate vasoconstriction through local production of angiotensin-converting enzyme (ACE), prostaglandins, and endothelin. Vasoconstriction is driven by high angiotensin II levels, inducing smooth-muscle activation and bradykinin breakdown mediated by high levels of ACE. Hyperglycemia disrupts normal production of nitric oxide, leading to decreased blood flow. In addition, elevated levels of nonesterified fatty acids, often present in type 2 diabetes, further contribute by impairing vasodilation.[24]

Hyperglycemia also induces inflammation through stimulation of adipokines and upregulation of toll-like receptors (TLRs) in the endothelium. The usual function of TLRs is triggering both innate and adaptive immune response against a broad range of pathogens. When inappropriately activated, they initiate an excessive white blood cell response, resulting in ischemic reperfusion injury, restenosis, and formation of atherosclerotic plaque.[24]

Hyperglycemia may also play a role in monocytes adhering to a vessel wall and differentiating into macrophages. Glucose modulates the ability of macrophages to take up lipids and become foam cells.[24] This accumulation of lipid cells results in fatty streaks, which later become necrotic in the center and rupture.[25] Matrix metalloproteinases are also induced by hyperglycemia and may be linked to intraplaque hemorrhage, which destabilizes plaque.

There is some evidence that changes in the extracellular matrix resulting from hyperglycemia may cause collagen-matrix remodeling and smooth-muscle cell proliferation, resulting in a protective response of stabilization of a plaque. The same mechanisms may also play a deleterious role in coronary vessel restenosis after intervention.

Furthermore, hyperglycemia, hyperinsulinemia, and hypertriglyceridemia may cause excessive platelet activation and an increase in plasminogen activator inhibitor (PAI-1) levels, a major inhibitor of fibrinolysis. These changes of normal metabolism lead to a prothrombotic state.

Hyperglycemia and an increased level of fatty acids are important factors in inducing oxidative stress and inflammation in the pathogenesis of atherosclerosis, but may not be the only ones. Insulin resistance on a vascular level and a high circulating concentration of insulin may also play a role in acceleration of atherogenesis in diabetes. All of these mechanisms are still not completely understood.

MITIGATING THE RISKS
Intensive Glycemic Control

It has been well established that good glycemic control decreases the risks of microvascular complications. With regard to macrovascular complications, the answer is not as clear. It seems that treating more aggressively early in the course of DM does decrease the risk of myocardial infarction and reduces mortality. In UKPDS, a large study of patients with type 2 DM early in the disease course, there was no difference found in cardiovascular outcomes during the first 10 years between diet-controlled and intensively managed, pharmacologically treated groups. The average HbA1c difference between groups was 7.0% versus 7.9%, which was sufficient to decrease the rate of microvascular complications.[26] During the additional decade of follow-up observation with no intervention, there was a significant reduction of myocardial infarctions and death noted in the original intensive treatment group, despite the fact that the difference in HbA1c levels was lost after the first year of the follow-up study, 11 years after enrollment.[27] Similar results were found in a study of patients with type 1 DM.[28] Reduction of HbA1c from 9.1% to 7.4% early in disease course significantly reduced the risks of any cardiovascular disease by 42% and decreased the risk of strokes, myocardial infarctions, and cardiovascular death by 57% over a 17-year follow-up period.[29]

However, attempts to treat hyperglycemia aggressively in patients with long-standing diabetes did not bring similar positive results. VADT, a study of older men with long-standing diabetes, showed that reduction of HbA1c from 8.4% to 6.9% did not improve cardiovascular outcomes.[30]

Two recent large trials involving populations with previous cardiovascular events or at significant risk are the ADVANCE and ACCORD trials. The ADVANCE trial showed no beneficial effect on the rate of macrovascular events, when HbA1c was brought to 6.5% rather than the standard 7.3%.[31] On the other hand, the ACCORD trial was stopped early because of a 22% higher mortality in intensive glycemic control group.[20] During a 5-year observational follow-up period, patients initially assigned to the intensive treatment group experience a decreased risk of myocardial infarctions, but the increased risk of mortality persisted[32]; this despite HbA1c increasing from 6.6% to 7.4% in the initial intensive control group while HbA1c remained stable in the standard group (rising from 7.7% to 7.8%). The patients in the intensive group did require a more complicated multidrug regimen. The mortality, however, did not appear to be a direct result of hypoglycemic events.[33] It is also interesting that in the intensive control group, there was a liner relationship between mortality and HbA1c: individuals with higher HbA1c had higher mortality, similarly to what was observed in the UKPDS and DCCT-EDIC trials. One possible explanation for this finding is that disproportionate mortality occurred in a group of individuals who enter the intensive arm with HbA1c higher than 8%, and whose HbA1c remains higher than 8% throughout the course of the trial despite all efforts.[34]

When these and other studies are compiled in a meta-analysis, the results are a little more reassuring. It appears that intensive glycemic control may decrease the risk of nonfatal myocardial infarction, with no positive or negative effect on mortality, strokes, and peripheral vascular disease. However, this reduction in myocardial infarcts carries a price of a 30% increased risk of hypoglycemia.[35-38]

These data indicate the need for individualization of glycemic goals. Intensive therapy may be helpful in reducing cardiovascular events and mortality when initiated in people with shorter, uncomplicated diabetes. In patients with diabetes of longer than 15 years and long-standing complications, risk of tight control may outweigh the benefit.[39] Some investigators suggest that for such patients, an HbA1c goal of 7% to 7.9% may be sufficient to optimize the risk profile for cardiovascular events (**Table 1**).[40]

There is still a significant amount of debate over what are the most appropriate goals and for whom. Part of this discussion also concerns the most beneficial manner of treating diabetes: that is, whether any particular medication or medication combination improves cardiovascular outcomes.

CHOOSING THE RIGHT AGENTS

Metformin is a first-line drug recommended by several professional associations.[41,42] Lactic acidosis is its most feared side effect, although the actual risk is likely overestimated.[43] The UKPDS trial showed that metformin was particularly efficacious, with a 33% risk reduction of myocardial infarctions and 27% reduction of death in comparison with diet therapy.[27] BARI 2D did not show a clear mortality advantage, although patients on insulin sensitizers developed less peripheral artery disease.[44,45] However, this study did not separate the effect of metformin from other sensitizers, so it is difficult to say if the beneficial effect of metformin could have been blunted by the negative effect of other drugs such as rosiglitazone. Metformin has also been associated with decreased mortality in patients with CHF, despite the fact that heart failure is listed as a relative contraindication on the insert package.[46]

Thiazolidinediones (TZDs) are another class of insulin sensitizers, but with a controversial risk profile. It is now well recognized that this class of drugs has a negative effect on heart failure, as it is associated with volume expansion through peroxisome proliferator-activated receptor (PPAR)-γ–dependent pathways. Rosiglitazone created headlines when a significantly increased risk of myocardial infarctions and cardiovascular mortality were discovered.[47] Although a follow-up study showed no mortality effect, the use of TZDs has declined.[48] Favorable data for pioglitazone with regard to decreased risk of myocardial infarctions, strokes, and death did little to restore the reputation of TZDs.[48,49]

Sulfonylureas also appear to have a less favorable profile in comparison with metformin. Although they did decrease myocardial infarctions by 15% and mortality by

Table 1
Major trials: effect of treatment of diabetes mellitus (DM) on cardiovascular (CV) outcomes

Study	Goal	Outcome	Notes
ACCORD[20,32]	Lowering HbA1c to <6% in intense vs standard therapy in high CV group	Increased mortality in intense therapy group	Study stopped prematurely Mortality not related to hypoglycemia
ADVANCE[31]	Lowering HbA1c to <6.5% vs standard therapy in high CV risk group	No decrease in mortality or rate of cardiovascular events	
BARI2D[44,45]	Use of insulin sensitizers vs insulin-provision therapy	No difference in CV outcomes	Analysis of events not broken down further into different class of drugs
DCCT[28]	Intense vs standard therapy (HbA1c of 7.4% vs 9.1%) in type 1 DM early in disease course	No difference in CV events during 7 y of follow-up	Low number of events in both groups (young volunteers: average age 27 y)
DCCT-EDIC[29]	17-y follow-up of patients from DCCT	Lower rates of events including death in intensive therapy group	HbA1c converged in both groups to 7.8%–7.9% at the end of study
Heart 2D 2009	Prandial vs basal insulin therapy	No difference in CV events	Stopped due to lack of efficacy. Less than expected prandial difference
LOOK AHEAD[94]	Intensive lifestyle intervention/weight loss	No effect on CV event rate at 10 y	Stopped prematurely due to futility. 6% in intervention group vs 3.5% body weight loss at the end of the study: difference may have been too small to show CV effect
UKPDS[26,27]	Diet vs medication for control of early diabetes	Lower rates of myocardial infarction and death from any cause in intense treatment group during 2nd decade of follow-up, no difference during the 1st decade	Low number of events during 1st decade of follow-up in both groups
VADT[30]	Lowering HbA1c to 1.5% below standard therapy in older men with long-standing DM and high CV risk	No difference in outcomes	

13% when compared with placebo in UKPDS, there are data indicating that sulfonyl-ureas may not be optimal medications for patients with preexisting CHD and CHF.[27,50] The evidence is far from clear, and there are multiple contradictory reports.[51] Compared with other agents, including insulin, sulfonylureas carry a significant risk of hypoglycemia. It is debatable whether a specific drug has a worse profile than others, but glyburide has shown, although not consistently, to have an increased risk of acute coronary syndrome and cardiovascular death.[52,53] Some investigators suggest that if sulfonylureas must be used, glimepiride is the safest choice.[54]

Insulin is a staple of diabetes treatment. However, treatment of diabetes with insulin leads to a much higher plasma levels of insulin, potentially leading to excessive smooth-muscle activation, which may play a role in atherogenesis.[55] There are also data suggesting worse outcomes in patients with heart failure who use insulin. It is unclear whether this is a function of more severe diabetes affecting mortality or if insulin is in fact a culprit.[56] In well-controlled studies there is no conclusive evidence that insulin administration has a direct beneficial or deleterious effect on the cardio-vascular system, apart from reducing hyperglycemia.[51,57]

It is possible that over the next few years clinicians may be encouraged away from insulin toward other classes of drugs. Dipeptidyl-peptidase 4 (DPP-4) inhibitors and glucagon-like peptide 1 (GLP-1) agonists are 2 classes of drugs with promising effects on cardiovascular disease. Preliminary data have suggested that there may be a lower rate of cardiovascular events and mild lipid reduction in patients on DDP-4 inhibitors. The recently published prospective trial SAVOR-TIMI53 found that saxagliptin was not cardioprotective when compared with placebo during a 2-year follow-up for patients with a high cardiovascular risk. On the other hand, there were slightly more hospital-izations for CHF in the saxagliptin group (3.5% vs 2.8% with hazard ratio of 1.27 and $P = .007$).[58] CAROLINA, a study comparing cardiovascular outcomes in patients on linagliptin versus glimepiride, is in progress and will be completed in 2018.

GLP-1 agonists induce weight loss, have a blood-pressure–lowering effect of 2 to 8 mm Hg, and improve lipids, in addition to being linked to decreased rates of cardio-vascular events and hospitalizations. In experimental animals, they also improve left ventricular function and reduce infarct size caused by reperfusion.[59] Prospective studies are being conducted to confirm that this is a true effect on the cardiovascular system: the larger among these are MAGNA VICTORIA and LEADER, which will be completed in 2015 and 2016, respectively.

The newest drugs arriving on the market are sodium-glucose cotransporter-2 (SGC-2) inhibitors. Their mechanism of inducing glucosuria promises benefits of modest weight loss and possible reduction in blood pressure of 3 to 9 mm Hg, likely because of its diuretic effect. The effect on lipids is not clear as yet: it appears that treatment with SGC-2 inhibitors may slightly increase high-density lipoprotein (HDL). Data sub-mitted to the Food and Drug Administration show a possible decreased risk of cardio-vascular death and events, but long-term data is not yet available.[60] CANVAS, a canagliflozin long-term cardiovascular outcomes trial, and DECLARE-TIMI58, a 6-year cardiovascular outcomes study of dapagliflozin, are both ongoing and will be completed in 2018 and 2019, respectively.

LIPIDS

Lipid-lowering therapy is another critical intervention in improving cardiovascular out-comes. In patients with diabetes it may actually have a more profound effect than intensive glycemic control on lowering mortality and cardiovascular risk.[61] Current standard of care is to treat patients with DM to the goal of a low-density lipoprotein

(LDL) level of less than 100 mg/dL, with an optional goal of less than 70 mg/dL. Patients with DM and CHD should have their LDL level lower than 70 mg/dL. Patients older than 40 years with additional risk factors should be treated with statins as well. Given the recent decline in the cost of statins and benefit of therapy, there is a debate as to whether people younger than 40 years, those with no other risk factors, and good lipid panel should also be treated with statins in the absence of CHD.[62] This proposal is prompted by data that there is a significant reduction in cardiovascular events and mortality with statin use. One study reports a 13% decline in mortality per 1 mmol/L (39 mg/dL) decrease in LDL, with a 21% reduction in major vascular events per 1 mmol/L reduction in LDL-cholesterol in people with diabetes over a period of 4 years.[63] There was no evidence of harm.[64] This treatment effect is consistent with what is observed in patients with no DM: risk reduction is effective. When results were adjusted for baseline risk, diabetic patients benefited more in both primary and secondary prevention, even though lipid reduction was similar in both groups.[65]

Fibrates have also been studied extensively, with mixed results.[66,67] In the FIELD study when fibrates were compared with placebo, there was no decrease in events, likely because of high statin use in the placebo arm, but men with low HDL and triglycerides higher than 200 mg/dL benefited from a reduction in cardiovascular events.[68] In ACCORD, fibrates as an add-on therapy to statins appeared to also have benefited men with low HDL with and without hypertriglyceridemia, whereas women might have been harmed.

Data on use of ezetimibe are still not clear. While it does lower LDL, as yet no results from prospective studies with regard to morbidity and mortality outcomes are available for ezetimibe alone or as add-on therapy. It is reassuring that at least one group found no difference in the rate of events on comparison with statins: results for patients with diabetes did not differ from the rest of the cohort.[69]

Fish oil and omega-3 fatty acid supplements enjoy popularity among physicians and lay public alike. Fish oil is an effective treatment for hypertriglyceridemia, a disorder frequently coexisting with type 2 diabetes. Earlier studies in the cardiovascular literature suggested a possible mortality decrease in patients with heart disease. However, patients with early diabetes and high cardiovascular risk did not reduce their risk of cardiovascular events or mortality by using 1 g of fish oil per day.[70]

HYPERTENSION

Hypertension is a frequent comorbidity in patients with diabetes, especially with type 2 diabetes or type 1 diabetes associated with renal disease. It significantly increases cardiovascular risks, especially strokes. Current American Diabetes Association (ADA) guidelines call for treatment of hypertension when blood pressure is higher than 140/80 mm Hg. Lowering blood pressure to less than 130/80 mm Hg is advised in younger patients if it "can be achieved without undue treatment burden."[41] This figure represents a change from previous guidelines whereby blood pressure goals were less than 130/80 mm Hg.[71] Such a change is a positive one and reflects current data, which show a clear benefit derived by lowering the blood pressure below the threshold of 140 mm Hg. ADVANCE is a clear example of this. Reduction of blood pressure from 141/77 to 135/75 mm Hg with a fixed dose of perindopril and a diuretic indapamide versus placebo resulted in an 18% reduction of cardiovascular death and a significantly lower number of coronary events.[72]

Another recent large prospective study, ACCORD, showed that lowering systolic blood pressure (SBP) to less than 120 mm Hg did not improve mortality. Risk of stroke was diminished, however, from 0.53% to 0.32% yearly, at the price of doubling the rate of serious side effects (from 1.3% to 3.3%) such as syncope and hyperkalemia.[73]

A recent meta-analysis of patients with DM and prediabetes suggested that an SBP of 130 to 135 mm Hg may be optimal. Compared with blood pressure of 140 mm Hg, SBP of less than 135 mm Hg reduced mortality by 10% and strokes by 17%. There was no further reduction in microvascualar complication, mortality or CV events, with exception of strokes when SBP was lowered to <130 mm Hg. Reducing blood pressure to less than 135 mm Hg carried a 20% increased risk of serious events, with a 40% increase with SBP lower than 130 mm Hg.[74]

Although patients with diabetes often require multiple medications to control blood pressure, blocking the renin-angiotensin system seems to decrease mortality and the risk of complications in comparison with other antihypertensive agents. Current guidelines recognize this, and recommend the use of ACE inhibitors or angiotensin receptor blockers in the treatment of hypertension in diabetes.[41] Enalapril has been shown to be superior to nisoldipine in reduction of myocardial infarctions in patients in with poorly controlled diabetes.[75]

ASPIRIN

The role of aspirin in the treatment of cardiovascular disease is well established. However, data on the use of aspirin for primary prevention is less clear. There are several prospective studies indicating to a lack of mortality benefit in the general diabetic population.[76,77] Results of subset data analysis and meta-analysis are somewhat inconsistent. Some studies find a decreased risk of fatal and nonfatal strokes and myocardial infarctions through use of low-dose aspirin only in older patients, whereas others show a similar risk reduction only in men.[75,78] One meta-analysis reported a decreased rate of major cardiovascular events and calculated that 92 patients would need to be treated to prevent 1 major cardiovascular event. There was also evidence of harm, mostly from bleeding, in 1 out of every 526 treated patients. Interestingly there was no benefit when each of the events (strokes, myocardial infarctions, mortality) was evaluated separately.[79] Decreased mortality with low-dose aspirin has been found in a study of patients with an average age of 60 years, with the most significant benefit in older and male participants.[80]

With such inconsistency in the literature, it is not surprising that various professional associations differ in their recommendations with regard to the most appropriate age at when to start aspirin in diabetes for primary prevention. Whereas the ADA recommends 75 to 162 mg aspirin for men older than 50 and women older than 60 with an additional major risk factor for cardiovascular disease, the American Heart Association advocates starting therapy for patients older than 40 with risk factors.[81] The results of ASCEND and ACCEPT-D are expected to clarify this issue.

DIAGNOSIS OF CHD IN ASYMPTOMATIC PATIENTS

There is no consensus on how to approach screening of a patient with diabetes and no symptoms of coronary artery disease, yet it is a relevant issue in practice when patients ask if they are safe to start an exercise program. Clinically significant CHD was reported in 20% to 25% of asymptomatic patients with type 2 diabetes when tested by various modalities.[82] However, whether testing is beneficial and which tests to use are unclear. Exercise stress testing with an electrocardiogram is relatively inexpensive and has a 97% negative predictive value. On the other hand, a positive predictive value is less helpful. There is also a practical limitation: some patients may not be able to complete a treadmill test because of obesity, deconditioning, or arthritis.[83]

Using coronary artery calcium scores (CACS) in patients with diabetes can have pitfalls. Asymptomatic patients with a low score of less than 100 had a 21% prevalence of CHD. When identified as low to intermediate risk by the Framingham Risk Score, a CACS score greater than 40 was an independent predictor for atherosclerotic events.[84] In the general diabetic population, an even lower CACS score of 10 or more has been shown to predict all-cause mortality and cardiovascular events with high sensitivity but low specificity. Conversely, a score of less than 10 has an excellent negative predictive value.[85]

Screening patients with adenosine-stress radionuclide myocardial perfusion imaging is widely accepted, although it does not appear to result in event reduction.[86] On the other hand, prompt revascularization in optimally medically managed patients did not result in improved outcomes or survival.[44] Of note, optimally medically managed patients with angina symptoms and those with silent ischemia did not fare any differently.[87]

REVASCULARIZATION

Although there were no differences in outcomes between patients receiving prompt revascularization and those on medical therapy in the BARI 2D trial, a group with the biggest improvement in survival was patients who had coronary artery bypass grafting (CABG).[44] The FREEDOM trial confirmed that for patients with DM and multivessel CHD, CABG was a better option than percutaneous coronary intervention (PCI) stenting. During a 5-year follow-up, the CABG group had a significantly lower mortality (10.9% vs 16.3%) and fewer myocardial infarctions (6.0% vs 13.9%). The downside was a significantly higher incidence of strokes in the postoperative period in the CABG group, 5.2% versus 2.4%.[88] Similar results were found in the past in a meta-analysis study.[89] Because the analysis incorporated studies using non–drug-eluting stents, as the technology improved the results were called to question. FREEDOM, however, compared CABG with PCI using mostly drug-eluting stents.

Men and women with diabetes treated with revascularization have similar risks of myocardial infarction, cardiovascular accidents, and death. Women, however, have more residual angina symptoms and poorer functional status even if they have less anatomic disease before revascularization.[90] After PCI stenting to a single lesion, diabetic patients have worse outcomes when compared with patients without DM. These patients are at increased risk for needing revascularization of the stented lesions during the first year after the procedure, and have an increased risk for cardiac death and myocardial infarctions during 5 years following the procedure.[91]

SUMMARY

Overall, the advanced made in care of patients with diabetes and patients with CHD are encouraging. The mean predicted risk for CHD in the entire population of 7.2% in 1999 to 2000 has dropped to 6.5% in 2009 to 2010. Risk of a cardiovascular event has also fallen from 9.2% to 8.7%, despite an increase in the prevalence of DM. Blood-pressure control, smoking cessation, and improvement in HDL-cholesterol appear to be linked to this improvement. On the other hand, minorities such as African Americans and Mexican Americans still appear to be vulnerable populations.[92]

Encouraging lifestyle modifications such as healthy diet, weight reduction, and exercise is a commonsense approach that has been a cornerstone of diabetes prevention and treatment for many years. Although as little as 5% weight loss results in improvement of metabolic parameters, the recently completed LOOK AHEAD trial

Box 1 **Treatment strategies proved to improve cardiovascular outcomes**
Lowering HbA1c to less than 8%: benefit of further lowering is controversial
Blocking angiotensin-renin system
Blood-pressure control to lower than 140/80 mm Hg
Low-dose aspirin in older individuals, especially men
Aggressive lipid-lowering therapy to low-density lipoprotein less than 100 mg/dL for primary prevention and less than 70 mg/dL for secondary prevention
Coronary artery bypass grafting is better that percutaneous coronary intervention in treatment of multivessel coronary artery disease

shows that it is not enough to decrease the risk for cardiovascular events in patients with diabetes.[93,94]

To date, it appears that multifactorial therapy including reduction of lipids, renin-angiotensin system suppression, personalized glycemic control, and the use of aspirin in selected patients may be the most effective way to reduce the cardiovascular complications of diabetes (**Box 1**).[61] Early diagnosis and interventions with a treat-to-target approach have been shown to be beneficial over the long term in patients with both type 1 and type 2 diabetes.

ACKNOWLEDGMENTS

Many thanks are extended to Dr Jose Enrique Garcia and Dr Zahid Ahmad for their invaluable input in editing this article.

REFERENCES

1. Centers for Disease Control and Prevention. National diabetes fact sheet: national estimates and general information on diabetes and prediabetes in the United States. 2011. Available at: http://www.cdc.gov/diabetes/pubs/factsheet11.htm. Accessed June 6, 2013.
2. Shaw JE, Sicree RA, Zimmet PZ. Global estimates of the prevalence of diabetes for 2010 and 2030. Diabetes Res Clin Pract 2010;87(1):4–14.
3. Gu K, Cowie CC, Harris MI. Mortality in adults with and without diabetes in a national cohort of the U.S. population, 1971-1993. Diabetes Care 1998;21(7): 1138–45.
4. Haffner SM, Lehto S, Ronnemaa T, et al. Mortality from coronary heart disease in subjects with type 2 diabetes and in nondiabetic subjects with and without prior myocardial infarction. N Engl J Med 1998;339(4):229–34.
5. Evans JM, Wang J, Morris AD. Comparison of cardiovascular risk between patients with type 2 diabetes and those who had had a myocardial infarction: cross sectional and cohort studies. BMJ 2002;324(7343):939–42.
6. Eberly LE, Cohen JD, Prineas R, et al. Impact of incident diabetes and incident nonfatal cardiovascular disease on 18-year mortality: the multiple risk factor intervention trial experience. Diabetes Care 2003;26(3):848–54.
7. Juutilainen A, Lehto S, Rönnemaa T, et al. Type 2 diabetes as a "coronary heart disease equivalent": an 18-year prospective population-based study in Finnish subjects. Diabetes Care 2005;28(12):2901–7.

8. Whiteley L, Padmanabhan S, Hole D, et al. Should diabetes be considered a coronary heart disease risk equivalent?: results from 25 years of follow-up in the Renfrew and Paisley survey. Diabetes Care 2005;28(7):1588–93.

9. Grundy SM, Benjamin IJ, Burke GL, et al. Diabetes and cardiovascular disease: a statement for healthcare professionals from the American Heart Association. Circulation 1999;100(10):1134–46.

10. The Emerging Risk Factors Collaboration. Diabetes mellitus, fasting blood glucose concentration, and risk of vascular disease: a collaborative meta-analysis of 102 prospective studies. Lancet 2010;375(9733):2215–22.

11. Seshasai SR, Kaptoge S, Thompson A, et al. Diabetes mellitus, fasting glucose, and risk of cause-specific death. N Engl J Med 2011;364(9):829–41.

12. Kanaya AM, Herrington D, Vittinghoff E, et al. Impaired fasting glucose and cardiovascular outcomes in postmenopausal women with coronary artery disease. Ann Intern Med 2005;142(10):813–20.

13. Ceriello A, Hanefeld M, Leiter L, et al. Postprandial glucose regulation and diabetic complications. Arch Intern Med 2004;164(19):2090–5.

14. Smith NL, Barzilay JI, Shaffer D, et al. Fasting and 2-hour postchallenge serum glucose measures and risk of incident cardiovascular events in the elderly: the Cardiovascular Health Study. Arch Intern Med 2002;162(2):209–16.

15. Sorkin JD, Muller DC, Fleg JL, et al. The relation of fasting and 2-h postchallenge plasma glucose concentrations to mortality: data from the Baltimore Longitudinal Study of Aging with a critical review of the literature. Diabetes Care 2005; 28(11):2626–32.

16. Khaw KT, Wareham N, Bingham S, et al. Association of hemoglobin A1c with cardiovascular disease and mortality in adults: the European prospective investigation into cancer in Norfolk. Ann Intern Med 2004;141(6):413–20.

17. Selvin E, Marinopoulos S, Berkenblit G, et al. Meta-analysis: glycosylated hemoglobin and cardiovascular disease in diabetes mellitus. Ann Intern Med 2004; 141(6):421–31.

18. Pai JK, Cahill LE, Hu FB, et al. Hemoglobin a1c is associated with increased risk of incident coronary heart disease among apparently healthy, nondiabetic men and women. J Am Heart Assoc 2013;2(2):e000077.

19. Pradhan AD, Rifai N, Buring JE, et al. Hemoglobin A1c predicts diabetes but not cardiovascular disease in nondiabetic women. Am J Med 2007;120(8): 720–7.

20. Gerstein HC, Miller ME, Byington RP, et al. Effects of intensive glucose lowering in type 2 diabetes. N Engl J Med 2008;358(24):2545–59.

21. Cosson E, Nguyen MT, Chanu B, et al. Cardiovascular risk prediction is improved by adding asymptomatic coronary status to routine risk assessment in type 2 diabetic patients. Diabetes Care 2011;34(9):2101–7.

22. Coleman RL, Stevens RJ, Retnakaran R, et al. Framingham, SCORE, and DECODE risk equations do not provide reliable cardiovascular risk estimates in type 2 diabetes. Diabetes Care 2007;30(5):1292–3.

23. van der Heijden AA, Ortegon MM, Niessen LW, et al. Prediction of coronary heart disease risk in a general, pre-diabetic, and diabetic population during 10 years of follow-up: accuracy of the Framingham, SCORE, and UKPDS risk functions: The Hoorn Study. Diabetes Care 2009;32(11):2094–8.

24. Pasterkamp G. Methods of accelerated atherosclerosis in diabetic patients. Heart 2013;99(10):743–9.

25. Chait A, Bornfeldt KE. Diabetes and atherosclerosis: is there a role for hyperglycemia? J Lipid Res 2009;50(Suppl):S335–9.

26. UK Prospective Diabetes Study (UKPDS) Group. Intensive blood-glucose control with sulphonylureas or insulin compared with conventional treatment and risk of complications in patients with type 2 diabetes (UKPDS 33). UK Prospective Diabetes Study (UKPDS) Group. Lancet 1998;352(9131):837–53.
27. Holman RR, Paul SK, Bethel MA, et al. 10-year follow-up of intensive glucose control in type 2 diabetes. N Engl J Med 2008;359(15):1577–89.
28. The Diabetes Control and Complications Trial Research Group. The effect of intensive treatment of diabetes on the development and progression of long-term complications in insulin-dependent diabetes mellitus. The Diabetes Control and Complications Trial Research Group. N Engl J Med 1993;329(14):977–86.
29. Nathan DM, Cleary PA, Backlund JY, et al. Intensive diabetes treatment and cardiovascular disease in patients with type 1 diabetes. N Engl J Med 2005; 353(25):2643–53.
30. Duckworth W, Abraira C, Moritz T, et al. Glucose control and vascular complications in veterans with type 2 diabetes. N Engl J Med 2009;360(2):129–39.
31. Patel A, MacMahon S, Chalmers J, et al. Intensive blood glucose control and vascular outcomes in patients with type 2 diabetes. N Engl J Med 2008; 358(24):2560–72.
32. Gerstein HC, Miller ME, Genuth S, et al. Long-term effects of intensive glucose lowering on cardiovascular outcomes. N Engl J Med 2011;364(9):818–28.
33. Bonds DE, Miller ME, Bergenstal RM, et al. The association between symptomatic, severe hypoglycaemia and mortality in type 2 diabetes: retrospective epidemiological analysis of the ACCORD study. BMJ 2010;340:b4909.
34. Riddle MC. Effects of intensive glucose lowering in the management of patients with type 2 diabetes mellitus in the Action to Control Cardiovascular Risk in Diabetes (ACCORD) trial. Circulation 2010;122(8):844–6.
35. Mannucci E, Monami M, Lamanna C, et al. Prevention of cardiovascular disease through glycemic control in type 2 diabetes: a meta-analysis of randomized clinical trials. Nutr Metab Cardiovasc Dis 2009;19(9):604–12.
36. Ma J, Yang W, Fang N, et al. The association between intensive glycemic control and vascular complications in type 2 diabetes mellitus: a meta-analysis. Nutr Metab Cardiovasc Dis 2009;19(9):596–603.
37. Ray KK, Seshasai SR, Wijesuriya S, et al. Effect of intensive control of glucose on cardiovascular outcomes and death in patients with diabetes mellitus: a meta-analysis of randomised controlled trials. Lancet 2009;373(9677):1765–72.
38. Hemmingsen B, Lund SS, Gluud C, et al. Targeting intensive glycaemic control versus targeting conventional glycaemic control for type 2 diabetes mellitus. Cochrane Database Syst Rev 2011;(6):CD008143.
39. Duckworth WC, Abraira C, Moritz TE, et al. The duration of diabetes affects the response to intensive glucose control in type 2 subjects: the VA Diabetes Trial. J Diabetes Complications 2011;25(6):355–61.
40. Hoogwerf BJ. Does intensive therapy of type 2 diabetes help or harm? Seeking accord on ACCORD. Cleve Clin J Med 2008;75(10):729–37.
41. American Diabetes Association. Standards of medical care in diabetes—2013. Diabetes Care 2013;36(Suppl 1):S11–66.
42. Garber AJ, Abrahamson MJ, Barzilay JI, et al. AACE comprehensive diabetes management algorithm 2013. Endocr Pract 2013;19(2):327–36.
43. Klachko D, Whaley-Connell A. Use of metformin in patients with kidney and cardiovascular diseases. Cardiorenal Med 2011;1(2):87–95.
44. Frye RL, August P, Brooks MM, et al. A randomized trial of therapies for type 2 diabetes and coronary artery disease. N Engl J Med 2009;360(24):2503–15.

45. Althouse AD, Abbott JD, Sutton-Tyrrell K, et al. Favorable effects of insulin sensitizers pertinent to peripheral arterial disease in type 2 diabetes: results from the bypass angioplasty revascularization investigation 2 diabetes (BARI 2D) trial. Diabetes Care 2013;36(10):3269–75.

46. Eurich DT, McAlister FA, Blackburn DF, et al. Benefits and harms of antidiabetic agents in patients with diabetes and heart failure: systematic review. BMJ 2007; 335(7618):497.

47. Nissen SE, Wolski K. Effect of rosiglitazone on the risk of myocardial infarction and death from cardiovascular causes. N Engl J Med 2007;356(24):2457–71.

48. Nissen SE, Wolski K. Rosiglitazone revisited: an updated meta-analysis of risk for myocardial infarction and cardiovascular mortality. Arch Intern Med 2010; 170(14):1191–201.

49. Lincoff AM, Wolski K, Nicholls SJ, et al. Pioglitazone and risk of cardiovascular events in patients with type 2 diabetes mellitus: a meta-analysis of randomized trials. JAMA 2007;298(10):1180–8.

50. Rao AD, Kuhadiya N, Reynolds K, et al. Is the combination of sulfonylureas and metformin associated with an increased risk of cardiovascular disease or all-cause mortality?: a meta-analysis of observational studies. Diabetes Care 2008;31(8):1672–8.

51. Sillars B, Davis WA, Hirsch IB, et al. Sulphonylurea-metformin combination therapy, cardiovascular disease and all-cause mortality: the Fremantle Diabetes Study. Diabetes Obes Metab 2010;12(9):757–65.

52. Gangji AS, Cukierman T, Gerstein HC, et al. A systematic review and meta-analysis of hypoglycemia and cardiovascular events: a comparison of glyburide with other secretagogues and with insulin. Diabetes Care 2007;30(2): 389–94.

53. Abdelmoneim AS, Eurich DT, Gamble JM, et al. Risk of acute coronary events associated with glyburide compared to gliclazide use in patients with type 2 diabetes: a nested case-control study. Diabetes Obes Metab 2013. [Epub ahead of print].

54. Breen DM, Giacca A. Effects of insulin on the vasculature. Curr Vasc Pharmacol 2011;9(3):321–32.

55. Chaitman BR, Hardison RM, Adler D, et al. The bypass angioplasty revascularization investigation 2 diabetes randomized trial of different treatment strategies in type 2 diabetes mellitus with stable ischemic heart disease: impact of treatment strategy on cardiac mortality and myocardial infarction. Circulation 2009; 120(25):2529–40.

56. Smooke S, Horwich TB, Fonarow GC. Insulin-treated diabetes is associated with a marked increase in mortality in patients with advanced heart failure. Am Heart J 2005;149(1):168–74.

57. The Origin Trial Investigators. Basal insulin and cardiovascular and other outcomes in dysglycemia. N Engl J Med 2012;367(4):319–28.

58. Scirica BM, Bhatt DL, Braunwald E, et al. Saxagliptin and cardiovascular outcomes in patients with type 2 diabetes mellitus. N Engl J Med 2013;369: 1317–26.

59. Umpierrez GE, Meneghini L. Reshaping diabetes care: the fundamental role of DPP-4 inhibitors and GLP-1 receptor agonists in clinical practice. Endocr Pract 2013;19(4):1–37.

60. Basile JN. The potential of sodium glucose cotransporter 2 (SGLT2) inhibitors to reduce cardiovascular risk in patients with type 2 diabetes (T2DM). J Diabetes Complications 2013;27(3):280–6.

61. Gæde P, Lund-Andersen H, Parving HH, et al. Effect of a multifactorial intervention on mortality in type 2 diabetes. N Engl J Med 2008;358(6):580–91.
62. Steinberg D, Grundy SM. The case for treating hypercholesterolemia at an earlier age: moving toward consensus. J Am Coll Cardiol 2012;60(25): 2640–2.
63. Kearney PM, Blackwell L, Collins R, et al. Efficacy of cholesterol-lowering therapy in 18,686 people with diabetes in 14 randomised trials of statins: a meta-analysis. Lancet 2008;371(9607):117–25.
64. Taylor F, Ward K, Moore TH, et al. Statins for the primary prevention of cardiovascular disease. Cochrane Database Syst Rev 2011;(1):CD004816.
65. Costa J, Borges M, David C, et al. Efficacy of lipid lowering drug treatment for diabetic and non-diabetic patients: meta-analysis of randomised controlled trials. BMJ 2006;332(7550):1115–24.
66. Ginsberg HN, Elam MB, Lovato LC, et al. Effects of combination lipid therapy in type 2 diabetes mellitus. N Engl J Med 2010;362(17):1563–74.
67. Keech A, Simes RJ, Barter P, et al. Effects of long-term fenofibrate therapy on cardiovascular events in 9795 people with type 2 diabetes mellitus (the FIELD study): randomised controlled trial. Lancet 2005;366(9500):1849–61.
68. Steiner G. How can we improve the management of vascular risk in type 2 diabetes: insights from FIELD. Cardiovasc Drugs Ther 2009;23(5):403–8.
69. Hayek S, Canepa Escaro F, Sattar A, et al. Effect of ezetimibe on major atherosclerotic disease events and all-cause mortality. Am J Cardiol 2013;111(4): 532–9.
70. Bosch J, Gerstein HC, Dagenais GR, et al. n-3 fatty acids and cardiovascular outcomes in patients with dysglycemia. N Engl J Med 2012;367(4): 309–18.
71. American Diabetes Association. Standards of medical care in diabetes—2012. Diabetes Care 2012;35(Suppl 1):S11–63.
72. Patel A. Effects of a fixed combination of perindopril and indapamide on macrovascular and microvascular outcomes in patients with type 2 diabetes mellitus (the ADVANCE trial): a randomised controlled trial. Lancet 2007;370(9590): 829–40.
73. Cushman WC, Evans GW, Byington RP, et al. Effects of intensive blood-pressure control in type 2 diabetes mellitus. N Engl J Med 2010;362(17):1575–85.
74. Bangalore S, Kumar S, Lobach I, et al. Blood pressure targets in subjects with type 2 diabetes mellitus/impaired fasting glucose: observations from traditional and bayesian random-effects meta-analyses of randomized trials. Circulation 2011;123(24):2799–810, 2799 p following 2810.
75. Estacio RO, Jeffers BW, Hiatt WR, et al. The effect of nisoldipine as compared with enalapril on cardiovascular outcomes in patients with non-insulin-dependent diabetes and hypertension. N Engl J Med 1998;338(10):645–52.
76. Ogawa H, Nakayama M, Morimoto T, et al. Low-dose aspirin for primary prevention of atherosclerotic events in patients with type 2 diabetes: a randomized controlled trial. JAMA 2008;300(18):2134–41.
77. Belch J, MacCuish A, Campbell I, et al. The prevention of progression of arterial disease and diabetes (POPADAD) trial: factorial randomised placebo controlled trial of aspirin and antioxidants in patients with diabetes and asymptomatic peripheral arterial disease. BMJ 2008;337:a1840.
78. De Berardis G, Sacco M, Strippoli GF, et al. Aspirin for primary prevention of cardiovascular events in people with diabetes: meta-analysis of randomised controlled trials. BMJ 2009;339:b4531.

79. Butalia S, Leung AA, Ghali WA, et al. Aspirin effect on the incidence of major adverse cardiovascular events in patients with diabetes mellitus: a systematic review and meta-analysis. Cardiovasc Diabetol 2011;10:25.

80. Ong G, Davis TM, Davis WA. Aspirin is associated with reduced cardiovascular and all-cause mortality in type 2 diabetes in a primary prevention setting: the Fremantle Diabetes study. Diabetes Care 2010;33(2):317–21.

81. Buse JB, Ginsberg HN, Bakris GL, et al. Primary prevention of cardiovascular diseases in people with diabetes mellitus: a scientific statement from the American Heart Association and the American Diabetes Association. Circulation 2007;115(1):114–26.

82. Scholte AJ, Schuijf JD, Kharagjitsingh AV, et al. Different manifestations of coronary artery disease by stress SPECT myocardial perfusion imaging, coronary calcium scoring, and multislice CT coronary angiography in asymptomatic patients with type 2 diabetes mellitus. J Nucl Cardiol 2008;15(4):503–9.

83. Upchurch CT, Barrett EJ. Clinical review: screening for coronary artery disease in type 2 diabetes. J Clin Endocrinol Metab 2012;97(5):1434–42.

84. Lau KK, Wong YK, Chan YH, et al. Prognostic implications of surrogate markers of atherosclerosis in low to intermediate risk patients with type 2 diabetes. Cardiovasc Diabetol 2012;11:101.

85. Kramer CK, Zinman B, Gross JL, et al. Coronary artery calcium score prediction of all cause mortality and cardiovascular events in people with type 2 diabetes: systematic review and meta-analysis. BMJ 2013;346:f1654.

86. Young LH, Wackers FJ, Chyun DA, et al. Cardiac outcomes after screening for asymptomatic coronary artery disease in patients with type 2 diabetes: the DIAD study: a randomized controlled trial. JAMA 2009;301(15):1547–55.

87. Dagenais GR, Lu J, Faxon DP, et al. Prognostic impact of the presence and absence of angina on mortality and cardiovascular outcomes in patients with type 2 diabetes and stable coronary artery disease: results from the BARI 2D (Bypass Angioplasty Revascularization Investigation 2 Diabetes) trial. J Am Coll Cardiol 2013;61(7):702–11.

88. Farkouh ME, Domanski M, Sleeper LA, et al. Strategies for multivessel revascularization in patients with diabetes. N Engl J Med 2012;367(25):2375–84.

89. Hlatky MA, Boothroyd DB, Bravata DM, et al. Coronary artery bypass surgery compared with percutaneous coronary interventions for multivessel disease: a collaborative analysis of individual patient data from ten randomised trials. Lancet 2009;373(9670):1190–7.

90. Tamis-Holland JE, Lu J, Korytkowski M, et al. Sex differences in presentation and outcome among patients with type 2 diabetes and coronary artery disease treated with contemporary medical therapy with or without prompt revascularization: a report from the BARI 2D Trial (Bypass Angioplasty Revascularization Investigation 2 Diabetes). J Am Coll Cardiol 2013;61(17):1767–76.

91. Lee TT, Feinberg L, Baim DS, et al. Effect of diabetes mellitus on five-year clinical outcomes after single-vessel coronary stenting (a pooled analysis of coronary stent clinical trials). Am J Cardiol 2006;98(6):718–21.

92. Ford ES. Trends in predicted 10-year risk of coronary heart disease and cardiovascular disease among U.S. Adults from 1999 to 2010. J Am Coll Cardiol 2013;61(22):2249–52.

93. Blackburn G. Effect of degree of weight loss on health benefits. Obes Res 1995;3(Suppl 2):211s–6s.

94. Look Ahead Research Group. Cardiovascular effects of intensive lifestyle intervention in type 2 diabetes. N Engl J Med 2013;369(2):145–54.

The Relationships Between Cardiovascular Disease and Diabetes: Focus on Pathogenesis

Jason C. Kovacic, MD, PhD[a,b], Jose M. Castellano, MD, PhD[a,b], Michael E. Farkouh, MD[a,b,c], Valentin Fuster, MD, PhD[a,b,d],*

KEYWORDS

- Cardiovascular disease • Diabetes • Obesity • Diabetic cardiomyopathy

KEY POINTS

- Diabetes has reached an epidemic level worldwide and patients suffering from this disease are at significantly higher risk for cardiovascular disease (CVD).
- The close relationship between diabetes and CVD together with the substantial projected rise in prevalence of diabetes will likely lead to a huge increase in the future demand for health care services at a global level.
- The economic force behind the continuing rise in the cost of health care derived from caring for the 300 million projected diabetic patients in 2025 will leave policy makers no choice but to devise efficient solutions to prevent the widespread surge of this disease.
- Focus should be placed back on the mechanisms that prevent the development of diabetes and related pathologies through the promotion of cardiovascular health by smoking cessation, exercising, following a healthy diet, and weight loss strategies, all of which will improve health outcomes and reduce costs.

INTRODUCTION

Diabetes mellitus currently affects 180 million people worldwide. The epidemic of obesity and sedentary lifestyle, however, is projected to result in more than 300 million

No specific funding or grant was used to prepare this article. Jason Kovacic is supported by National Institutes of Health Grant K08HL111330 and has received research support from AstraZeneca.

[a] Zena and Michael A. Wiener Cardiovascular Institute, Mount Sinai School of Medicine, One Gustave L. Levy Place, Box 1030, New York, NY 10029, USA; [b] Marie-Josée and Henry R. Kravis Cardiovascular Health Center, Mount Sinai School of Medicine, One Gustave L. Levy Place, Box 1030, New York, NY 10029, USA; [c] Peter Munk Cardiac Centre and Heart and Stroke Richard Lewar Centre of Excellence, Cardiovascular Research, University of Toronto, MaRS Building 101 College Street, 3rd Floor, Toronto, ON M5G 1L7, Canada; [d] The Centro Nacional de Investigaciones Cardiovasculares (CNIC), Melchor Fernández Almagro, 3.Código Postal 28029, Madrid, Spain
* Corresponding author. Mount Sinai School of Medicine, One Gustave L. Levy Place, Box 1030, New York, NY 10029.
E-mail address: valentin.fuster@mountsinai.org

people with diabetes in 2025.[1,2] Developing countries, in particular, will be hit by this increase, with an expected 170% rise from 84 million to 228 million affected individuals. This projection is of particular importance in developing nations, where diabetes tends to arise earlier in life (at ages 40–64 years) compared with developed countries, where diabetes often occurs at age 65 years or older. The onset of diabetes at an earlier age in developing nations inevitably causes a longer duration of exposure to diabetes and, therefore, carries a potentially greater risk of diabetes-associated morbidity and mortality in later life. Although a developed nation, the projections in the United States are somber, with the number of Americans with diabetes projected to increase by 165%, from 11 million in 2000 to 29 million in 2050.[2]

Diabetes is a major risk factor for CVD and cardiovascular complications are the leading cause of mortality among diabetic patients. Recent data from the World Health Organization suggest that 50% of diabetic patients die from heart-related causes and heart disease is noted on more than two-thirds of diabetes-related death certificates among people 65 years or older.[3] Diabetes predisposes to aggressive obstructive coronary artery disease (CAD), which leads to ischemic heart disease, heart failure, and death. There is consensus in the literature about an increased prevalence of coronary plaques in diabetic hearts, with such plaques bearing a higher propensity for rupture. Furthermore, diabetes also predisposes to heart failure independent of valvular heart disease, underlying CAD, or hypertension[4]—a condition known as diabetic cardiomyopathy (DCM).[5] Nevertheless, although remaining an enormous public health burden, recent progress has been made in the ways that diabetic patients with CVD are clinically approached and treated. This article reviews some of the recent advances in the understanding of the relationships between CVD and diabetes at the vascular, cardiac, and clinical levels.

DIABETES AND THE VASCULATURE

Of the major burden of morbidity and mortality associated with diabetes, a significant proportion is attributable to vascular manifestations. In many instances these vascular manifestations are obvious, for example, when a diabetic patient presents with myocardial infarction (MI) or thromboembolic stroke, the underlying pathology is readily traceable to rampant and diffuse diabetic atherosclerosis. Beyond increased atherosclerosis, however, many of the numerous disease-related end-organ effects of diabetes include a vascular contribution. For example, although diabetic neuropathy involves direct nerve damage, microvascular changes leading to secondary neural ischemia also play a major role in the neuropathic process.[6] Similarly, alterations in the microvasculature and glomerular endothelial changes are an important aspect of diabetic nephropathy and macroalbuminuria,[7] whereas microvascular changes in the retina may lead to diabetic retinopathy and blindness. So pervasive are the effects of diabetes, that it is impossible to review in this article all of the many pathologic diabetic pathways and effects on the vascular system and, conversely, all the effects that the diabetic vasculature has on the resulting clinical end-organ phenotype. Several of the major mechanisms of interaction between diabetes and the vasculature are discussed, including oxidative stress, progenitor cell dysfunction, microvascular dysfunction, and impaired reverse cholesterol transport (**Fig. 1**).

Oxidative Stress and the Vasculature

Oxidative stress and the accumulation of reactive oxygen species (ROS) are key aspects in the development of diabetic complications and diabetic vascular disease and perhaps the most important initiating events in the cascade of diabetic vascular

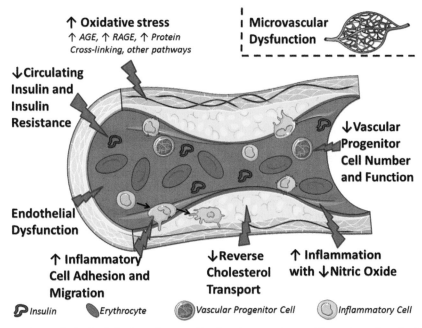

↑ Oxidative stress
↑ AGE, ↑ RAGE, ↑ Protein Cross-linking, other pathways

↑ Microvascular Dysfunction

↓Circulating Insulin and Insulin Resistance

↓Vascular Progenitor Cell Number and Function

Endothelial Dysfunction

↑ Inflammatory Cell Adhesion and Migration

↓Reverse Cholesterol Transport

↑ Inflammation with ↓Nitric Oxide

Insulin   *Erythrocyte*   *Vascular Progenitor Cell*   *Inflammatory Cell*

Fig. 1. Key pathologic diabetic pathways affecting the vasculature. Figure 1 produced using Servier Medical Art.

pathology. There are multiple targets of oxidative damage in the vasculature, with both endothelial and vascular smooth muscle cells (VSMCs) exposed to oxidative modifications of proteins, lipids, and nucleic acids. In turn, there are numerous consequences of this increased vascular ROS generation and oxidative damage. Impaired endothelial function is one of the key pathologic disturbances in diabetic patients, which seems due primarily to loss of nitric oxide bioactivity.[8] This is thought a seminal event in the rampant atherosclerotic process that typifies diabetes and other lipodystrophic conditions.[9]

There are multiple sources of ROS in the diabetic vasculature, including the mitochondrial electron transport chain, NADPH oxidase, xanthine oxidase, endothelial nitric oxide synthase, and cytochrome P450. The pathologic changes in these pathways that lead to increased ROS generation are diverse, but are thought to ultimately arise due to hyperglycemia or altered glucose utilization. Although debate is ongoing,[10] a popular theory to explain these vascular damage pathways was put forward in 2001 by Brownlee.[11] Referred to as the "unifying hypothesis," Brownlee argued that hyperglycemia leads to overproduction of superoxide by the mitochondrial electron transport chain, which is an upstream and central event in 4 key damage pathways: increased polyol pathway flux, increased formation of advanced glycation end-products (AGEs), activation of protein kinase C, and increased flux through the hexosamine pathway.[10,11]

Among these damage pathways, AGE accumulation has received particular attention and is linked to multiple vascular pathologies.[12] AGE formation occurs due to several nonenzymatic reactions of glucose with lipids, proteins, and nucleic acids (glycation). This leads to the formation of a network of poorly characterized AGEs that typifies both diabetes and older age.[12] The adverse vascular effects of AGEs are multifactorial. AGEs act directly to induce cross-linking of proteins, such as vascular collagen and elastin. AGE-linked collagen and elastin are stiffer and less amenable to physiologic turnover, leading to the pathologic accumulation of structurally dysfunctional vascular proteins and a structurally rigid vascular scaffolding.[12,13] In addition to direct effects, AGE and various other ligands, such as S100B, can activate the AGE receptor, termed *RAGE*. With ligand binding to RAGE, activation of signal transduction machinery occurs, triggering further up-regulation of inflammatory and other detrimental vascular pathways, such as nuclear factor κB.[14] RAGE is expressed by endothelial cells,[15] and RAGE activation or other direct AGE effects on endothelial cells lead to multifactorial vascular dysfunction that includes increased vascular cell adhesion molecule-1 expression and inflammatory cell transmigration,[14,16,17] increased vascular permeability,[18,19] quenching of nitric oxide leading to defective endothelium-dependent vasodilatation,[20] endothelial progenitor cell (EPC) dysfunction,[21] and endothelial cell apoptosis.[22] Linking several of these aspects at the clinical level, Virmani and coworkers[23] have shown that compared with nondiabetics, plaques from diabetic subjects who died suddenly have larger mean necrotic cores and greater plaque load, increased inflammation, greater expression of RAGE, and increased VSMC apoptosis.

Diabetic Microvascular Dysfunction

Pathologic microvascular changes are a hallmark of the diabetic process and may precede the clinical diagnosis of diabetes.[24] Vascular changes seen with microvascular disease include cellular morphologic alterations, reduced cell mitochondrial content, and attenuated capillaries with thickened and fibrotic basement membranes.[12] In a meta-analysis of clinical studies, Muris and colleagues[24] identified several factors related to microvascular dysfunction that predicted a subsequent diagnosis of diabetes, including higher levels of soluble plasma E-selectin and intercellular adhesion molecule-1, a lower response to acetylcholine-mediated peripheral vascular reactivity testing, a lower retinal arteriole-to-venule ratio, and a higher albumin-to-creatinine ratio.

As an emerging but seemingly critical pathobiological disease mechanism, the authors and colleagues previously reviewed the major role played by microvascular disease in the pathology of Alzheimer disease and vascular cognitive impairment.[25] Although epidemiologic studies have documented an association between diabetes and Alzheimer disease,[26] autopsy studies have failed to find a positive relationship between diabetes and the characteristic Alzheimer pathologic changes of neurofibrillary plaques and tangles.[27] Rather, a consistent association between diabetes and ischemic cerebral vascular pathologies has been found.[27] Although other diabetes-related vascular mechanisms are also implicated, such as increased atherosclerotic burden, accumulation of ROS, and large-vessel stroke, it is now increasingly appreciated that diabetic microvascular damage is one of the fundamental pathologic pathways that culminates in degenerative brain disease.[28] Specific pathologic insults that arise due to cortical microvascular dysfuction include disruption of the blood-brain barrier and dysregulated cerebral blood flow. Given the aging of the population and concurrent obesity epidemic, the important role played by diabetic microvascular dysfunction in neurocognitive decline is certain to attract increasing research interest in the years ahead.

Vascular Progenitor Cell Dysfunction and Diabetes

Striking at the core of the vascular system, diabetes exerts a major toll on several vascular stem and vascular progenitor cell (VPC) populations. Although controversy exists regarding the precise definitions of these populations,[29] the detrimental effects of diabetes are widespread and affect both the number and functionality of VPCs.[30] This has led to the hypothesis that defective endothelial and vascular repair, arising due to these progenitor cell deficiencies, may play a role in the diabetic vascular phenotype.

The bone marrow (BM) is an important reservoir for VPCs, specifically, EPCs, in addition to its function as a reservoir for hematopoietic stem cells. Here, in this nurturing-ground for VPCs, an array of adverse changes has been described. As an example, Spinetti and colleagues[31] studied BM samples from patients with type 2 diabetes mellitus and identified a reduction of hematopoietic tissue, increased apoptosis and fat deposition, and microvascular rarefaction. Moreover, in addition to this anatomic evidence, hematopoietic and VPC numbers were reduced and molecular cell survival pathways were adversely affected in BM progenitor cells from diabetic subjects.[31]

Impaired Reverse Cholesterol Transport

Therapeutic interventions to reduce plaque burden are beginning to appear in the clinical arena. Although not all of these have lived up to expectations, therapies, such as high-dose statins and high-density lipoprotein (HDL)-raising agents, are thought to hold promise for reversing the atherosclerotic disease process. Several studies have indicated that diabetes impairs atherosclerotic regression and lipid egress from plaques. Parathath and colleagues[32] made use of a unique mouse model to show that during atherosclerotic regression there were lower reductions in plaque cholesterol (approximately 30%) and macrophages (approximately 41%) in diabetic mice compared with control mice. Diabetic (vs control) plaque macrophages also exhibited increased oxidant stress and a cellular phenotype more consistent with enhanced inflammation.[32] These findings were corroborated in humans in the prospective Reduction in Yellow Plaque by Aggressive Lipid-lowering Therapy (YELLOW) trial, in which 87 patients with multivessel CAD undergoing percutaneous coronary intervention (PCI) were randomized to intensive lipid-lowering therapy (rosuvastatin 40 mg daily) or standard-of-care lipid-lowering therapy.[33] These investigators identified that the mean reduction in plaque lipid with statin therapy was significantly greater in nondiabetic compared with diabetic subjects over an 8-week period. It was concluded that although high-dose statin therapy can reduce lipid content in obstructive coronary lesions, the magnitude of this effect is attenuated in those with diabetes versus those without diabetes, suggesting an impaired pattern for short-term regression in diabetic atherosclerosis.[33]

Summary of Relationships Between Diabetes and the Vasculature

This article reviews only a few of the many relationships between diabetes, the vasculature, and CVD. Space limitations have not permitted discussion of many other aspects, such as the role of insulin and insulin resistance,[34] altered platelet function, or the diabetes-associated circulating lipid disturbances that drive vascular disease, consisting of low HDL, increased triglycerides, and postprandial lipemia (diabetic dyslipidemia). Without question, the unifying theme of these pathways is the broad and multifaceted nature of these disease-causing insults that culminate in the diabetic vascular phenotype.

DIABETES AND THE HEART: DIABETIC CARDIOMYOPATHY

Moving from the vessels to the heart, the possibility that diabetes directly causes cardiomyopathy was first suggested more than 4 decades ago by Rubler and colleagues,[35] who reported postmortem observations from 4 patients with diabetes and congestive heart failure (CHF), where no other reason for heart failure could be determined. In the ensuing years, and not without controversy, accumulating data from experimental, pathologic, epidemiologic, and clinical studies have indicated that diabetes results in specific cardiac functional and structural changes.[36] This has led to the contemporary outlook on this disease, whereby DCM is defined as the specific cardiac dysfunction and damage present in diabetic patients, which is characterized by myocardial dilatation, hypertrophy, and decreased left ventricular (LV) systolic and diastolic functions, and which is independent of the coexistence of ischemic heart disease, MI, or hypertension.[37] Robust data now support the existence of DCM, with one of the largest epidemiologic studies, involving more than 800,000 patients, concluding that diabetes is independently associated with the occurrence of CHF after adjusting for ventricular hypertrophy, hypertension, CAD, and atrial fibrillation.[38]

Mechanisms of Disease

A clear understanding of the pathobiology of DCM is lacking at the present time. Several pathophysiologic mechanisms have been proposed, however, to explain the structural and functional changes associated with DCM that likely act in a synergistic fashion, and which include hyperglycemia, lipotoxicity, inflammation, autonomic neuropathy, and both microvascular and macrovascular changes.[39] Recent evidence has also identified mitochondrial dysfunction and epigenetic changes (alteration in gene function without changes in nucleotide sequence) as pathogenic contributors to DCM.[40] Importantly, hyperglycemia is considered a critical driver of DCM because it has the ability to trigger several adaptive and maladaptive responses that are evident during the evolution of cardiac dysfunction. In addition to the vascular effects discussed previously, hyperglycemia contributes to the generation of ROS, connective tissue damage, systemic and local cytokine elaboration, renin-angiotensin-aldosterone system activation, cardiac hypertrophy, and fibrosis. Furthermore, AGEs formed in diabetic patients not only harm the vasculature but also accumulate in cardiac tissues and are implicated in the morphologic changes that result in myocardial stiffness and impaired contractility with DCM (**Fig. 2**).[41]

Altered Substrate Metabolism

In healthy individuals, equivalent proportions of energy required for cardiac performance come from glucose metabolism and free fatty acids (FFAs). In a hyperglycemic state, increased insulin resistance leads to reductions in the glucose transporter proteins 1 and 4. Consequently, myocardial cells rely less on glucose metabolism (which accounts for only approximately 10% of myocardial energy production) and more on β-oxidation of FFAs for energy production. FFA metabolism generates several toxic intermediates that accumulate in myocardial cells, a phenomenon termed *lipotoxicity*. Lipotoxicity disrupts cellular function in several ways. First, it impairs myocyte calcium handling through reduced activity of ATPases, decreased ability of the sarcoplasmic reticulum to take up calcium, and reduced activities of other exchanges, such as sodium-calcium and the sarcolemmal calcium ATPase.[42] This impairment in calcium regulation seems to cause an overload of calcium ions in the cytosol and increased ventricular stiffness in the early stages of DCM.[43] Second, it causes increased production and release of ROS, which in turn cause oxidative stress and abnormal gene expression, resulting in cardiomyocyte death, cardiac fibrosis, and myocardial dysfunction.[44] In addition, FFAs inhibit pyruvate dehydrogenase, which leads to the accumulation of glycolytic intermediates and ceramide, which are known to enhance

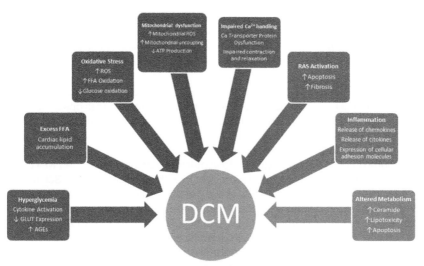

Fig. 2. Pathophysiologic triggers of DCM in diabetic patients. In addition to hyperglycemia, the combination of ROS, increased β-oxidation with elevated FFAs leading to myocardial lipotoxicity, cytokine damage, and the activation of the renin-angiotensin system (RAS) lead to the molecular and structural changes that characterize diabetic cardiomyopathy. GLUT, glucose transporter.

apoptosis.[45] FFAs have also been shown to enhance peripheral insulin resistance and trigger cell death. Abnormalities in FFA metabolism have been demonstrated in idiopathic dilated cardiomyopathy, in which the rate of FFA uptake by myocardium is inversely proportional to the severity of the myocardial dysfunction.[46] It is possible, therefore, that similar effects may be contributing to the development of DCM.

Activation of the Renin-angiotensin System

Activation of the renin-angiotensin system can exert deleterious effects on the myocardium through different mechanisms. Angiotensin II receptor density and mRNA expression are elevated in the diabetic heart.[47] Furthermore, activation of the renin-angiotensin system in the setting of diabetes is strongly associated with increased oxidative damage and cardiomyocyte and endothelial cell apoptosis and necrosis in diabetic hearts, contributing to accelerated interstitial fibrosis.[48]

Cardiac Autonomic Neuropathy

Diabetic cardiac autonomic neuropathy (CAN) occurs in 17% of patients with type 1 diabetes mellitus and 22% of patients with type 2 diabetes mellitus and is strongly associated with mortality.[39] Over time, hyperglycemia results in impaired sympathetic innervation and increases both adrenergic receptor expression and catecholamine levels.[49] One of the earliest signs of CAN is an increased resting heart rate and associated loss of heart rate variability. Resting tachycardia causes an increase in myocardial work, increased oxygen demand, reduced ventricular filling time, and reduced cardiac efficiency. These effects collectively lead to myocyte apoptosis and myocardial fibrosis, culminating in ventricular hypertrophy and dysfunction. These pathologic processes seem to increase with age, high glucose levels, and duration of disease. Not surprisingly, several studies have shown that CAN plays an important role in the deleterious effects of diabetes on the heart, causing impaired LV systolic function with reduced ejection fraction and decreased diastolic filling.[39,49] There is also evidence that autonomic neuropathy, in combination with vascular endothelial dysfunction and inflammation, leads to further insulin resistance, resulting in a vicious cycle of worsening hyperglycemia and its effects on the myocardium.[5]

Myocardial Fibrosis

Myocardial fibrosis and collagen deposition are the primary changes observed in DCM and arise in the interstitium, perivascular region, or in a combined manner. In addition to fibrosis, pathologic examination of the diabetic heart typically reveals myocardial hypertrophy, capillary endothelial changes, and capillary basal laminar thickening.[50] The pathomolecular changes that lead to ventricular stiffening have been well characterized. Increased collagen deposition interacts with glucose, forming Schiff bases, and which are reorganized into so called Amadori products (glycated collagen). Further chemical modification of the Amadori products results in the formation of AGEs, which has a profound effect on diastolic function. Furthermore, AGEs have the ability to cross-link with circulating proteins and cause impaired nitric oxide signaling and increased intracellular oxidative stress, all of which contribute to cell damage. Therefore, impaired LV function in the setting of diabetes, both diastolic and systolic, can be the result of fibrosis and altered collagen structure, specifically through the mechanisms of cross-linking and AGE formation.

Cardiovascular Findings

The complex pathogenesis of DMC ultimately leads to altered cardiac structure and function. Furthermore, frequent coexisting conditions, such as hypertension and CAD, further complicate the diabetic cardiac phenotype. Recently, in an effort to consolidate these factors into a cohesive description of the structural phenotype, a categorization of the DCM has been proposed.[39] According to this categorization, stage 1 DCM is diastolic heart failure with normal ejection fraction in the absence of other causes of heart disease. It is found in 75% of asymptomatic diabetic patients.[51] Stage 2 is defined by both diastolic and systolic dysfunction, in the absence of other contributing comorbidities for structural heart disease. Stage 3 is diastolic and/or systolic dysfunction, but in the setting of microvascular disease, uncontrolled hypertension, or other direct myopathic processes, such as infection or inflammation. Stage 4 is diastolic and/or systolic dysfunction in the setting of CAD. The advantages of the proposed scheme are 2-fold. First, it separates clinical phenotypes into those that are primarily due to DCM (stages 1 and 2) and those where other pathologies are also contributory (stages 3 and 4). Second, this classification has prognostic implications. Patients with stage 1 DCM have a 5% to 8% mortality compared with normal controls. Moreover, 37% of patients in stage 1, compared with 16.8% of normal controls, progress to symptomatic heart failure, which usually precedes the development of stage 2 DCM and systolic dysfunction.[39]

Diagnosing DCM

The diagnosis of DCM currently relies on noninvasive imaging that can demonstrate myocardial dysfunction across the continuum of ventricular dysfunction found in these patients. Although currently a consensus on the imaging definition of DCM is lacing, it is generally accepted that hypertrophy and diastolic dysfunction are responsible for (although not specific to) the clinical presentation of DCM.

Cardiac hypertrophy is a hallmark in the morphologic manifestations of DCM and can be quantified through conventional echocardiography.[52] The advent of MRI and its ability to qualitatively assess the myocardium has broadened understanding of the processes that lead to DCM and can demonstrate the presence of fatty or fibrotic infiltrates in the hypertrophied myocardium. Studies of myocardial geometry have also shown altered torsion dynamics in asymptomatic patients that could represent a subclinical phenotype with a higher propensity to develop cardiac dysfunction in the future.[53]

Changes in diastolic function have been reported in up to 75% of diabetic patients without evidence of heart disease caused by other factors, whereas it is a rare condition in healthy, nonobese individuals (where the incidence approaches 1%).[54] Consistent with this, additional studies have shown a correlation between altered transmitral Doppler inflow patterns and poor glycemic control.[54] Using tissue Doppler imaging techniques, recent studies have also shown that the prevalence of diastolic dysfunction in diabetic subjects may be as high as 50%.[55] Diastolic variables have proved especially useful in predicting the prognosis of diabetic patients without overt heart failure. A retrospective study of 486 diabetic patients demonstrated that echocardiographically derived parameter of the E/e' ratio was associated with an increase in global mortality after adjusting for age, gender, CAD, hypertension, LV ejection fraction, and left atrial volume.[56] Newer echocardiographic markers, such as total ejection isovolumic (TEI) index, are emerging as additional useful tools in the diagnosis of DCM. In a recent study of patients with type 2 diabetes mellitus without macrovascular complications, TEI index was significantly and independently associated with the presence of DCM.[37] Other modern echocardiographic techniques, such as transmitral pulsed Doppler and its applications (strain and strain rate), have recently demonstrated good sensitivity in the diagnosis of DCM.

DIABETES AND THE CARDIOVASCULAR PATIENT

Moving from the heart and DCM to the patient as a whole, the clinical implications of the association between diabetes and CVD have been well described.

Coronary Artery Disease Risk Factors

There is a strong association and overlap between diabetes and the metabolic syndrome. For patients who have developed diabetes, the strongest associations are with dyslipidemia and hypertension.

Dyslipidemia

A large number of studies both for primary and secondary prevention in diabetes have evaluated the use of statin medications. What is remarkable is that statins not only reduce coronary events by relative risk proportions equal to the nondiabetic population but also in many cases demonstrate that relative risk reduction is higher. This is one of the first demonstrations that not only is absolute risk reduction higher but also relative risk reduction.[57] This speaks to the pleotrophic effects of statins, such as reduced inflammation and thrombosis.[58] The American Diabetes Association has recommended that patients with diabetes be treated with a statin medication even if their low-density lipoprotein (LDL) cholesterol is on target. At present, for patients without coronary disease, the LDL target is less than 100 mg/dL, whereas for patients with advanced CAD and prior events, the recommended target is less than 70 mg/dL.[57] Because of the association of diabetes with hypertriglyceridemia and reduced levels of HDL, investigations are under way to find novel therapies. Fibrates have not reduced risks in diabetics in the ACCORD (Action to Control Cardiovascular Risk in Diabetes) trial,[59] however, and published data regarding the CETP inhibitors have been disappointing.[60,61] Recently, studies of niacin have also been negative for elevating HDL levels in the setting of low LDL levels.[62] As a result, statin therapy has become the gold standard therapy for hyperlipidemia in diabetic patients, with recommended LDL targets lower than those for nondiabetic patients.

Hypertension

With regards to hypertension, important recent information has shown that the goals for blood pressure control need to be carefully evaluated. In the ACCORD trial, which evaluated patients with type 2 diabetes mellitus and high cardiovascular risk, patients achieving a systolic blood pressure less than 120 mm Hg had outcomes similar to patients who achieved a systolic blood pressure less than 140 mm Hg, the traditional standard.[63] There were small reductions in stroke but for the primary cluster of death, MI, and stroke, there was no significant difference. Similar analyses from the INVEST (International Verapamil-Trandolapril Study) trial have demonstrated that the cardiovascular event rates are comparable in those patients with a systolic blood pressure less than 130 mm Hg compared with those achieving between 130 mm Hg and 140 mm Hg.[64] This speaks to the importance of less-aggressive blood pressure control than has been advocated in the past. In INVEST, it was also shown that patients with a systolic blood pressure less than 110 mm Hg experienced increased cardiovascular event rates. As a result, according to the new Eighth Report of the Joint National Committee on Prevention, Detection, Evaluation, and Treatment of High Blood Pressure guidelines and other expert opinions, it is questionable whether a blood pressure target of 130/80, as opposed to 140/90, is justified.

Glycemic control

Several pivotal trials have demonstrated that tight glycemic control (target hemoglobin A_{1c} approximately 6.0%) is not associated with improved cardiovascular outcomes.[65] This has led to a general relaxing of how aggressively physicians are treating glycemic control in their diabetic patients. Beyond this, one of the major problems with antidiabetic medications is their association with weight gain and hypoglycemia. Recently, incretin drugs in the form of glucagon-like peptide-1 agonists and dipeptidyl peptidase-4 inhibitors have entered the market. The promise of incretin therapy is the association with favorable weight changes and the relative lack of hypoglycemia.[66] Several key cardiovascular outcomes trials in type 2 diabetes mellitus are near completion and will report in the next 2 years.

Diabetes and Coronary Artery Disease

At the clinical level, the association between diabetes and CAD is well established and has been documented in several large observational cohort studies.[67,68]

Dating back to the BARI trial from the early 1990s, there has been a demonstration that patients with multivessel CAD and diabetes have improved outcomes with coronary artery bypass graft (CABG) surgery compared with PCI.[69] After BARI, researchers speculated that these findings may be related to the balloon angioplasty used in the percutaneous arm and later raised the question of whether the advent of stenting would change this outcome. Several important studies have ensued. The ARTS trial showed that there was still an increased cardiovascular event rate for diabetic patients undergoing PCI with bare metal stents compared with coronary artery bypass surgery.[70] Later, the SYNTAX trial, recruiting more than 400 diabetic patients and using drug-eluting stents (DES) (paclitaxel) with percutaneous coronary intervention (PCI) (DES-PCI), showed no difference in hard cardiovascular endpoint data at 1 year but did demonstrate and reaffirm very high repeat revascularization rates. With long-term follow-up out to 5 years, the SYNTAX study showed a clear advantage of CABG over PCI for left main and triple vessel disease.[71]

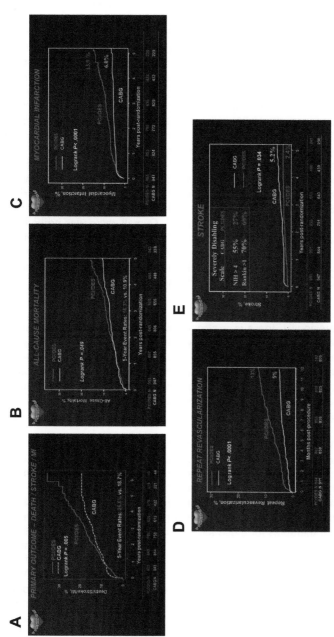

Fig. 3. Kaplan-Meier estimates from the FREEDOM study of the proportion of subjects with a clinical event by treatment assignment, as indicated: (A) primary endpoint (death/stroke/MI), (B) all-cause mortality, (C) MI, (D) repeat revascularization to 1 year, and (E) stroke. (*Reprinted with permission AHA Scientific Sessions 2012* © 2012 American Heart Association, Inc.)

The FREEDOM Trial, published in the *New England Journal of Medicine* in December 2012, provided a comprehensive insight into diabetes and multivessel CAD because it exclusively studied diabetic patients in a 1900-patient international randomized trial of DES-PCI versus CABG.[72] The majority of patients enrolled had multivessel CAD (84% had triple vessel disease). The median patient age was 63 years, with the majority having preserved LV function and an average SYNTAX score of approximately 26. FREEDOM patients were approximately 70% elective stable CAD patients, with the remainder having suffered a recent acute coronary syndrome. In the FREEDOM study, 20% of patients had off-pump CABG in the surgical arm and the mean number of treated lesions was greater than 5. For the primary endpoint, the composite of death, MI, and stroke at 5 years, there was an 8% absolute difference from 26.6% in the DES-PCI arm compared with 18.7% in the CABG arm (**Fig. 3**A). There was also an associated increase in all-cause mortality at 5 years in the DES-PCI arm, which was marginally significant ($P = .049$) (see **Fig. 3**B) as well as an increased rate of MI, which continued to accrue over the 5 years of trial ($P<.001$) (see **Fig. 3**C). Further counting against PCI, there was a significantly lower rate of repeat revascularization in the CABG arm (see **Fig. 3**D). On the other hand, there was a greater stroke rate in the bypass arm at 5 years (5.2% vs 2.4%, $P = .03$), which was most apparent in the first 30 days after the index procedure (see **Fig. 3**E). Overall, there was no heterogeneity across important subgroups, including SYNTAX score.[73] The FREEDOM trial was confirmation of the BARI findings and other meta-analysis data based on earlier trials with and without stenting,[74] and collectively these studies have clearly documented the benefits of CABG in diabetic patients with advanced CAD.

Heart Failure

As discussed previously, there is a strong relationship between diabetes and the development of CHF. In order to simplify the prescription of a clinical treatment plan, it is convenient to define heart failure as 3 distinct entities. First is systolic heart failure, which is almost always related to ischemic heart disease and is defined as an LV ejection fraction of less than 45%. Second is heart failure with preserved LV function. This is associated with diastolic abnormalities, largely related to the strong association between diabetes and hypertension. The third is DCM, as described previously.[44]

The treatment of heart failure has evolved over the past several years. In systolic heart failure, the use of β-blockers and angiotensin-converting enzyme (ACE) inhibitors has been the mainstay. Coronary revascularization for CAD with associated myocardial ischemia and CHF has also been recommended. For diastolic or preserved LV ejection fraction CHF, several therapies have been evaluated in addition to ACE inhibitors and β-blockers. This is an area of fruitful investigation at present, although targeted therapies for these forms of diabetic CHF remain to be identified.

SUMMARY

Diabetes has reached an epidemic level worldwide, and patients suffering from this disease are at significantly higher risk for CVD. Moreover, cardiovascular complications are the leading cause of diabetes-related morbidity and mortality.

The close relationship between diabetes and CVD together with the substantial rise in prevalence of diabetes will ultimately lead to a huge increase in the demand for health care services at a global level. Although FREEDOM and other studies have clarified how best to manage patients at the individual level, there are enormous challenges and opportunities in addressing the growing diabetes epidemic at the population level. Ultimately, the economic force behind the continuing rise in the cost of health care derived from caring for the 300 million projected diabetic patients in 2025 will leave policy makers no choice but to deeply revise, and come up with, efficient solutions to prevent the widespread surge of this disease. In a health care system that is continually becoming more complex, and where efficacious drugs and sophisticated devices continue to improve clinical outcomes, part of the focus should be placed back on the mechanisms that prevent the development of diabetes and related pathologies through the promotion of cardiovascular health by smoking cessation, exercising, following a healthy diet, and weight loss strategies, all of which will improve health outcomes and reduce costs.

REFERENCES

1. King H, Aubert RE, Herman WH. Global burden of diabetes, 1995-2025: prevalence, numerical estimates, and projections. Diabetes Care 1998;21: 1414–31.
2. Boyle JP, Honeycutt AA, Narayan KM, et al. Projection of diabetes burden through 2050: impact of changing demography and disease prevalence in the U.S. Diabetes Care 2001;24:1936–40.
3. New WHO statistics highlight increases in blood pressure and diabetes, other noncommunicable risk factors. Cent Eur J Public Health 2012;20(134):149.
4. Chiha M, Njeim M, Chedrawy EG. Diabetes and coronary heart disease: a risk factor for the global epidemic. Int J Hypertens 2012;2012:697240.
5. Tillquist MN, Maddox TM. Update on diabetic cardiomyopathy: inches forward, miles to go. Curr Diab Rep 2012;12:305–13.
6. Johnson PC, Doll SC, Cromey DW. Pathogenesis of diabetic neuropathy. Ann Neurol 1986;19:450–7.
7. Weil EJ, Lemley KV, Mason CC, et al. Podocyte detachment and reduced glomerular capillary endothelial fenestration promote kidney disease in type 2 diabetic nephropathy. Kidney Int 2012;82:1010–7.
8. Tang Y, Li GD. Chronic exposure to high glucose impairs bradykinin-stimulated nitric oxide production by interfering with the phospholipase-C-implicated signalling pathway in endothelial cells: evidence for the involvement of protein kinase C. Diabetologia 2004;47:2093–104.
9. Kovacic JC, Martin A, Carey D, et al. Influence of rosiglitazone on flow-mediated dilation and other markers of cardiovascular risk in HIV-infected patients with lipoatrophy. Antivir Ther 2005;10:135–43.
10. Schaffer SW, Jong CJ, Mozaffari M. Role of oxidative stress in diabetes-mediated vascular dysfunction: unifying hypothesis of diabetes revisited. Vascul Pharmacol 2012;57:139–49.
11. Brownlee M. Biochemistry and molecular cell biology of diabetic complications. Nature 2001;414:813–20.
12. Kovacic JC, Moreno P, Nabel EG, et al. Cellular senescence, vascular disease, and aging: part 2 of a 2-part review: clinical vascular disease in the elderly. Circulation 2011;123:1900–10.
13. Konova E, Baydanoff S, Atanasova M, et al. Age-related changes in the glycation of human aortic elastin. Exp Gerontol 2004;39:249–54.
14. Kislinger T, Fu C, Huber B, et al. N(epsilon)-(carboxymethyl)lysine adducts of proteins are ligands for receptor for advanced glycation end products that activate cell signaling pathways and modulate gene expression. J Biol Chem 1999; 274:31740–9.

15. Brett J, Schmidt AM, Yan SD, et al. Survey of the distribution of a newly characterized receptor for advanced glycation end products in tissues. Am J Pathol 1993;143:1699–712.

16. Giri R, Shen Y, Stins M, et al. beta-amyloid-induced migration of monocytes across human brain endothelial cells involves RAGE and PECAM-1. Am J Physiol Cell Physiol 2000;279:C1772–81.

17. Kunt T, Forst T, Harzer O, et al. The influence of advanced glycation endproducts (AGE) on the expression of human endothelial adhesion molecules. Exp Clin Endocrinol Diabetes 1998;106:183–8.

18. Otero K, Martinez F, Beltran A, et al. Albumin-derived advanced glycation endproducts trigger the disruption of the vascular endothelial cadherin complex in cultured human and murine endothelial cells. Biochem J 2001;359:567–74.

19. Svensjo E, Cyrino F, Michoud E, et al. Vascular permeability increase as induced by histamine or bradykinin is enhanced by advanced glycation endproducts (AGEs). J Diabet Complications 1999;13:187–90.

20. Bucala R, Tracey KJ, Cerami A. Advanced glycosylation products quench nitric oxide and mediate defective endothelium-dependent vasodilatation in experimental diabetes. J Clin Invest 1991;87:432–8.

21. Scheubel RJ, Kahrstedt S, Weber H, et al. Depression of progenitor cell function by advanced glycation endproducts (AGEs): potential relevance for impaired angiogenesis in advanced age and diabetes. Exp Gerontol 2006;41:540–8.

22. Xiang M, Yang M, Zhou C, et al. Crocetin prevents AGEs-induced vascular endothelial cell apoptosis. Pharmacol Res 2006;54:268–74.

23. Burke AP, Kolodgie FD, Zieske A, et al. Morphologic findings of coronary atherosclerotic plaques in diabetics: a postmortem study. Arterioscler Thromb Vasc Biol 2004;24:1266–71.

24. Muris DM, Houben AJ, Schram MT, et al. Microvascular dysfunction is associated with a higher incidence of type 2 diabetes mellitus: a systematic review and meta-analysis. Arterioscler Thromb Vasc Biol 2012;32:3082–94.

25. Kovacic JC, Fuster V. Atherosclerotic risk factors, vascular cognitive impairment, and Alzheimer disease. Mt Sinai J Med 2012;79:664–73.

26. Centers for Disease Control and Prevention. Leading causes of death reports. Available at: http://webappa.cdc.gov/sasweb/ncipc/leadcaus10.html. Accessed May 19, 2011.

27. Beeri MS, Silverman JM, Davis KL, et al. Type 2 diabetes is negatively associated with Alzheimer's disease neuropathology. J Gerontol A Biol Sci Med Sci 2005;60:471–5.

28. Nelson PT, Smith CD, Abner EA, et al. Human cerebral neuropathology of Type 2 diabetes mellitus. Biochim Biophys Acta 2009;1792:454–69.

29. Kovacic JC, Moore J, Herbert A, et al. Endothelial progenitor cells, angioblasts, and angiogenesis–old terms reconsidered from a current perspective. Trends Cardiovasc Med 2008;18:45–51.

30. Tepper OM, Galiano RD, Capla JM, et al. Human endothelial progenitor cells from type II diabetics exhibit impaired proliferation, adhesion, and incorporation into vascular structures. Circulation 2002;106:2781–6.

31. Spinetti G, Cordella D, Fortunato O, et al. Global remodeling of the vascular stem cell niche in bone marrow of diabetic patients: implication of the microRNA-155/FOXO3a signaling pathway. Circ Res 2013;112:510–22.

32. Parathath S, Grauer L, Huang LS, et al. Diabetes adversely affects macrophages during atherosclerotic plaque regression in mice. Diabetes 2011;60:1759–69.

33. Kini A, Baber U, Kovacic JC, et al. Impact of diabetes mellitus on atherosclerotic plaque lipid regression: results from the prospective. Randomized YELLOW Trial Circulation 2012;126:A17291.
34. Mather KJ, Steinberg HO, Baron AD. Insulin resistance in the vasculature. J Clin Invest 2013;123:1003–4.
35. Rubler S, Dlugash J, Yuceoglu YZ, et al. New type of cardiomyopathy associated with diabetic glomerulosclerosis. Am J Cardiol 1972;30:595–602.
36. Fang ZY, Prins JB, Marwick TH. Diabetic cardiomyopathy: evidence, mechanisms, and therapeutic implications. Endocr Rev 2004;25:543–67.
37. Voulgari C, Papadogiannis D, Tentolouris N. Diabetic cardiomyopathy: from the pathophysiology of the cardiac myocytes to current diagnosis and management strategies. Vasc Health Risk Manag 2010;6:883–903.
38. Movahed MR, Hashemzadeh M, Jamal MM. Diabetes mellitus is a strong, independent risk for atrial fibrillation and flutter in addition to other cardiovascular disease. Int J Cardiol 2005;105:315–8.
39. Maisch B, Alter P, Pankuweit S. Diabetic cardiomyopathy–fact or fiction? Herz 2011;36:102–15.
40. Singh GB, Sharma R, Khullar M. Epigenetics and diabetic cardiomyopathy. Diabetes Res Clin Pract 2011;94:14–21.
41. Avendano GF, Agarwal RK, Bashey RI, et al. Effects of glucose intolerance on myocardial function and collagen-linked glycation. Diabetes 1999;48:1443–7.
42. Cesario DA, Brar R, Shivkumar K. Alterations in ion channel physiology in diabetic cardiomyopathy. Endocrinol Metab Clin North Am 2006;35:601–10, ix–x.
43. Falcao-Pires I, Leite-Moreira AF. Diabetic cardiomyopathy: understanding the molecular and cellular basis to progress in diagnosis and treatment. Heart Fail Rev 2012;17:325–44.
44. Aneja A, Tang WH, Bansilal S, et al. Diabetic cardiomyopathy: insights into pathogenesis, diagnostic challenges, and therapeutic options. Am J Med 2008;121: 748–57.
45. Park TS, Hu Y, Noh HL, et al. Ceramide is a cardiotoxin in lipotoxic cardiomyopathy. J Lipid Res 2008;49:2101–12.
46. Yazaki Y, Isobe M, Takahashi W, et al. Assessment of myocardial fatty acid metabolic abnormalities in patients with idiopathic dilated cardiomyopathy using 123I BMIPP SPECT: correlation with clinicopathological findings and clinical course. Heart 1999;81:153–9.
47. Peti-Peterdi J, Kang JJ, Toma I. Activation of the renal renin-angiotensin system in diabetes–new concepts. Nephrol Dial Transplant 2008;23:3047–9.
48. Kawasaki D, Kosugi K, Waki H, et al. Role of activated renin-angiotensin system in myocardial fibrosis and left ventricular diastolic dysfunction in diabetic patients–reversal by chronic angiotensin II type 1A receptor blockade. Circ J 2007;71:524–9.
49. Mytas DZ, Stougiannos PN, Zairis MN, et al. Diabetic myocardial disease: pathophysiology, early diagnosis and therapeutic options. J Diabet Complications 2009;23:273–82.
50. Asbun J, Villarreal FJ. The pathogenesis of myocardial fibrosis in the setting of diabetic cardiomyopathy. J Am Coll Cardiol 2006;47:693–700.
51. Boyer JK, Thanigaraj S, Schechtman KB, et al. Prevalence of ventricular diastolic dysfunction in asymptomatic, normotensive patients with diabetes mellitus. Am J Cardiol 2004;93:870–5.
52. Lang RM, Bierig M, Devereux RB, et al. Recommendations for chamber quantification: a report from the American Society of Echocardiography's Guidelines

and Standards Committee and the Chamber Quantification Writing Group, developed in conjunction with the European Association of Echocardiography, a branch of the European Society of Cardiology. J Am Soc Echocardiogr 2005; 18:1440–63.

53. Chung J, Abraszewski P, Yu X, et al. Paradoxical increase in ventricular torsion and systolic torsion rate in type I diabetic patients under tight glycemic control. J Am Coll Cardiol 2006;47:384–90.

54. Galderisi M. Diastolic dysfunction and diabetic cardiomyopathy: evaluation by Doppler echocardiography. J Am Coll Cardiol 2006;48:1548–51.

55. Kiencke S, Handschin R, von Dahlen R, et al. Pre-clinical diabetic cardiomyopathy: prevalence, screening, and outcome. Eur J Heart Fail 2010;12:951–7.

56. From AM, Scott CG, Chen HH. The development of heart failure in patients with diabetes mellitus and pre-clinical diastolic dysfunction a population-based study. J Am Coll Cardiol 2010;55:300–5.

57. American Diabetes Association. Standards of medical care in diabetes–2013. Diabetes Care 2013;36(Suppl 1):S11–66.

58. Puccetti L, Santilli F, Pasqui AL, et al. Effects of atorvastatin and rosuvastatin on thromboxane-dependent platelet activation and oxidative stress in hypercholesterolemia. Atherosclerosis 2011;214:122–8.

59. Group AS, Ginsberg HN, Elam MB, et al. Effects of combination lipid therapy in type 2 diabetes mellitus. N Engl J Med 2010;362:1563–74.

60. Barter PJ, Caulfield M, Eriksson M, et al. Effects of torcetrapib in patients at high risk for coronary events. N Engl J Med 2007;357:2109–22.

61. Schwartz GG, Olsson AG, Abt M, et al. Effects of dalcetrapib in patients with a recent acute coronary syndrome. N Engl J Med 2012;367:2089–99.

62. Investigators AH, Boden WE, Probstfield JL, et al. Niacin in patients with low HDL cholesterol levels receiving intensive statin therapy. N Engl J Med 2011; 365:2255–67.

63. Reboldi G, Gentile G, Angeli F, et al. Effects of intensive blood pressure reduction on myocardial infarction and stroke in diabetes: a meta-analysis in 73,913 patients. J Hypertens 2011;29:1253–69.

64. Cooper-DeHoff RM, Gong Y, Handberg EM, et al. Tight blood pressure control and cardiovascular outcomes among hypertensive patients with diabetes and coronary artery disease. JAMA 2010;304:61–8.

65. Macisaac RJ, Jerums G. Intensive glucose control and cardiovascular outcomes in type 2 diabetes. Heart Lung Circ 2011;20:647–54.

66. Ussher JR, Drucker DJ. Cardiovascular biology of the incretin system. Endocr Rev 2012;33:187–215.

67. Roger VL, Go AS, Lloyd-Jones DM, et al. Heart disease and stroke statistics–2012 update: a report from the American Heart Association. Circulation 2012; 125:e2–220.

68. Smith SC Jr, Faxon D, Cascio W, et al. Prevention Conference VI: Diabetes and Cardiovascular Disease: Writing Group VI: revascularization in diabetic patients. Circulation 2002;105:e165–9.

69. Comparison of coronary bypass surgery with angioplasty in patients with multivessel disease. The Bypass Angioplasty Revascularization Investigation (BARI) Investigators. N Engl J Med 1996;335:217–25.

70. Serruys PW, Ong AT, van Herwerden LA, et al. Five-year outcomes after coronary stenting versus bypass surgery for the treatment of multivessel disease: the final analysis of the Arterial Revascularization Therapies Study (ARTS) randomized trial. J Am Coll Cardiol 2005;46:575–81.

71. Mohr FW, Morice MC, Kappetein AP, et al. Coronary artery bypass graft surgery versus percutaneous coronary intervention in patients with three-vessel disease and left main coronary disease: 5-year follow-up of the randomised, clinical SYNTAX trial. Lancet 2013;381:629–38.
72. Farkouh ME, Domanski M, Sleeper LA, et al. Strategies for multivessel revascularization in patients with diabetes. N Engl J Med 2012;367:2375–84.
73. Sianos G, Morel MA, Kappetein AP, et al. The SYNTAX Score: an angiographic tool grading the complexity of coronary artery disease. EuroIntervention 2005;1:219–27.
74. Hlatky MA, Boothroyd DB, Bravata DM, et al. Coronary artery bypass surgery compared with percutaneous coronary interventions for multivessel disease: a collaborative analysis of individual patient data from ten randomised trials. Lancet 2009;373:1190–7.

Interventions for Coronary Artery Disease (Surgery vs Angioplasty) in Diabetic Patients

Darryl M. Hoffman, MD, FRCS*, Robert F. Tranbaugh, MD

KEYWORDS

- Coronary artery disease • Diabetes mellitus • Coronary artery bypass graft
- Drug-eluting stent • Percutaneous coronary intervention • FREEDOM trial
- Coronary revascularization

KEY POINTS

- Coronary artery disease is common and anatomically and physiologically worse in patients with diabetes than in patients without diabetes.
- For patients with diabetes, surgical revascularization (coronary artery bypass grafting [CABG]) is superior to percutaneous coronary intervention (PCI).
- The pivotal Future Revascularization Evaluation in Patients with Diabetes Mellitus: Optimal Management of Multivessel Disease (FREEDOM) trial confirms the superiority of CABG compared with PCI for patients with diabetes and multivessel coronary artery disease.
- The main role for PCI in patients with diabetes is in acute coronary syndromes.

INTRODUCTION

An estimated 22.3 million people in the United States were living with type 1 or type 2 diabetes in 2012, up 28% from 17.5 million in 2007. Medical and indirect costs for their care were $245 billion in 2012, up 41% from $174 billion in 2007.[1]

Diabetes exerts major effects on the cardiovascular system via many pathways. Endothelin, angiotensin, and tissue factor activity are increased, whereas nitric oxide and prostacyclin production is reduced.[2] Platelet activation and aggregation are increased with overexpression of glycoprotein IIb/IIIa receptors. The net effect is coronary atherosclerosis. Diabetic patients develop early coronary atherosclerosis, diffuse disease within the course of each diseased coronary artery, multivessel involvement, frequent left main coronary artery stenosis, and more frequently have total coronary occlusions. The patient's disease burden is greater and there are more lipid-rich and macrophage-rich plaques, more fissured plaque, and more intracoronary thrombi,

No disclosures.

Division of Cardiothoracic Surgery, Beth Israel Medical Center, 317 East 17th Street, 11th Floor, New York, NY 10003, USA

* Corresponding author.

E-mail address: dhoffman@chpnet.org

as well as an impaired ability to develop collateral circulation compared with patients without diabetes.[3]

The unique pathophysiology of atherosclerosis in patients with diabetes mellitus (DM) modifies the response to revascularization of the coronary arteries, whether by surgical grafting (coronary artery bypass grafting [CABG]) or percutaneous coronary intervention (PCI). Hyperglycemia promotes inflammation, causing the advanced glycosylation end products to accumulate in vascular tissues as part of normal aging but at an accelerated rate in patients with diabetes. Formation of these end products is proportional to both the glucose concentration and the duration of exposure to hyperglycemia. The advanced glycosylation end products interact with specific receptors on inflammatory cells, smooth muscle cells, and the vessel wall, producing inflammation, smooth muscle proliferation, and extracellular matrix production, which together can generate intimal hyperplasia and also restenosis.

There is a compelling need to provide effective, up-to-date, and evidence-based treatment of coronary artery disease (CAD) in patients with DM. This article considers the relative merits of surgical (CABG) and percutaneous (PCI) revascularization for patients with DM and CAD.

REVASCULARIZATION TREATMENT OPTIONS

Early medical management clinical trials established the superiority of CABG compared with medical management for patients with DM and CAD.[4] Patients with diabetes have an increased risk with CABG: compared with patients without DM in the Society of Thoracic Surgeons (STS) Registry, patients with DM had worse 30-day mortality and a higher rate of major complications (stroke, renal failure, and deep sternal wound infection [DSWI]). Inferior outcomes for patients with DM can only partly be explained by their greater rate of comorbidities (obesity, hypertension, renal insufficiency, peripheral vascular, and cerebrovascular disease.) Long-term survival after CABG is also worse for patients with DM, likely because of a combination of the burden of comorbidities, more rapid progression of atherosclerosis, as well as the reduced long-term patency of their saphenous vein grafts.

Percutaneous transluminal coronary angioplasty (PTCA), pioneered by Gruentzig, promised a less invasive approach to revascularization. The first such intervention was balloon angioplasty in what is now considered the prestent era. The pivotal BARI (Bypass Angioplasty Revascularization Investigation)[5] compared CABG and PTCA in patients with multivessel coronary disease. Major findings were the superiority of CABG compared with PCI and the high rate of target vessel revascularization (TVR) after PTCA (76.8% vs 20.3%; $P<.001$).

For patients with DM, survival was better after CABG.[6] These findings prompted an National Heart, Lung and Blood Institute alert recommending that patients with diabetes and multivessel disease undergo CABG as the preferred mode of revascularization. Despite this, clinical practice did not change appreciably after the alert or the subsequent publication.

Cardiovascular practice evolved as new techniques (bare-metal stents [BMSs], drug-eluting stents [DES], glycoprotein IIb/IIIa inhibitors, and oral antiplatelet agents) were introduced for PCI, adopted enthusiastically, and deployed in patients with DM. Surgical techniques have also evolved since the era of the BARI trial.

To combat the high rate of restenosis after PTCA, BMSs were introduced, and DES were later developed. Hlatky and colleagues[7] (2009) analyzed 10 randomized controlled trials (RCTs; PTCA or BMS vs CABG). Of 7812 patients, 1233 were diabetic (CABG, n = 615; PCI, n = 618). Although restenosis was reduced by BMSs, mortality for patients with DM remained substantially lower for CABG versus PCI (hazard ratio [HR], 0·70, 0·56–0·87) and the lower mortality after CABG was still evident at 8 years (22% vs 34% for PCI).

Multiple small, single-institution studies have been published comparing DES with CABG, and usually show CABG to be superior.[8,9] Five major trials provided important information and created a compelling platform for the evidence-based approach to revascularization for the patient with DM and CAD.

The American College of Cardiology Foundation (ACCF)–STS Database Collaboration on the Comparative Effectiveness of Revascularization Strategies (ASCERT) study[10] was a unique collaboration between the ACCF and the STS that compared outcomes of PCI versus CABG, using records from their respective databases, correlated with follow-up data from Centers for Medicare and Medicaid Services (CMS). The study included 190,000 patients from the years 2004 to 2007. Among these, more than one-third were patients with DM and 10% in each arm were on insulin therapy. PCI followed contemporary practice, using DES in 80%, whereas only 6% of patients having PCI had no stent placed (PTCA only.). There was a strong survival benefit from CABG. In the CABG cohort, mortality was 20% lower at 4 years. The survival advantage for CABG persisted across all subgroups analyzed (sex, age, body mass index [BMI], chronic lung disease, left ventricular function, renal function, and presence or absence of diabetes).

The Synergy Between PCI with Taxus and Cardiac Surgery[11] (SYNTAX) trial was a multicenter study of 3-vessel or left main CAD and randomized patients to treatment by PCI with DES or CABG. The most important contribution of SYNTAX was to create a standardized score allowing comparisons of the anatomic extent and severity of CAD. At 4 years, all-cause mortality and cardiac mortality were each lower after CABG. The mortality differences were mainly caused by differences in those patients with moderate or high SYNTAX scores.

A prespecified subgroup of SYNTAX[12] patients had DM (n = 452). In SYNTAX, patients having PCI had significantly more cardiac deaths at 5 years, but the patients with DM after PCI had twice as many deaths as after CABG (mortality in patients without DM was 62% higher for PCI than for CABG.) TVRs were more frequent after PCI than after CABG: HRs were 2.75 (patients with DM) and 1.82 (patients without DM.) Major adverse cardiovascular and cerebrovascular event (MACCE) rates were higher for PCI at 1, 3, and 5 years. The composite of death, stroke, or myocardial infarction (MI) approached significance at 3 years. The difference in MACCE rates between PCI and CABG treatments was wider for the patients with DM than for patients without DM.

Patients requiring insulin fared poorly with PCI, with the MACCE rate double that for CABG, and mortality almost tripled (12.6% vs 4.5%).

For the patients with DM who were not on insulin, differences were more modest. After CABG, outcomes were similar for cohorts with or without DM but, after PCI, outcomes were worse for patients with DM than for patients without DM. Mortality was lower for CABG in those patients with a high SYNTAX score (4.1% vs 13.5%; $P \leq .04$). SYNTAX scores did not predict stroke or MI; they correlated with outcomes after PCI but not after CABG. Because of the more distal location of bypass grafts, new or progressive atherosclerotic disease or plaque rupture in segments of coronary arteries proximal to the bypass graft anastomosis site are protected against by CABG.

Coronary Artery Revascularization in Diabetes (CARDIA)[13] was an RCT that enrolled 510 patients with proximal left anterior descending or multivessel coronary disease and compared PCI and CABG. PCI used DES in 71% and BMS in 29% of cases. The primary outcome specified a composite end point of death, MI, or cerebrovascular accident. At 1 year the composite was not significantly different, but mortality approached statistical significance and both MI and TVR were significantly less common after CABG. PCI outcomes were worse at 1 year for insulin-dependent patients.

The Veterans Affairs Coronary Artery Revascularization in Diabetes Study (VA CARDS) 2013[14] randomized patients with DM and proximal left anterior descending or multivessel CAD to CABG or PCI with DES. A composite end point (death or MI) was specified. However, the study was terminated because of slow recruitment (25% of intended sample) and was underpowered as a result. Mortality in patients having PCI was quadrupled by 2 years and the PCI rate of MI was triple that of CABG.

The need for a definitive randomized trial designed to identify an optimal revascularization strategy for patients with DM and multivessel CAD was perceived and the Future Revascularization Evaluation in Patients with Diabetes Mellitus: Optimal Management of Multivessel Disease (FREEDOM) trial was undertaken.

The FREEDOM trial[15] was a multicenter study of patients with DM who had double-vessel (17%) or triple-vessel CAD (83%) without left main stenosis. Patients were randomized to CABG or PCI (DES, 94%). From 2005 to 2010, 33,000 patients were screened; 3300 were eligible and 1900 consented and were randomized. The primary outcome was a composite of all-cause death, MI, and stroke.

Most patients had normal left ventricular function (mean ejection fraction, 66%) and the mean age was 63.1 ± 9.1 years. Mean hemoglobin A1C (HbA1c) was 7.8% and the mean SYNTAX score was 26.2 ± 8.6 (middle tercile.) As in the original SYNTAX study, the SYNTAX score did not predict outcomes after CABG but did predict worse outcomes after PCI.

At 30 days, the primary outcome favored PCI. However, at all times after 30 days the primary outcome favored CABG (PCI 26.6% vs CABG 18.7%; $P = .005$.) The relative risk reduction was 30% for CABG. Results were driven by differences in MI (13.9% vs 6.0%; $P<.001$) and death from any cause (16.3% vs 10.9%; $P<.049$).

The 5-year stroke rate was higher for CABG (5.3% vs 2.4%; $P = .03$) but the higher relative risk of stroke for CABG (which included preoperative strokes in the intent-to-treat analysis) occurred only in the first 30 days after the procedure.

Median follow-up was 3.8 years but only a quarter of patients were followed beyond 4 years. MACCE at 1 year significantly favored CABG (11.8% vs 16.8% PCI; $P = .004$) but this was largely driven by the difference in TVR. All-cause mortality at 5 years was worse after PCI (although underpowered for statistical analysis) and patients having PCI had more MI. The benefit of CABG compared with PCI was consistent across all prespecified subgroups.

In summary, in FREEDOM patients with diabetes and advanced CAD, CABG was unequivocally superior to PCI in reducing late MI and death. The findings correspond with other studies of patients with diabetes and multivessel CAD (since BARI), which have consistently reported worse outcomes after PCI compared with CABG. The contention that newer stents than those used in FREEDOM may improve PCI outcome is undermined by studies comparing outcomes of newer versus older stents, which show only slight improvement in outcomes. These improvements were too small to undermine the conclusions of FREEDOM.[16] An editorial from a cardiologist in *The New England Journal of Medicine* opined that, "The results of the FREEDOM trial suggest that the comparative effectiveness of CABG and PCI on hard outcomes remains similar whether PCI is performed without stents, with bare-metal stents, or with drug-eluting stents. Mortality has been consistently reduced by CABG, as compared with PCI, in more than 4000 patients with diabetes who have been evaluated in 13 clinical trials. The controversy should finally be settled."[17]

To assess cost-effectiveness, the FREEDOM[18] investigators used several models to calculate the life-years added by CABG. Calculated cost ranged from $8100 to

$27,000 per quality-adjusted life-year added, all less than the commonly used $50,000 benchmark. CABG for patients with DM and multivessel CAD saved an additional 5 lives for every 100 patients treated, at an additional cost versus PCI of just $3600 per patient over 5 years.

GUIDELINES AND OTHER ISSUES

Major professional societies have collaborated in the compilation of evidence-based guidelines for management of CAD, and these have included diabetic patients and their specific issues.[19] However, compliance with such guidelines has been shown to be poor. After the BARI study was halted in patients with DM because of excess mortality in the PCI arm, and after publication of the study, clinical practice was not much altered to conform with the recommendations.

New York State tested application of guidelines (from American College of Cardiology [ACC]/AHA) 2005–2007[20]:

Of those with:

- Indications for CABG, 53% were recommended CABG and 34% PCI.
- Indications for PCI, 94% were recommended PCI.
- Indications for both, 93% were recommended PCI and only 5% CABG.

More recently in Europe, despite recommendations by both cardiology and cardiac surgical societies and widespread publicity, a significant number of patients in one single-center study were still not receiving optimal treatment according to guidelines.[21] The large, mandatory New York State Registry[22] confirmed the benefit of CABG compared with DES at 18 months for mortality and for the composite of death/MI for patients with triple-vessel or double-vessel disease. CABG also generated lower rates of TVR.

Patients with DM usually have extensive CAD and require multiple grafts. Incomplete revascularization (by DES) was associated with higher 18-month mortality (HR, 1.23) and MI.[23] A study of CAD remaining after successful PCI found that even a mildly increased residual SYNTAX score calculated after PCI was successfully correlated with increased 1-year mortality, MI, and MACCE.[24] Incomplete revascularization was especially likely among insulin-treated patients. There was a strong correlation between CAD severity at baseline and completeness of revascularization. Of patients in the middle and highest SYNTAX score terciles at baseline, 90% were incompletely revascularized after PCI, strongly arguing for CABG for all patients in these two terciles. Even focusing on the lowest tercile, a third of the patients were incompletely revascularized by PCI. Thus, for patients with DM, factoring their greater disease burden and their likelihood of incomplete revascularization by PCI, CABG is the preferred technique.

CHOICE OF CONDUIT

Choice of conduit in patients with DM is an important determinant of long-term outcomes because saphenous vein grafts are more prone to failure in patients with DM. Diabetes is a risk factor for wound infection and mediastinitis, but the impact of bilateral internal thoracic artery (BITA) on wound complications (from sternal devascularization) is still not known and there is only observational evidence that using both internal thoracic arteries improves outcomes without compromising sternal stability. In the only RCT comparing BITA with single internal thoracic artery (SITA) grafting, Taggart and colleagues[25] found a 3.24-times increase in the relative risk of DSWI after BITA (1.9%) versus SITA (0.6%).

For patients with DM, BITA versus PCI (nonrandomized) improved outcomes but not survival.[26,27] In a recent large registry report, patients with BITA and SITA had similar rates of DSWI (1.2% vs 1.0%) but BITA reduced mortality by 35% for patients with and without DM. Among patients with DM, although the incidence of DSWI was double that for patients without DM (1.5% vs 0.7%), DSWI was not predicted by graft choice (BITA 1.7% vs SITA 1.5%).[28]

If 2 arterial grafts are superior, might even more be better still? Testing this strategy showed a trend toward survival benefit for patients with DM (relative risk [RR], 0.77; but 95% CI, 0.56–1.07) and clear benefit for patients without diabetes (RR, 0.50; 95% CI, 0.37–0.69).[29]

Patients with DM did just as well as patients without DM at 5 years after total arterial off-pump revascularization for multivessel coronary disease (by angiographic results, long-term survival, and clinical events).[29] Completeness of revascularization emerged as an important long-term determinant of survival by multivariate analysis.[30]

We reported a strong survival benefit of radial artery (RA) compared with saphenous vein grafts in patients with DM.[31,32] The RA is an attractive alternative arterial conduit to the right internal thoracic artery (RITA), achieving for patients with DM the survival benefit of multiple arterial grafting without the added risk of DSWI, which is now defined by the US Center for Medicare and Medicaid as a so-called never event that is not covered by payments. There are no published studies directly comparing RITA with RA grafting in patients with DM. We are currently analyzing our experience.[33] Long-term survival was the same in 200 propensity-matched pairs of patients with diabetes who received either the RITA or RA as the second arterial conduit during CABG, but patients receiving RAs had significantly fewer sternal wound infections and fewer episodes of postoperative respiratory failure.

In summary, for CABG in patients with diabetes:

- Multiple arterial grafts (left internal thoracic artery plus either RITA or RA) improves survival
- RA and RITA grafts produce equivalent survival benefit
- RA generates fewer major adverse events than RITA
- RA is ideal for the multiple arterial graft strategy

Regarding off-pump versus on-pump CABG, questions about the completeness of revascularization and more frequent TVR have reduced enthusiasm but New York State data (2010) show that 25% of CABGs are off-pump coronary artery bypass (OPCAB). Three-year mortality was not different for on-pump or off-pump CABG; however, OPCAB had higher TVR (HR, 1.55).[34] There is clear support in the literature for off-pump CABG compared with DES.[35]

A strategy advocating PCI first, relying on later CABG, has been shown to be flawed in multiple studies in Europe and the United States. Operative risks increase and short-term and long-term survival are inferior if CABG is performed after PCI.[36,37] Prior PCI is an independent risk factor for CABG.[38] A microsimulation study estimated that prior PCI worsened 10-year survival after CABG by 3.3%.[39] Increased HbA1c (measured as a continuous variable) was associated with worse outcomes after CABG and with reduced long-term survival.[40,41]

Risk Scoring for CABG

The New York State analysis of risk factors is summarized in **Table 1**.[42–44]

Data from the mandatory New York State Cardiac Reporting System for 2002 were used to construct a risk prediction tool for in-hospital mortality. Multivariable analysis generated 10 risk factors but not diabetes. The 30-day mortality score was updated in

Table 1		
New York State mortality risk prediction		
In Hospital Mortality		**Long Term**
1990	**2013**	**2000**
Age	Age	Age
Hemodynamic state	Hemodynamic state	Hemodynamic state
Ejection fraction	Ejection fraction	Ejection fraction
Renal failure	Renal failure	Renal failure
—	CHF	CHF
Peripheral arterial disease	—	Peripheral arterial disease
Previous open heart surgery	—	Previous open heart surgery
—	BMI	BMI
COPD	—	COPD
—	—	Left main disease
—	—	Malignant ventricular arrhythmia
Female sex	—	—
—	—	Cerebrovascular disease
Previous MI	—	—
Calcified ascending aorta	—	—
—	DM	DM

Abbreviations: BMI, body mass index; CHF, chronic heart failure; COPD, chronic obstructive pulmonary disease; DM, diabetes mellitus.
Data from Refs.[42–44]

2013[43] with only 7 risk factors, now including diabetes. The streamlined 2013 scoring system was tested and validated in 5 western states.

A risk score for predicting long-term mortality was also developed; significant predictors of long-term death included diabetes (see **Table 1**).[44]

Why is CABG Better than PCI?

Although all trials have not confirmed a uniform survival advantage for CABG, this is usually explained by trial designs that enrolled highly selected and low-risk populations, not representative of patients in clinical practice.[45] However, patients with DM still have worse outcomes from revascularization, whether by PCI or CABG. Most coronary disease is located proximal in the epicardial arteries, and therefore bypass grafts to the midcoronary vessels (usual graft sites) also protect against new disease that might develop later in the coronary artery proximal to the graft anastomosis. Surgical revascularization by CABG is also usually more complete.

Although PCI can treat proximal CAD effectively, the long-term benefits of PCI are compromised by new disease in the native vessels proximal or distal to the stent, as well as within the stented segment (the only segment where DES have been less vulnerable). By contrast, for patients having CABG, only new disease within the graft (uncommon in arterial conduits) or in the native artery beyond the graft is important.

It follows that the SYNTAX score, based on extent of proximal stenoses, does not predict CABG outcomes but does predict PCI. The same pathoanatomic explanation predicts the substantially lower incidence of MI and TVR that has been observed after

CABG versus PCI, and explains why newer generations of stents reduce angiographic rates of restenosis, but consistently fail to reduce mortality.

Conclusions

For patients with DM and multivessel coronary disease, CABG improves survival compared with PCI and consistently lowers combined rates of death or MI and TVR.

Current ACC guidelines[19] for revascularization of multivessel disease that describe diabetes as an important factor when deciding on a strategy are likely to be strengthened in their next iteration.

On the basis of the current body of evidence, CABG should be preferred to PCI in patients with diabetes and multivessel disease with complex anatomy exemplified by SYNTAX scores greater than 22, and perhaps even all patients with diabetes with multivessel disease.[17]

FREEDOM results are clear and support wide indications for CABG.

The complementary results of SYNTAX and FREEDOM are likely to stand the test of time because CABG and PCI achieve their benefits in different ways.

Important Aspects of Perioperative Care: Glucose Control

Hyperglycemia before, during, or immediately after CABG predicts increased perioperative morbidity and mortality in patients with (and without) diabetes. Hospital length of stay and long-term survival are affected. An excellent executive summary from the STS[46] set out guidelines for perioperative management. Important recommendations are summarized later.

Glycemic control (<180 mg/dL) is best achieved with continuous insulin infusions[45]; however, extremely tight control (<140 md/dL) is not recommended.

Normoglycemia in intensive care evaluation and surviving using glucose algorithm regulation found increased 90-day mortality in surgical and medical patients in the intensive care unit (ICU) managed with tight blood glucose control.[47] The following approach to the perioperative management of patients is suggested[48]:

- All patients with DM having cardiac surgery should be on an insulin infusion in the operating room, and for at least 24 hours after surgery to maintain serum glucose 180 mg/dL (evidence level B)
- Before surgery, it is reasonable to maintain blood glucose concentration 180 mg/dL (evidence level B)
- For persistently increased serum glucose (>180 mg/dL) during CABG, start insulin drip and obtain an endocrinology consult (evidence level B)
- Any patient with (or without) DM who has persistently increased serum glucose greater than 180 mg/dL should receive intravenous insulin infusion to maintain serum glucose less than 180 mg/dL for the duration of the ICU care (evidence level A)
- Before insulin infusion is discontinued, patients should be transitioned to subcutaneous insulin using institutional protocols (evidence level B)

Lower initial blood glucose values immediately after CABG, which reflect an impaired stress response, have been associated with increased mortality and a significant delay in achieving tight glycemic control with intensive insulin.[49]

For primary PCI, increased blood glucose on admission predicts early and long-term mortality.[50]

Administration of insulin or glucose insulin potassium has not improved outcome after PCI for ST elevation myocardial infarction (STEMI).[51] After CABG, glucose insulin potassium (GIK) infusion reduced atrial fibrillation, myocardial injury, wound infection, and hospital stay in reports from Boston[52] and the United Kingdom,[53] but enthusiasm for GIK is limited to a few centers.

WHAT IS THE CURRENT ROLE FOR PCI?

In non–ST elevation acute coronary syndrome an early invasive strategy with PCI is indicated. Diabetes does not diminish the outcomes of myocardial revascularization[54] in the acute setting and in The Treat angina with Aggrastat and determine Cost of Therapy with an Invasive or Conservative Strategy—Thrombolysis in Myocardial Infarction 18 (TACTICS-TIMI 18)[55] study the benefit was greater for patients with DM. For ST elevation MI, the PCAT-2112 collaborative[56] analysis of 19 randomized trials showed that patients with DM benefit as much as patients without DM from primary PCI compared with fibrinolysis. After the acute phase, PCI of a totally occluded artery is not beneficial (also true for patients without DM). The Veterans Administration AWESOME (Angina With Extremely Serious Operative Mortality Evaluation) trial randomized patients with unstable angina (one-third with diabetes) to PCI or CABG but only 144 patients with DM were randomized.[57] At 3 years, they reported no significant difference in mortality but, of those treated with CABG, 39% were reoperations, so this study offers no information that can be generalized. In meta-analysis[58] and in a real-world population of patients with DM subject to mandatory reporting and follow-up, DES were superior to BMS in reducing mortality, MI, and TVR.[59] All currently used DES reduce the need for TVR (37%–69%) in patients with DM (as well as in patients without diabetes).[60] High MACCE and stent thrombosis rates remain a concern.[10] Outcomes of PCI are generally worse for patients with DM than for patients without DM, including higher mortality after PCI (in a registry of >100,000 PCIs),[61] more MACCE, more in-stent restenosis (ISR),[62] and more TVR for restenosis (although DES reduced ISR).[54] Diabetes remains an independent predictor of acute stent thrombosis.[63]

The Fractional Flow Reserve Versus Angiography in Multivessel Evaluation (FAME) study of angioplasty for multivessel PCI showed improved results when stent use was restricted to coronary lesions with objective confirmation of flow restriction compared with visual assessment of stenosis.[64] Wider application of this technique to determine hemodynamically significant stenoses should improve outcomes for PCI (as already shown) but also after CABG (by limiting the competitive flow, which promotes early graft closure).[65]

Antithrombotic drugs[66] used as a mandatory adjunct to PCI are no different for patients with DM versus patients without DM whether undergoing elective PCI or PCI for acute coronary syndromes.[54] Patients with DM do not benefit from the routine addition of glycoprotein IIb/IIIa inhibitors to antiplatelet agents. Diabetes almost doubles the risk of 9-month mortality and predicts more MACCE after PCI.[67,68] The risk is greatest in insulin-treated patients. However, diabetes is no longer a strong risk factor for adverse outcomes after PCI in women. However, in BARI 2D (Bypass Angioplasty Revascularization Investigation 2 Diabetes), women remained more symptomatic with more angina and poorer functional status than men.[69,70] Patients with DM had a higher frequency of new coronary lesions at 9 months (30% vs 26%), mainly in the treated vessel rather than in nontreated vessels,[67] perhaps caused by endothelial damage during PCI.

Newer stents are not better according to a post hoc analysis of 4 trials.[71] PCI is generally preferable to reoperative CABG, but PCI for vein graft disease in patients with DM may be less effective, because insulin-treated DM is associated with calcific vein graft degeneration.[72] Restenosis in patients with DM is associated pathologically with excess intimal fibrosis and reduced cell content.[73]

Vein graft PCI with DES significantly reduced TVR (vs BMS), but did not provide clear benefits for mortality or MI.[74]

BMI and metabolic control affect outcomes after PCI. Higher HbA1c predicts increased cardiovascular disease and mortality; however, there is no risk increase at low HbA1c levels even in those patients with longer duration of diabetes. Patients achieving HbA1c less than 7% showed risk reduction[75] but, after PCI, HbA1c greater than 7% predicts[75] increases in TVR (odds ratio [OR], 2.87), readmission (OR, 2.44), and recurrent angina (OR, 4.03). Metabolic syndrome is not prognostically significant after adjusting for its constituent components.[76] Diabetes is common in obesity, whereas low BMI is associated with advanced age, smoking, and peripheral vascular disease. However, obesity is not associated with severity of CAD. In Arterial Revascularization Therapies Study (ARTS), BMI had no effect for PCI but, after CABG, increasing BMI predicted reduced MACCE (HR, 0.59).[77] Reduced BMI predicts restenosis in patients with DM, so perhaps low BMI with short stature and small vessels negates the metabolic advantage of reduced body fat. Small-caliber arteries are common in patients with DM, and smaller diameter predicts restenosis after PCI.[78]

Patients with DM experience the pleiotropic effects of statins,[79] independently of the low-density lipoprotein cholesterol–lowering effects. The issue of acetylsalicylic acid (ASA) resistance is significant in revascularized patients with DM.[80] More than 20% of patients with DM seem to be ASA resistant.[81] Colchicine may reduce ISR and TVR in BMS used for patient with DM who have contraindications to dual antiplatelet therapy.[82] However, patients having CABG were less likely than patients having PCI to fill prescriptions for secondary preventive medications (statin, angiotensin-converting enzyme, angiotensin receptor blocker, or β-blocker) and to use those medications consistently in the first year after the procedure.[83] The benefit of surgical revascularization should be compounded by postoperative lifelong, evidence-based medical therapy.

SUMMARY

In patients with DM, atherosclerotic CAD is common and usually diffuse and progressive. Despite refinements, PCI has not significantly reduced the rates of death or MI. For all forms of revascularization, patients with DM have a higher rate of mortality and complications than similar patients without DM.

Surgical revascularization by CABG (on or off pump) consistently yields superior results for patients with diabetes and CAD. Level 1 evidence from the FREEDOM trial mandates that CABG is the appropriate strategy for the patient with diabetes and multivessel CAD. Improvements in CABG with important benefits for the patient with diabetes include meticulous perioperative glucose control and the wider use of multiple arterial grafts, for which the RA offers an attractive advantage.

The main role for PCI in patients with diabetes and CAD is in the management of acute coronary syndromes (STEMI and NSTEMI.) Patients with diabetes benefit from the same medical management and secondary risk factor modification as patients without diabetes.

REFERENCES

1. American Diabetes Association. Economic costs of diabetes in the U.S. 2012. Diabetes Care 2013;36:1033–46.
2. Rask-Madsen C, King GL. Mechanisms of disease: endothelial dysfunction in insulin resistance and diabetes. Nat Clin Pract Endocrinol Metab 2007;3:46–56.

3. Silva JA, Escobar A, Collins TJ, et al. Unstable angina: a comparison of angioscopic findings between diabetic and non-diabetic patients. Circulation 1995; 92:1731–6.
4. Flaherty JD, Davidson CJ. Diabetes and coronary revascularization. JAMA 2005;293:1501–8.
5. BARI Investigators. Comparison of coronary bypass surgery with angioplasty in patients with multivessel disease. N Engl J Med 1996;335:217–25.
6. BARI Investigators. The final 10-year follow-up results from the BARI randomized trial. J Am Coll Cardiol 2007;49:1600–6.
7. Hlatky MA, Boothroyd DE, Bravata DM, et al. Coronary artery bypass surgery compared with percutaneous coronary interventions for multivessel disease: a collaborative analysis of individual patient data from ten randomized trials. Lancet 2009;373:1190–7.
8. Lee MS, Jamal F, Kedia G, et al. Comparison of bypass surgery with drug eluting stents for diabetic patients with multivessel disease. Int J Cardiol 2007;123:34–42.
9. Javaid A, Steinberg DH, Buch AN. Outcomes of coronary artery bypass grafting versus percutaneous coronary intervention with drug-eluting stents for patients with multivessel coronary artery disease. Circulation 2007;116: I200–6.
10. Weintraub WS, Grau-Sepulveda MV, Weiss JM, et al. Comparative effectiveness of revascularization strategies. N Engl J Med 2012;366:1467–76.
11. Mack MJ, Banning AP, Serruys PW, et al. Bypass versus drug-eluting stents at three years in SYNTAX patients with diabetes mellitus or metabolic syndrome. Ann Thorac Surg 2011;92:2140–6.
12. Kappetein P, Head SJ, Morice MC, et al. Treatment of complex coronary artery disease in patients with diabetes: 5-year results comparing outcomes of bypass surgery and percutaneous coronary intervention in the SYNTAX trial. Eur J Cardiothorac Surg 2013;43:1006–13.
13. Kapur A, Hall RJ, Malik IS, et al. Randomized comparison of percutaneous coronary intervention with coronary artery bypass grafting in diabetic patients: 1-year results of the CARDIA (Coronary Artery Revascularization in Diabetes) trial. J Am Coll Cardiol 2010;55:432–40.
14. Kamalesh M, Sharp TG, Tang XC, et al. Percutaneous coronary intervention versus coronary bypass surgery in United States veterans with diabetes. J Am Coll Cardiol 2013;61:808–16.
15. Farkouh ME, Domanski M, Sleeper LA, et al. Strategies for multivessel revascularization in patients with diabetes. N Engl J Med 2012;367:2375–84.
16. Bangalore S, Kumar S, Fusaro M, et al. Short- and long-term outcomes with drug-eluting and bare-metal coronary stents: a mixed treatment comparison analysis of 117 762 patient-years of follow-up from randomized trials. Circulation 2012;125:2873–91.
17. Hlatky MA. Compelling evidence for coronary-bypass surgery in patients with diabetes. N Engl J Med 2012;367:2437–8.
18. Magnuson EA, Farkouh ME, Fuster V, et al. Cost-effectiveness of percutaneous coronary intervention with drug eluting stents versus bypass surgery for patients with diabetes mellitus and multivessel coronary artery disease: results from the FREEDOM trial. Circulation 2013;127:820–31.
19. Hillis LD, Smith PK, Anderson JL, et al. ACC Foundation/American Heart Association Task Force on choice of revascularization. J Am Coll Cardiol 2011;58: e123–210.

20. Hannan EL, Racz MJ, Gold J, et al. Adherence of catheterization laboratory cardiologists to American College of Cardiology/American Heart Association guidelines for percutaneous coronary interventions and coronary artery bypass graft surgery: what happens in actual practice? Circulation 2010;121:267–75.
21. Yates MT, Soppa GK, Valencia O, et al. Impact of European Society of Cardiology and European Association for Cardiothoracic Surgery Guidelines on Myocardial Revascularization on the activity of percutaneous coronary intervention and coronary artery bypass graft surgery for stable coronary artery disease. J Thorac Cardiovasc Surg 2014;147(2):606–10.
22. Hannan EL, Wu C, Walford G, et al. Drug-eluting stents vs. coronary-artery bypass grafting in multivessel coronary disease. N Engl J Med 2008;24:331–41.
23. Hannan EL, Wu C, Walford G, et al. Incomplete revascularization in the era of drug-eluting stents: impact on adverse outcomes. JACC Cardiovasc Interv 2009;2(1):17–25.
24. Genereux P, Palmerini R, Caixeta A, et al. Quantification and impact of untreated coronary artery disease after percutaneous coronary intervention. J Am Coll Cardiol 2012;59:2165–74.
25. Taggart DP, Altman DG, Gray AM, et al. Randomized trial to compare bilateral vs. single internal mammary coronary artery bypass grafting: 1-year results of the Arterial Revascularisation Trial (ART). Eur Heart J 2010;31(20):2470–81.
26. Toumpoulis IK, Swistel DG, Balaram S, et al. Does bilateral internal thoracic artery grafting increase long-term survival of diabetic patients? Ann Thorac Surg 2006;81:599–607.
27. Locker C, Mohr R, Lev-Ran O, et al. Comparison of bilateral thoracic artery grafting with percutaneous coronary interventions in diabetic patients. Ann Thorac Surg 2004;78:471–5.
28. Puskas JD, Sadiq A, Vassiliades TA, et al. Bilateral internal thoracic artery grafting is associated with significantly improved long-term survival, even among diabetic patients. Ann Thorac Surg 2012;94:710–6.
29. Zacharias A, Schwann TA, Riordan CJ, et al. Late results of conventional versus all-arterial revascularization based on internal thoracic and radial artery grafting. Ann Thorac Surg 2009;87:19–26.
30. Hwang HY, Choi JS, Ki KB. Diabetes does not affect long-term results after total arterial off-pump coronary revascularization. Ann Thorac Surg 2010;90:1180–6.
31. Tranbaugh RF, Dimitrova KR, Friedmann P, et al. Coronary artery bypass grafting using the radial artery: clinical outcomes, patency, and need for reintervention. Circulation 2012;126:S170–5.
32. Hoffman DM, Dimitrova KR, DeCastro H, et al. Improving long term outcome for diabetic patients undergoing surgical revascularization by use of the radial artery conduit: a propensity matched study. J Cardiovasc Surg 2013;8:27.
33. Hoffman et al. Abstract accepted for presentation at Society of Thoracic Surgeons annual meeting. The optimal arterial conduit for diabetic patients: a propensity analysis of the radial artery versus the right internal thoracic artery. Orlando (FL), January 27, 2014.
34. Hannan EL, Wu C, Smith CR, et al. Off-pump versus on-pump coronary artery bypass graft surgery: differences in short-term outcomes and in long-term mortality and need for subsequent revascularization. Circulation 2007;4(116):1145–52.
35. Briguori C, Condorelli G, Airoldi F. Comparison of coronary drug-eluting stents versus coronary artery bypass grafting in patients with diabetes mellitus. Am J Cardiol 2007;99:779–84.

36. Tran HA, Barnett SD, Hunt SL, et al. The effect of previous coronary artery stenting on short- and intermediate-term outcome after surgical revascularization in patients with diabetes mellitus. J Thorac Cardiovasc Surg 2009;138:316–23.

37. Chocron S, Baillot R, Rouleau JL, et al, The IMAGINE Investigators. Impact of previous percutaneous transluminal coronary angioplasty and/or stenting revascularization on outcomes after surgical revascularization: insights from the IMAGINE study. Eur Heart J 2008;29:673–9.

38. Thielmann M, Neuhäuse M, Stephan Knipp S, et al. Prognostic impact of previous percutaneous coronary intervention in patients with diabetes mellitus and triple-vessel disease undergoing coronary artery bypass surgery. J Thorac Cardiovasc Surg 2007;134:470–6.

39. Rao C, Stanbridge RD, Chikwe M, et al. Does previous percutaneous coronary stenting compromise the long-term efficacy of subsequent coronary artery bypass surgery? A microsimulation study. Ann Thorac Surg 2008;85:501–7.

40. Halkos ME, Puskas JD, Lattouf OM, et al. Elevated preoperative hemoglobin A1c level is predictive of adverse events after coronary artery bypass surgery. J Thorac Cardiovasc Surg 2008;136:631–40.

41. Halkos ME, Lattouf OM, Puskas JD, et al. Elevated preoperative hemoglobin A1c level is associated with reduced long-term survival after coronary artery bypass surgery. Ann Thorac Surg 2008;86:1431–7.

42. Hannan EL, Wu C, Bennett EV, et al. Risk stratification of in-hospital mortality for coronary artery bypass graft surgery. J Am Coll Cardiol 2006;47:661–8.

43. Hannan EL, Farrell LS, Wechsler A, et al. The New York risk score for in-hospital and 30-day mortality for coronary artery bypass graft surgery. Ann Thorac Surg 2013;95:46–52.

44. Wu C, Camacho FT, Wechsler AS, et al. Risk score for predicting long-term mortality after coronary artery bypass graft surgery. Circulation 2012;125:2423–30.

45. Taggart D. Thomas B. Ferguson Lecture. Coronary artery bypass grafting is still the best treatment for multivessel and left main disease, but patients need to know. Ann Thorac Surg 2006;82:1966–75.

46. Lazar HL, McDonnell M, Chipkin SR, et al. The Society of Thoracic Surgeons Practice Guideline Series: blood glucose management during adult cardiac surgery. Ann Thorac Surg 2009;87:663–9.

47. Furnary AP, Gao GQ, Grunkemeier GL, et al. Continuous insulin infusion reduces mortality in patients with diabetes undergoing coronary artery bypass grafting. J Thorac Cardiovasc Surg 2003;125:1007–21.

48. Finfer S, Chittock DR, Su SY, et al. Intensive versus conventional glucose control in critically ill patients. N Engl J Med 2009;360:1283–97.

49. Via MA, Scurlock C, Adams DH, et al. Impaired postoperative hyperglycemic stress response associated with increased mortality in patients in the cardiothoracic surgery intensive care unit. Endocr Pract 2010;16:798–804.

50. Straumann E, Kurz DJ, Muntwyler J, et al. Admission glucose concentrations independently predict early and later mortality in patients with acute myocardial infarction treated by primary or rescue percutaneous coronary intervention. Am Heart J 2005;150:1000–6.

51. Mehta SR, Yusuf S, Diaz R, et al. Effect of glucose-insulin-potassium infusion on mortality in patients with acute ST-segment elevation myocardial infarction: the CREATE-ECLA randomized controlled trial. JAMA 2005;293:437–46.

52. Lazar HL, Chipkin SR, Fitzgerald CA, et al. Tight glycemic control in diabetic coronary artery bypass graft patients improves perioperative outcomes and decreases recurrent ischemic events. Circulation 2004;109:1497–502.

53. Quinn DW, Pagano D, Bonser RS, et al. Improved myocardial protection during coronary artery surgery with glucose-insulin-potassium: a randomized controlled trial. J Thorac Cardiovasc Surg 2006;131:34–42.
54. West NE, Ruygrok PN, Disco CM, et al. Clinical and angiographic predictors of restenosis after stent deployment in diabetic patients. Circulation 2004;109:867–73.
55. Roffi M. Early invasive strategy in the diabetic patient with non-ST-segment elevation acute coronary syndromes. Eur Heart J Suppl 2005;7(Suppl K):K19–22.
56. Timmer JR, Ottervanger JP, de Boer MJ, et al. Primary percutaneous coronary intervention compared with fibrinolysis for myocardial infarction in diabetes mellitus: results from the Primary Coronary Angioplasty vs Thrombolysis-2 trial. Arch Intern Med 2007;167(13):1353–9.
57. Sedlis SP, Morrison DA, Lorin JD, et al. Percutaneous coronary intervention versus coronary bypass graft surgery for diabetic patients with unstable angina and risk factors for adverse outcomes with bypass: outcome of diabetic patients in the AWESOME randomized trial and registry. J Am Coll Cardiol 2002;40:1555–66.
58. Stettler C, Allemann S, Wandel S, et al. Drug eluting and bare metal stents in people with and without diabetes: collaborative network meta-analysis. BMJ 2008;337:a1331.
59. Garg P, Normand ST, Silbaugh TS, et al. Drug-eluting or bare-metal stenting in patients with diabetes mellitus. Results from the Massachusetts Data Analysis Center registry. Circulation 2008;118:2277–85.
60. Bangalore S, Kumar S, Fusaro F, et al. Outcomes with various drug eluting or bare metal stents in patients with diabetes mellitus: mixed treatment comparison analysis of 22 844 patient years of follow-up from randomised trials. BMJ 2012;345:e5170.
61. Anderson HV, Shaw RE, Brindis RG, et al. A contemporary overview of percutaneous coronary interventions: the American College of Cardiology-National Cardiovascular Data Registry (ACC-NCDR). J Am Coll Cardiol 2002;39:1096–103.
62. Sukhija R, Aronow WS, Sureddi R, et al. Predictors of in-stent restenosis and patient outcome after percutaneous coronary intervention in patients with diabetes mellitus. Am J Cardiol 2007;100:777–80.
63. Iakovou I, Schmidt T, Bonizzoni E, et al. Incidence, predictors, and outcome of thrombosis after successful implantation of drug-eluting stents. JAMA 2005;293:2126–30.
64. Tonino PA, De Bruyne B, Pijls NH, FAME Study Investigators, et al. Fractional flow reserve versus angiography for guiding percutaneous coronary intervention. N Engl J Med 2009;360:213–24.
65. Botman CJ, Schonberger J, Koolen S, et al. Does stenosis severity of native vessels influence bypass graft patency? A prospective fractional flow reserve-guided study. Ann Thorac Surg 2007;83:2093–7.
66. Rihal CS, Flather M, Hirsh J, et al. Advances in antithrombotic drug therapy for coronary artery disease. Eur Heart J 1995;16:D10–21.
67. Mathew V, Gersh BJ, Williams BA, et al. Outcomes in patients with diabetes mellitus undergoing percutaneous coronary intervention in the current era: a report from the Prevention of REStenosis with Tranilast and its Outcomes (PRESTO) Trial. Circulation 2004;109:476–80.
68. Laskey WK, Selzer F, Vlachos HA, et al. Comparison of in-hospital and one-year outcomes in patients with and without diabetes mellitus undergoing percutaneous catheter intervention (from the National Heart, Lung, and Blood Institute Dynamic Registry). Am J Cardiol 2002;90:1062–7.

69. Champney KP, Veledar E, Klein M, et al. Sex-specific effects of diabetes on adverse outcomes after percutaneous coronary intervention: trends over time. Am Heart J 2007;153:97028.

70. Tamis-Holland JE, Lu J, Korytkowski M, et al. Sex differences in presentation and outcome among patients with type 2 diabetes and coronary artery disease treated with contemporary medical therapy with or without prompt revascularization: a report from the BARI 2D trial (Bypass Angioplasty Revascularization Investigation 2 Diabetes). J Am Coll Cardiol 2013;61:1767–76.

71. Stone GW, Kedhi E, Kereiakes DJ. Differential clinical responses to everolimus-eluting and paclitaxel-eluting coronary stents in patients with and without diabetes mellitus. Circulation 2011;124:893–900.

72. Castagna MT, Mintz GS, Ohlmann P, et al. Incidence, location, magnitude, and clinical correlates of saphenous vein graft calcification: an intravascular ultrasound and angiographic study. Circulation 2005;111:1148–52.

73. Moreno PR, Murcia AM, Palacios IF, et al. Coronary composition and macrophage infiltration in atherectomy specimens from patients with diabetes mellitus. Circulation 2000;102:2180–4.

74. Lupi A, Navarese EP, Lazzero M, et al. Drug-eluting stents vs. bare metal stents in saphenous vein graft disease–insights from a meta-analysis of 7,090 patients. Circ J 2011;75:280–9.

75. Eeg-Olofsson K, Cederholm J, Nilsson PM, et al. New aspects of HbA1c as a risk factor for cardiovascular diseases in type 2 diabetes: an observational study from the Swedish National Diabetes Register (NDR). J Intern Med 2010; 268:471–82.

76. Corpus RA, George PB, House JA, et al. Optimal glycemic control is associated with a lower rate of target vessel revascularization in treated type II diabetic patients undergoing elective percutaneous coronary intervention. J Am Coll Cardiol 2004;43:8–14.

77. Maron DJ, Boden WE, Spertus JA, et al, The COURAGE Trial Research Group. Impact of metabolic syndrome and diabetes on prognosis and outcomes with early percutaneous coronary intervention in the COURAGE (Clinical Outcomes Utilizing Revascularization and Aggressive Drug Evaluation) trial. J Am Coll Cardiol 2011;58:131–7.

78. Gruberg L, Mercado N, Milo S, et al. Impact of body mass index on the outcome of patients with multivessel disease randomized to either coronary artery bypass grafting or stenting in the ARTS trial: the obesity paradox II? Am J Cardiol 2005; 95:439–44.

79. Kojim S, Sakamoto T, Ogawa H, et al. Standard-dose statin therapy provides incremental clinical benefits in normocholesterolemic diabetic patients. Circ J 2010;74:779–85.

80. Ajjan R, Storey RF, Grant PJ. Aspirin resistance and diabetes mellitus. Diabetologia 2008;51:385–90.

81. Mehta SS, Silver RJ, Aaronson A. Comparison of aspirin resistance in type 1 versus type 2 diabetes mellitus. Am J Cardiol 2006;97:567–70.

82. Deftereos S, Giannopoulos G, Konstantinos R. Colchicine treatment for the prevention of bare-metal stent restenosis in diabetic patients. J Am Coll Cardiol 2013;61:1679–85.

83. Hlatky MA, Solomon MD, Shilane D, et al. Use of medications for secondary prevention after coronary bypass surgery compared with percutaneous coronary intervention. J Am Coll Cardiol 2013;61:295–301.

Mechanisms of Glucocorticoid-Induced Insulin Resistance

Focus on Adipose Tissue Function and Lipid Metabolism

Eliza B. Geer, MD[a],*, Julie Islam, MD[b], Christoph Buettner, MD, PhD[a]

KEYWORDS

- Glucocorticoids • Cushing syndrome • Adipose tissue • Lipolysis • Lipids
- Insulin resistance

KEY POINTS

- Glucocorticoids (GCs) are critical in the regulation of energy homeostasis. GCs liberate energy substrates during stress by enhancing muscle protein breakdown, adipose tissue lipolysis, hepatic gluconeogenesis, and reducing glucose utilization, all of which elevate circulating glucose concentrations.
- Chronic excessive GC exposure results in whole-body insulin resistance and the development of abdominal adiposity in humans.
- The ability of GCs to induce adipose tissue lipolysis depends on their concentration, duration of exposure, and the specific adipose tissue depot.
- 11β-Hydroxysteroid dehydrogenase 1 is a gatekeeper for intracellular GC availability through the local activation of GCs within tissues.
- Prevalent forms of subtle GC excess include exogenous exposure as treatment of autoimmune and rheumatologic diseases, or chronic stress with resultant activation of the hypothalamic-pituitary-adrenal axis.

INTRODUCTION

Chronic glucocorticoid (GC) exposure in humans is well known to result in whole-body insulin resistance and obesity. Cushing syndrome, an endocrine disorder characterized by chronic endogenous or exogenous GC overexposure, increases visceral

Funding: This work was completed with the support of NIH grants K23 DK082617 and DK083658.

The authors have no relevant conflicts of interest to disclose.

[a] Division of Endocrinology, Mount Sinai Medical Center, One Gustave Levy Place, Box 1055, New York, NY 10029, USA; [b] Division of Endocrinology and Metabolism, Beth Israel Medical Center, 317 East 17th Street, 8th Floor, New York, NY 10003, USA

* Corresponding author.

E-mail address: eliza.geer@mssm.edu

and trunk subcutaneous adipose tissue and causes insulin resistance.[1,2] Likewise, abdominal obesity associated with the metabolic syndrome is linked with insulin resistance, cardiovascular risk, and decreased survival. Although endogenous Cushing syndrome is rare, the current prevalence of oral GC use in as high as 2.5% of the population makes insulin resistance and obesity resulting from exogenous GC exposure an important public health problem.[3] Moreover, subtle forms of endogenous GC excess are seen in the setting of chronic stress owing to activation of the hypothalamic-pituitary-adrenal (HPA) axis, leading to increased production of adrenal cortisol. Furthermore, so-called common obesity is believed to be associated with abnormalities in the HPA axis including the presence of increased local production of GCs in the adipose tissue, alterations in cortisol circadian rhythm, and enhanced susceptibility of the HPA axis to be activated, all of which result in greater GC exposure over time. Thus, the study of GC-induced obesity and its adverse metabolic profile has become increasingly important.

Adipose tissue is a complex endocrine and immune organ, responding to and, in turn, releasing signals that represent or reflect metabolic and cardiovascular risk factors.[4] A consensus statement published by the American Diabetes Association and the American Heart Association stated that "obesity is a visible marker of other underlying risk factors that can be addressed."[5] These underlying risks include the metabolic syndrome (abdominal obesity, hypertension, elevated triglycerides, decreased high-density lipoprotein [HDL], and insulin resistance/impaired fasting glucose) as well as a low-grade proinflammatory state[6] that confers an increased risk for atherosclerosis and cardiovascular events.[7,8] Individuals with hypercortisolism have a 4-fold higher mortality rate than the general population because of cardiovascular complications, likely related to the associated obesity and insulin resistance.[9] This article reviews the mechanisms by which supraphysiologic GC exposure promotes insulin resistance, focusing in particular on the effects on adipose tissue function and lipid metabolism.

MECHANISMS OF GC-INDUCED INSULIN RESISTANCE

Insulin resistance, the common thread between obesity, the metabolic syndrome, and type 2 diabetes mellitus, is defined as the impaired ability of insulin to control nutrient partitioning in target organs. In adipose tissue, insulin fails to restrain lipolysis and increase glucose uptake; in liver, to inhibit hepatic gluconeogenesis and glycogenolysis; and in muscle, to induce glucose uptake. A critical function of GCs is to liberate energy substrates (ie, glucose, amino acids, and fatty acids [FA]), and thus ensure their availability in fight-or-flight conditions. Thus, GCs enhance muscle protein breakdown, adipose tissue lipolysis, and hepatic gluconeogenesis, and reduce glucose utilization, effects which elevate circulating glucose concentrations (summarized in **Fig. 1**). Chronic GC overexposure alters body composition, which includes expansion of trunk adipose tissue depots, and impairs metabolism and insulin action, resulting in hyperglycemia and dyslipidemia.

TISSUE-SPECIFIC REGULATION OF INSULIN RESISTANCE
GC Regulation of Adipose Tissue Functionality, Mass, and Distribution

GC regulation of white adipose tissue lipolysis
Adipose tissue function is a key determinant of whole-body glucose and lipid homeostasis. The role of GCs in regulating adipose tissue function is complex and context dependent. GCs induce preadipocyte differentiation,[10] but also adipose tissue lipolysis[11–14] in some settings. Specifically, some,[11,12] but not all[15] in vitro data show

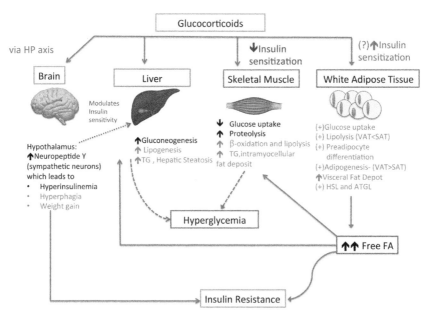

Fig. 1. GCs promote whole-body insulin resistance via visceral adipogenesis, mobilization and release of free fatty acids into the circulation, and development of hepatic steatosis. Whereas in muscle GCs impair insulin action, they may enhance insulin action in adipose tissue, thus promoting expansion of adipose tissue. ATGL, adipose triglyceride lipase; FA, fatty acids; HP, hypothalamic-pituitary-adrenal; HSL, hormone-sensitive lipase; SAT, subcutaneous adipose tissue; TG, triglycerides; VAT, visceral adipose tissue.

that when dexamethasone is added to rat adipocyte cultures, glycerol (a product of lipolysis) increases, in the context of increased mRNA expression of the 2 key lipolytic enzymes hormone-sensitive lipase (HSL)[12] and adipose triglyceride lipase.[16] Of note, one study showed that cortisol removal increased basal lipolytic rates of 3T3-L1 cells, suggesting that GC deficiency can increase basal lipolysis,[11] an unstudied potential mechanism that could underpin the cachexia of adrenal insufficiency. Physiologic doses of GCs maintain many biological functions such as vascular tone, and lipolysis may be another such function. Thus, the permissive effects of physiologic doses of GCs in maintaining normal lipolysis should not be confused with the effects of hypercortisolemia. Indeed, a single dose of high GCs induces lipolysis in vivo in rats and humans, although it remains unclear as to whether chronic GC exposure does the same.[11,13,14] Increased lipolysis will result in elevated circulating free FA (unless FA utilization is increased), and elevated circulating FA in turn can induce insulin resistance.[12,17] Thus, the diabetogenic effects of GCs are likely due to not only enhanced hepatic gluconeogenesis and impaired glucose uptake in muscle but also increased circulating free FA levels originating from increased adipose tissue lipolysis.

The role of GCs in the regulation of lipolysis also varies based on species, the specific adipose tissue depot,[18] and concentration and chronicity of GC exposure. For instance, chronic GCs increase circulating insulin, a potent antilipolytic hormone, but also decrease its action in some tissues. On the other hand, chronic GC exposure is associated with adipose tissue expansion, suggesting an increase in total body lipogenesis and, despite a possible increase in lipolysis, a positive balance of lipid storage in adipose tissue. To date, only 2 small studies have investigated lipolysis in chronic endogenous GC exposure caused by Cushing syndrome, and the results point to distinct differences between direct effects of GCs on adipose tissue and in vivo effects. Specifically, glycerol release was reduced in adipose tissue from individuals with active Cushing syndrome when assessed ex vivo from a biopsy,[19] consistent with decreased lipolysis in active Cushing syndrome.[19] However, in vivo adipose tissue glycerol release as studied through microdialysis[20] was increased, signifying augmented lipolysis. Thus it is likely that GCs regulate factors such as hormones, cytokines, or neuronal signals in tissues other than adipose, which indirectly control adipose tissue functionality and may override the direct effects of GCs on adipose tissue. Further clinical investigation is needed to dissect these factors.

GC regulation of de novo lipogenesis in white adipose tissue

Our understanding of the role of de novo lipogenesis in adipose tissue and its role in whole-body energy homeostasis is still evolving. Although adipose tissue expansion caused by chronic GCs suggests an increase in total body lipogenesis, recent data suggest that de novo lipogenesis in adipose tissue is a marker of metabolic health and may be reduced in human obesity.[21–24] In the human adipocyte (Chub-S7) cell line, but also in primary cultures of human subcutaneous and omental adipocytes, cortisol and cortisone treatment decreased lipogenesis, demonstrated by decreased ^{14}C-acetate incorporation into lipid, in the context of reductions in acetyl coenzyme A carboxylase (ACC) mRNA expression and increases in the inactivating phosphorylation of the ACC protein.[25] Furthermore, inhibition of 11β-hydroxysteroid dehydrogenase 1 (11β-HSD1), which prevents conversion of inactive cortisone to active cortisol, prevented cortisone-mediated suppression of lipogenesis. In this study, low-dose dexamethasone pretreatment of Chub-S7 cells enhanced the ability of insulin to stimulate de novo lipogenesis, suggesting that insulin concentrations are critical for GC regulation of lipogenesis.[25] Whether the enhanced total body lipogenesis that occurs in humans in response to chronic GC exposure reflects adipose tissue or hepatic lipogenesis is not known but, based on the higher contribution of hepatic lipogenesis to whole-body lipogenesis,[26] one would expect GC-induced lipogenesis to be primarily hepatic in origin.

GC regulation of insulin sensitivity in white adipose tissue

Although GCs result in whole-body insulin resistance, this does not necessarily mean that they impair insulin action in each tissue. Recent work has shown that both endogenous and synthetic GCs may in fact enhance insulin signaling and action in human adipose tissue.[25,27–29] For example, short-term (24 hours) pretreatment with GCs enhanced insulin-stimulated tyrosine phosphorylation of insulin receptor (IR) substrate protein 1 (IRS1) and protein kinase B/akt phosphorylation in human adipocytes derived from a subcutaneous adipose tissue biopsy.[27] These effects, which were dose dependent and time dependent, occurred in the context of increased expression of IR, IRS2, and the p85 regulatory subunit of phopshoinositide-3-kinase.[27,28] Subsequent work showed that both short-term (24 hours) and long-term (7 days) exposure of immortalized differentiated human adipocytes (Chub-S7 cells) to dexamethasone,[29] enhanced insulin signaling, and seemed to prevent the insulin resistance caused by chronic high-dose insulin treatment.[29] This finding is in agreement with a recent in vivo study performed in humans, whereby overnight administration of hydrocortisone resulted in systemic insulin resistance, but enhanced insulin action in subcutaneous adipose tissue.[30]

These findings suggest that GCs may regulate insulin action in a tissue-dependent manner, sensitizing subcutaneous adipose tissue to insulin but doing the opposite in muscle, although this has not been confirmed by all studies.[31–33] This GC-mediated enhancement of adipose tissue insulin sensitivity could in turn drive its expansion, leading to obesity, because insulin and GCs are critical factors in adipocyte differentiation and lipid accumulation. Thus, although it seems somewhat paradoxical, increased adiposity caused by excessive GC exposure may in fact be due to enhanced insulin sensitivity of adipose tissue. This process can be understood as a compensatory adaptation whereby, by favoring storage of lipids in adipose tissue, GCs ameliorate the lipotoxicity that would otherwise arise from the increased caloric intake and whole-body lipogenesis observed in Cushing syndrome. However, these findings need to be explored in vivo in animal and human studies in the setting of chronic GC exposure where obesity, global insulin resistance, and hyperinsulinemia may eventually exhaust the ability of adipose tissue to expand and function properly, which in turn may impair insulin action in adipose tissue.

Finally, the biology of adipose tissue has important depot-specific differences, and it is not known to what extent the GC effects are depot dependent. The aforementioned findings elucidate the expansion of subcutaneous but not visceral adipose tissue. For example, one study showed that in omental but not subcutaneous cells, GCs decreased insulin-stimulated glucose uptake,[32] but whether this was due to decreased insulin signaling remains to be determined. Thus, the effects of GCs on insulin sensitivity may differ between visceral and subcutaneous adipose tissue.

Chronic in vivo GC effects on adipogenesis and white adipose tissue mass and distribution in humans: studies on Cushing syndrome

By numerous potential mechanisms, including the production of proinflammatory cytokines and increased portal FA delivery to the liver,[34] abdominal obesity, the accumulation of visceral and trunk subcutaneous fat, is closely linked to the development of insulin resistance, dyslipidemia, and cardiovascular risk.[35–40] Of importance are not only the absolute increases in abdominal fat mass but also the proportion of adipose to muscle mass. For example, an elevated ratio of both visceral to total fat and visceral fat to thigh muscle have been linked to insulin resistance, hepatic steatosis, and the metabolic syndrome.[41]

Chronic excessive GC exposure also increases the ratio of visceral fat to both total fat and muscle. These effects of GCs manifest most clearly in patients with Cushing syndrome, in whom profound increases in total and visceral adipose tissue mass is commonly observed[1,19,42–49] while increases in the subcutaneous depots are moderate.[1] Specifically, although the mass of the total subcutaneous adipose tissue is not different between patients and controls, trunk subcutaneous adipose tissue is enlarged, which, similarly to visceral adipose tissue, is associated with adverse metabolic sequelae.[1] Although some studies have reported lower limb subcutaneous adipose tissue mass in Cushing patients,[46] when quantified by whole-body magnetic resonance imaging (MRI) (the gold standard for assessment of body composition), limb subcutaneous adipose tissue in Cushing patients was not different in comparison with controls.[1]

Normalization of cortisol concentrations in patients with Cushing disease significantly reduces the mass of the total, trunk, subcutaneous, and visceral adipose tissue.[2] Furthermore, cortisol normalization alters adipose tissue distribution, resulting in decreased visceral/total fat and visceral fat/skeletal muscle ratios.[2] Thus, successful treatment of Cushing disease results in redistribution of adipose tissue that is associated with a reduced cardiovascular risk. However, some cardiovascular risk markers, including C-reactive protein (CRP) and high molecular weight adiponectin, do not seem to normalize despite the restoration of physiologic cortisol concentrations, suggesting that exposure to excess GCs has lasting adverse effects on cardiovascular risk.[2] Furthermore, the increased incidence of the metabolic syndrome and cardiovascular disease seen in Cushing patients may not normalize after remission.[50–52] In fact, the duration of the GC exposure in Cushing disease has been shown to increase the hazard of death in patients even after long-term treatment.[53] Prospective studies are needed to understand whether, despite long-term Cushing remission, previous exposure to GCs will result in elevated trunk and ectopic fat when compared with controls. Persistent obesity and ectopic fat distribution, in turn, could contribute to the elevated mortality risk seen after GC exposure.

GC exposure could enhance lipoprotein lipase (LPL) activity, which mediates the hydrolysis and uptake of circulating triglycerides and FA into adipocytes,[19] and this could occur preferentially in the visceral and trunk subcutaneous adipose tissue depots,[54] although what accounts for this depot-specific LPL activity is unknown. The role of altered lipolytic rates in response to GCs, as previously mentioned, is controversial, although it has been suggested that abdominal depots show reduced lipolysis, which could play a role in their expansion in humans exposed to chronic GCs.[19] Finally, the GC receptor (GR) α is more highly expressed in visceral than in subcutaneous adipose tissue,[55] and because activation or repression of GC-sensitive genes is mediated by GCs through the GR, differential expression of this receptor is another potential mechanism for preferential accumulation of abdominal adipose tissue.

Accumulation of adipose tissue involves not only hypertrophy of adipocytes but also expansion of the extracellular matrix and nonadipocyte cells, including stromal vascular cells, endothelial cells, monocytes, and macrophages. Obesity and insulin resistance are associated with adipose tissue remodeling, characterized by increases in macrophages (discussed further in the section on anti-inflammatory and diabetogenic actions of GCs), fibrosis, and the extracellular matrix.[56–58] A recent study has demonstrated that in comparison with lean insulin-sensitive subjects, adipose tissue from obese insulin-sensitive individuals had decreased capillary density but larger blood vessels, suggesting a role for altered angiogenesis and oxygen delivery in the setting of obesity.[59] The role of GCs in the regulation of these nonadipocyte components in the adipose tissue in the setting of increasing adipose tissue mass and whole-body insulin resistance has not been investigated, and represents an important area of future research.

GC regulation of the secretory profile of white adipose tissue

Adipokines such as leptin and adiponectin are hormones secreted by adipose tissue that regulate metabolism in other tissues, thereby exerting control of systemic glucose and lipid homeostasis, appetite regulation, and energy expenditure. Leptin levels are elevated in human obesity and diabetes, which are characterized by leptin resistance. Cortisol is known to increase leptin production[60] and high circulating leptin concentrations are seen in patients with active Cushing syndrome, which in turn decrease during remission.[2,61] Cushing remission also reduces the leptin/total adipose tissue and leptin/subcutaneous adipose tissue ratios, but not leptin/visceral adipose tissue ratio, suggesting that the hypercortisolemia in active Cushing syndrome enhances leptin production preferentially in subcutaneous over visceral adipose tissue,[2] consistent with data on healthy individuals showing higher leptin expression in subcutaneous than in visceral adipose tissue.[62]

Adiponectin levels, particularly the biologically more active high molecular weight adiponectin, tightly correlate with insulin sensitivity,[63] and levels and are lower in obesity and diabetes. Values in active Cushing patients were similar to those of nondiabetic healthy women from the Nurses' Health Study[64] and, in contrast to leptin, both high molecular weight[2] and total[42] adiponectin do not change during Cushing remission. GCs reduce adiponectin gene expression,[65] so it is unclear as to why adiponectin does not increase with Cushing remission. A potential explanation could be provided by the observation that in the subcutaneous adipose tissue of rats, corticotropin increases adiponectin gene expression, whereas dexamethasone decreases it.[66] Thus, the elevated circulating corticotropin concentrations that are present during active Cushing disease could counterbalance the effects of GCs on adiponectin secretion.

Cytokines such as interleukin (IL)-6 and tumor necrosis factor (TNF)-α can be considered adipokines because they also have systemic metabolic effects. Of importance is that adipose tissue inflammation, which manifests through increased expression of proinflammatory cytokines such as IL-6, IL-1, and TNF-α, and increased infiltration of macrophages in adipose tissue, is believed to play an important role in the pathogenesis of insulin resistance and diabetes. In keeping with their anti-inflammatory actions, GCs decrease adipose tissue inflammatory cytokines ex vivo, which are mainly produced in nonadipocyte cells within the adipose tissue.[67–69] The anti-inflammatory actions of GCs could be another mechanism through which GCs increase insulin sensitivity of adipose tissue in the context of whole-body insulin resistance.[70] In humans, investigations of the proinflammatory state after chronic GC exposure have been limited to measurement of circulating cytokines, which may or may not reflect the degree of adipose tissue inflammation. A cross-sectional study has demonstrated that patients with active as well as "cured" Cushing syndrome had elevated circulating proinflammatory markers, including soluble TNF-α receptor 1 and IL-6, in comparison with controls, suggesting a persistent state of chronic low-grade inflammation in both active and treated Cushing syndrome,[42] but whether the source of these proinflammatory cytokines is adipose tissue remains to be determined. Furthermore, whether exogenous or endogenous GCs reduce adipose tissue inflammation in an obese insulin-resistant individual is presently not known. In fact, some in vitro data suggest that GCs restrain the lipolytic effects of inflammatory cytokines produced in adipose tissue. Specifically, the addition of dexamethasone to cultured adipocytes blocked the induction of lipolysis and insulin resistance induced by TNF-α treatment.[15] In contrast to these data, however, one 11β-HSD1 inhibitor currently in development was found to decrease adipose tissue expression of TNF-α and macrophage infiltration,[71] suggesting that limiting adipose tissue GC exposure could prevent the inflammation that occurs with the development of obesity. These apparent contradictions again are likely explained by the complex physiology of GC action in vivo, in particular by the many secondary effects that occur through altered metabolism and insulin action induced by GCs.

GC regulation of brown adipose tissue

In contrast to white adipose tissue, brown adipose tissue primarily functions as a thermogenic tissue through uncoupled β-oxidation.[72] Murine data show that increasing brown adipose tissue can enhance energy expenditure and reduce adiposity.[73] Accordingly, brown adipose tissue ablation promotes the development of an obese phenotype in response to high-fat diets.[74] In contrast to previous belief, recent studies using positron emission tomography combined with computed tomography have shown the presence of brown adipose tissue in adult humans in the paracervical and supraclavicular region[75–77]; thus, its potential role in metabolism and energy homeostasis has gained recent attention. GCs have been shown to downregulate expression of mitochondrial uncoupling protein 1 (UCP-1), which is the protein that confers the exceptional thermogenic capacity and the ability to uncouple β-oxidation from adenosine triphosphate production in brown adipose tissue. Transgenic mice that overexpress 11β-HSD1 selectively in white adipose tissue had decreased UCP-1 expression in the interscapular brown adipose tissue.[54] Both pharmacologic 11β-HSD1 inhibition and genetic knockout of 11β-HSD1 lead to increased expression of brown adipose tissue–specific genes, whereas overexpression of 11β-HSD1 in mice leads to decreased expression of these genes in brown adipose tissue.[78] These data suggest that GCs reduce the function of brown adipose tissue, while 11β-HSD1 inhibition could represent a therapeutic strategy to increase such function and prevent obesity.

Mechanisms of GC-Induced Insulin Resistance in Muscle

The ability of GCs to increase insulin sensitivity of adipose tissue contrasts with their effects on muscle where GCs decrease insulin-mediated glucose uptake. As shown in primary cell culture and cell lines, this may occur via stimulation of serine kinases, resulting in phosphorylation and inactivation of IR and IRS molecules.[27,79] Accumulation of intramyocellular lipids (droplets of triglyceride in skeletal muscle fibers) is similarly associated with insulin resistance.[80–84] Thus, intramyocellular lipid accumulation is thought to represent an early defect in the development of type 2 diabetes mellitus.[85] Excessive accumulation of intramyocellular lipid could represent another mechanism by which GCs affect metabolism, but as yet it remains unclear as to whether this occurs during GC exposure in humans. However, a recent study using cell lines and rodent models demonstrated that GCs dysregulate lipid metabolism in skeletal muscle by enhancing β-oxidation and lipolysis.[86] Furthermore, inhibition of 11β-HSD1, which is expressed in muscle,[79] decreased lipogenic and lipolytic gene expression. Thus, GCs regulate both carbohydrate and lipid metabolism in skeletal muscle, which could play an important role in regulating muscle and whole-body insulin sensitivity.

Another recently characterized ectopic adipose depot is called intermuscular adipose tissue, which should not be confused with the already described intramyocellular lipid, and is defined as fat that is located beneath the muscle fascia but between the muscle groups (ie, fat "marbling" within the muscle). Intermuscular adipose tissue has been associated with development of insulin resistance,[87] but was not found to be different in patients with Cushing disease in comparison with weight-matched controls,[1] nor decreased after remission[2] when measured by whole-body MRI.

Although a direct relationship between GC-induced skeletal muscle atrophy and development of insulin resistance in muscle has not been established, myopathy is another well-described adverse consequence of GC exposure. In humans with Cushing syndrome, skeletal muscle mass is reduced in comparison with weight-matched controls.[1] Surprisingly, skeletal muscle mass continued to decrease significantly over time after surgical remission, possibly in part related to the weight loss that these patients experience (which results in loss of both fat and lean tissue). Of note, the skeletal muscle mass in remission was inversely correlated with duration of oral GC exposure, suggesting that even exposure to physiologic-range exogenous GCs may have an effect on reducing skeletal muscle mass. This finding underscores the gap in knowledge surrounding what constitutes the least amount of GC exposure, in both dose and duration, that will not result in adverse body composition and metabolic consequences.

Mechanisms of GC-Induced Hepatic Insulin Resistance: Lipogenesis, Steatosis, and Circulating Lipids

Intrahepatic lipids have been shown to be associated with insulin resistance and obesity, and to represent an important marker of cardiovascular risk, possibly even more so than visceral fat.[80–84,88] Several mechanisms have implicated GCs in the stimulation of hepatic lipogenesis and insulin resistance. GCs enhance insulin-stimulated hepatic lipogenesis by upregulation of acetyl-CoA carboxylase and FA synthase.[89,90] GCs also increase very low-density lipoprotein (VLDL) production and secretion due to inhibition of hepatic lipolysis.[91] Several indirect mechanisms also likely play a role in the accumulation of hepatic lipids in response to GCs, including accumulation and lipolysis of visceral adipose tissue, with delivery of free FA to the liver, and systemic hyperinsulinemia and hyperglycemia, which drive hepatic de novo lipogenesis.[92] Finally, GCs induce hepatic insulin resistance by stimulating hepatic gluconeogenesis via induction of phosphoenolpyruvate carboxykinase (PEPCK) and glucose-6-phosphatase. The critical role of GCs in hepatic lipid metabolism is demonstrated in vivo by improvements in hepatic steatosis and normalization of hepatic triglyceride concentrations in a fatty liver mouse model after liver-specific GR disruption.[93]

Clinical data implicating GCs in the pathogenesis of hepatic steatosis are limited, however. Obese patients with hepatic steatosis (quantified by ultrasonography) had higher post–dexamethasone-suppressed cortisol values compared with patients without steatosis,[94] and altered cortisol metabolism has been shown in patients with hepatic steatosis,[95–97] suggesting a relationship between hepatic fat and altered cortisol sensitivity and regulation in the general population. Although the development of hepatic steatosis is recognized as a sequela of chronic excess GC exposure in humans, only one report has demonstrated hepatic steatosis in Cushing syndrome by computed tomography,[98] and only a few clinical reports have described the effect of exogenous GCs to promote hepatic steatosis.[99,100] Intrahepatic lipid as assessed by ^{1}H-magnetic resonance spectroscopy, the gold standard for assessing hepatic lipid, has never been investigated in states of chronic GC exposure in humans. Thus, while existing data suggest a role for GCs in the development and progression of hepatic steatosis and its metabolic consequences, this hypothesis needs to be confirmed in clinical studies.

GC Regulation of Circulating Lipids

It is widely recognized that GCs result in dyslipidemia, although good-quality clinical data characterizing the prevalence and degree of lipid abnormalities are lacking. Surprisingly, a large survey of patients exposed to exogenous GCs did not show an association with an adverse lipid profile; in fact, higher HDL levels were seen in patients older than 60 years.[101] In keeping with this finding, daily low-dose dexamethasone given to healthy people for 3 weeks increased HDL cholesterol.[102] By contrast, an association between GC exposure and triglyceride, total cholesterol (TC), and low-density lipoprotein (LDL) concentrations was seen in a large cohort of hypopituitary patients on replacement GCs.[103] Some data suggest that corticotropin itself exerts hypolipidemic effects, introducing the potential importance of the route of GC exposure (eg, endogenous vs exogenous) and suggesting that hyperlipidemia in individuals treated with GCs may in part result from corticotropin deficiency, in addition to GC excess.[104–106]

In active Cushing syndrome dyslipidemia has been described, possibly as a result of an increase in VLDL and LDL but not HDL, resulting in an elevation of triglyceride and TC.[51,107,108] Accordingly, morning plasma cortisol and cortisol concentration after low-dose dexamethasone correlated with TC and LDL cholesterol in a series of patients with active Cushing syndrome.[109] However, one report did not find reduced HDL-cholesterol concentrations in active Cushing syndrome,[109] and in another series mean TC/HDL and LDL/HDL values were in the desirable range (<4.5 for TC/HDL and <3.0 for LDL/HDL) in active disease.[2] Furthermore, a prospective study of patients with Cushing disease studied before and over time after surgical remission demonstrated a decrease in only TC, whereas LDL, HDL, triglyceride, and the ratios (TC/HDL and LDL/HDL) did not change.[2] In fact, HDL decreased in 11 of the 14 patients, but the mean change was not significant.[2] Other longitudinal Cushing studies have also not shown a change in lipid profile with remission.[51,108] The fact that many Cushing patients remain either overweight or obese despite remission could play a role in the lack of change in the lipid profile.[2] These findings also suggest the possibility that GC exposure has lasting effects on lipid profiles even after eucortisolism has been restored.

Potential Effects of Brain GCs on Metabolic Homeostasis

An understanding of the role of brain GCs in whole-body metabolic homeostasis is needed, in part given the widely prevalent use of nasal GCs, which potentially could, depending on the formulation and dose, result in central nervous system (CNS) GC exposure via transport along the olfactory and trigeminal nerve fibers, although this is yet to be studied specifically for GCs. A few studies have suggested a role for brain GCs in the regulation of metabolic homeostasis, although data are still very limited in this area.

Brain GC levels are a function of GC uptake and local GC activation through 11β-HSD1, which is present in hippocampal neurons as well as neurons in the hypothalamic arcuate and paraventricular hypothalamic nuclei.[110–112] A recent human brain-bank study found wide expression of 11β-HSD1 mRNA in the suprachiasmatic nucleus, which is the biological clock of the brain, as well as the supraoptic, paraventricular, and infundibular nuclei. In the paraventricular nucleus, neuronal 11β-HSD1 immunoreactivity colocalized with corticotropin-releasing hormone, suggesting that modulation of brain GC availability could play a role in the regulation of the HPA axis with regard to metabolism, appetite, and circadian rhythms.[113]

Several central and peripheral GC effects are mediated via neuropeptide Y (NPY), which is an abundantly expressed peptide involved in the regulation of the stress response, including appetite, anxiolysis, and vasoconstriction. Animal studies have shown that central (intracerebroventricular) administration of dexamethasone enhances NPY content in the arcuate nucleus of the hypothalamus, a key regulator of the HPA axis, and results in hyperphagia, hyperinsulinemia, insulin resistance, and weight gain in rats.[114,115] Specifically, using euglycemic-hyperinsulinemic clamps, continuous central dexamethasone infusion resulted in weight gain and insulin resistance, manifested by decreased insulin-stimulated glucose utilization.[114,116] These effects were shown to be mediated by the activation of the parasympathetic nervous system, as they were abolished in vagotomized animals.[116] Another study demonstrated that hypothalamic GC action modulates hepatic insulin sensitivity via NPY and the sympathetic nervous system.[117] In the periphery, excess GCs caused by chronic stress in mice upregulated the expression of NPY in sympathetic neurons and the expression of its receptor on abdominal adipocytes, leading to angiogenesis and adipogenesis, thus contributing to the development of abdominal obesity and insulin resistance.[118]

Another potential mechanism for many GC-induced effects is through tissue-specific regulation of adenosine monophosphate–activated kinase (AMPK), a regulator of cellular and systemic energy homeostasis, which acts through enzyme phosphorylation and regulation of gene and protein expression.[119,120] Activation of hypothalamic AMPK may be associated with an increase in appetite, whereas in adipose tissue it may inhibit lipogenesis. One study demonstrated reduced adipose tissue AMPK activity in insulin-resistant subjects in comparison with insulin-sensitive individuals.[121] In the liver, AMPK activation is suggested to play a role in inhibiting gluconeogenesis and FA and cholesterol synthesis. A recent study using a rat model of Cushing showed that GC treatment was associated with inhibition of AMPK activity in the adipose tissue and heart, but stimulation in the liver and hypothalamus. Similar activity patterns were observed in vitro in adipose, hypothalamic, and liver cells. These data suggest that GC-induced changes in AMPK could underpin the increase in appetite, the accumulation of visceral and hepatic fat, and the cardiovascular risk that characterizes GC excess.[122] Furthermore, the regulation of AMPK through GCs may occur, at least in part, via endocannabinoids and their cognate receptor cannabinoid receptor 1 (CB1), a widely expressed receptor in the CNS and the hypothalamus, but which is also present at low levels in adipose tissue, liver, and muscle.[123] In the hypothalamus, activation of CB1 enhances appetite, whereas in adipose tissue it may increase lipogenesis.[124] GC stimulation of endocannabinoid tone in the hypothalamus[125,126] also altered hypothalamic AMPK,[122] and this may be dependent on the CB1 receptor because GC-treated CB1 knockout mice did not gain weight in the setting of a lack of increase in hypothalamic and hepatic AMPK.[127] Whether the effects of GCs indicate a specific role of CB1, or if the reduced weight gain after GCs is secondarily due to the impaired ability of CB1 knockout mice to gain weight on a high-fat diet or in the setting of genetic forms of obesity,[128] is unclear.

11β-HSD1 AS A GATEKEEPER FOR INTRACELLULAR GC AVAILABILITY

Intracellular GC availability is regulated by the activity of 11β-HSD1, a widely expressed NADP(H)-dependent enzyme that acts predominantly as a reductase in vivo to convert inactive cortisone to cortisol.[129–135] Tissue-specific actions of 11β-HSD1 are shown in **Table 1**. Overexpression of 11β-HSD1 in the adipose tissue of mice promotes abdominal obesity, insulin resistance, hepatic steatosis, and

Table 1 Tissue-dependent actions of 11β-hydroxysteroid dehydrogenase 1		
Tissue	**Overexpression**	**Inhibition or Knockout**
White adipose tissue	Hyperglycemia and insulin resistance Dyslipidemia: elevated circulating TG and FA Increased adiposity: visceral > subcutaneous adipose tissue	Enhanced insulin sensitivity Improved hepatic insulin action Decreased TG and FA Resistance to development of obese phenotype
Brown adipose tissue	Decreased UCP-1 expression	Increased UCP-1 expression
Liver (highest expression)	Insulin resistance Elevated circulating TC and TG Hepatic steatosis Stimulation of HPA axis leading to adrenal hypertrophy	Increased hepatic insulin action Decreased fasting glucose and glucose output Decreased expression of gluconeogenic enzymes PEPCK and G6P
Brain	Expression seen in hippocampus and hypothalamus, suggesting a role in the regulation of metabolism and appetite	Needs further exploration
Muscle	Needs further exploration	Decreased lipogenic and lipolytic gene expression

Abbreviations: FA, fatty acids; G6P, glucose-6-phosphatase; HPA, hypothalamic-pituitary-adrenal; PEPCK, phosphoenolpyruvate carboxykinase; TC, total cholesterol; TG, triglyceride; UCP-1, mitochondrial uncoupling protein 1.

elevated circulating free FA and triglyceride concentrations.[54,136] Similarly, in vitro studies have shown that 11β-HSD1 inhibition reduces adipogenesis in human adipose cells.[137] Knockout of 11β-HSD1 in mice improves hepatic insulin action and results in a phenotype that is resistant to overfeeding-induced obesity and diabetes.[138–141]

As liver is the site of highest 11β-HSD1 expression and a major cortisol producer,[134,135,142,143] liver-selective 11β-HSD1 disruption has profound effects on whole-body metabolism, resulting in HPA-axis activation and adrenal hypertrophy.[144] Similar to that seen in adipose tissue, overexpression of 11β-HSD1 in the liver is associated with hepatic steatosis, insulin resistance, and elevated TC and triglyceride levels.[145,146] In fact, an animal model of obesity and the metabolic syndrome had increased hepatic (but reduced adipose tissue) 11β-HSD1 levels,[147] suggesting a possible role for selective hepatic 11β-HSD1 inhibition to reduce GC-mediated hepatic glucose output.[148] However, although some murine liver-specific knockout models of 11β-HSD1 lack significant metabolic abnormalities, highlighting the important compensatory role of HPA-axis activation and extrahepatic 11β-HSD1 activity,[144] these mice are protected from the obesity and insulin resistance that develop in the setting of chronic 11-dehydrocorticosterone administration.[149]

In humans, local production of excess GCs by upregulation of 11β-HSD1 in abdominal adipose tissue[131,150,151] has been suggested to cause visceral adiposity and the metabolic syndrome,[132,133] as 11β-HSD1 activity is higher in visceral than in subcutaneous adipose stromal cells,[134,142] and higher in adipose tissue from obese subjects compared with lean controls.[130,152] Studies in obesity and diabetes, however, are mixed, with both similar[153–157] and increased[130,151,158–161] adipose tissue 11β-HSD1 expression in obese diabetics when compared with lean insulin-sensitive individuals. Human obesity may be associated with decreased hepatic 11β-HSD1 activity, which is speculated to be a compensatory mechanism aimed to decrease hepatic glucose output and preserve insulin sensitivity.[54,162,163] By contrast, decreased 11β-HSD1 activity was not demonstrated in patients with diabetes, suggesting that higher cortisol hepatic exposure could contribute to the progression to diabetes in some obese individuals.[156]

Expression of 11β-HSD1 is increased by GCs and insulin.[164] However, patients with Cushing syndrome had levels of 11β-HSD1 mRNA similar to those of lean controls and lower than those of obese individuals, possibly because of downregulation from chronic hypercortisolemia.[151,165] 11β-HSD1 expression is also induced by leptin and proinflammatory cytokines. Thus, the increases in local or systemic proinflammatory cytokines seen in obesity may further enhance adiposity by increasing 11β-HSD1 expression and local generation of GCs.

The Potential Role of 11β-HSD1 Inhibition in Humans

11β-HSD1 inhibition is a potentially promising novel therapeutic approach for the treatment of obesity and diabetes. In healthy people, carbenoxolone (a nonselective 11β-HSD inhibitor) improves whole-body insulin sensitivity[166]; in diabetic subjects, it decreases production rates of hepatic glucose during hyperinsulinemic-euglycemic clamp but does not augment glucose disposal.[167] Carbenoxolone has also been shown to limit GC-induced lipolysis in subcutaneous fat[168] and decrease circulating TC.[167] These data have provided a rationale for the development of selective 11β-1HSD1 inhibitors.

In rodent models, inhibition of 11β-HSD1 improves insulin sensitivity; decreases hepatic steatosis and the expression of the hepatic gluconeogenic enzymes PEPCK and glucose-6-phosphatase; reduces TC, free FA, and triglycerides; and results in a phenotype that is resistant to obesity and diabetes.[140,169–175] A confounding factor is the reduction in food intake seen in many studies, which could be due to nonspecific toxic effects of these compounds. However, some studies have shown similar results with pair-fed groups,[79] supporting the notion that 11β-HSD1 inhibition improves insulin action that at least in part is independent of alterations in caloric intake.

Initial studies in humans have been encouraging. One compound, which has been administered to diabetic patients in combination with metformin, was shown to have beneficial effects on weight, lipid profile, and glycemic control.[176] However, another compound had more modest beneficial effects on glycemic control and, despite a moderate decrease in weight, increased both LDL and HDL concentrations.[177] Some compounds also lower blood pressure.[178] Concerns regarding clinical use of 11β-HSD1 inhibitors include compensatory HPA-axis upregulation, resulting in adrenal hypertrophy and corticotropin-driven adrenal androgen excess.[179] Additional effects on the immune system, as 11β-HSD1 may play a role in limiting the acute inflammatory response, are unknown, as are effects of longer-term treatment in humans. The magnitude of the effect of inhibition in humans is also questionable, as there may be species differences in the extent of the role of GC metabolism in obesity and metabolic disease.

THE ROLE OF GCS IN THE DEVELOPMENT OF COMMON OBESITY

Given the striking phenotypic and metabolic similarities between so-called common obesity (and associated insulin resistance) with Cushing syndrome, endogenous GCs have been implicated in the pathogenesis of this condition. However, data are limited by variability of serum and urine cortisol measures and their lack of reflection of true cellular and tissue GC action. Subtle GC abnormalities, including reduced endogenous cortisol suppression to dexamethasone[180,181] and tissue-specific alterations in cortisol metabolism,[150,152] have been associated with obesity and insulin resistance. The abdominal obesity phenotype, in particular, may be associated with alterations in GC activity,[182,183] as well as increased cortisol response to food and other HPA-axis stimulators including corticotropin, vasopressin, and corticotropin-releasing hormone.[184–188] Other abnormalities, including higher salivary cortisol level in response to stress,[189,190] different GR polymorphisms,[191–193] and chronic low-dose oral GCs,[103] have also been associated with obesity, higher waist circumference,[194,195] insulin resistance, the metabolic syndrome, and increased mortality. A recent study showed that long-term elevations in cortisol, measured in scalp hair, were associated with higher risk for diabetes, cardiovascular disease,[196] and the metabolic syndrome among community dwellers.[197] However, some studies show decreased salivary and serum cortisol levels in obesity; moreover, circulating GC concentrations and their response to stimulation or suppression are well known to be variable, and often do not predict their effects or function in target tissues.[198] Thus, the mechanisms for altered GC activity, and the precise tissue and cellular actions of GCs in obesity and metabolism, need further elucidation. As circulating cortisol is normal in obesity, further work should also explore the role of local tissue GC exposure via 11β-HSD1, and alterations in HPA-axis sensitivity and circadian rhythm in the pathogenesis of obesity.

THE PARADOX OF GC ANTI-INFLAMMATORY YET DIABETOGENIC ACTIONS: DURATION, LOCATION, OR CONTEXT?

Inflammation of white adipose tissue is believed to play an important role in the development of obesity-related adverse metabolic sequelae.[70,199] Chronic activation of proinflammatory pathways within white adipose tissue and other insulin target tissues may impair metabolic control, possibly by impairing insulin signaling. For instance, adipocytes from obese individuals exhibit higher basal lipolysis,[200] in part because of elevated TNF-α,[201] an inflammatory cytokine that can impair insulin signaling through serine phosphorylation of IRS proteins.[202] Lipolysis results in the release of free FA which, in turn, leads to macrophage infiltration of adipose tissue.[203,204] Thus, a popular model of how obesity leads to insulin resistance is that inflammation within adipose tissue causes insulin resistance, and increases the risk for atherosclerosis and cardiovascular events.[7,8] By contrast, GCs have potent anti-inflammatory and immunosuppressive actions, and as such are used to treat states of abnormal immune activation, including many autoimmune and rheumatologic diseases. GCs suppress proinflammatory cytokine expression in vitro[205–207] and in vivo,[208] with the most pronounced effect on TNF-α and the least effect on IL-6.[209] States of chronic GC excess consistently predispose patients to the adverse effects of immune suppression, such as the increased fungal infections seen in Cushing syndrome.[210] It might follow that Cushing syndrome would be characterized by a lower degree of inflammation, in particular adipose tissue inflammation, thereby reducing insulin resistance and improving metabolic regulation. Clinically, however, Cushing syndrome induces glucose intolerance, dyslipidemia, and cardiovascular mortality, all of which are usually associated with inflammation, suggesting that chronic in vivo exposure to GCs may in fact result in systemic inflammation.[6,51,211,212] Thus, there is a paradox between the anti-inflammatory properties of GCs and their dysmetabolic effects, which presents an important caveat to the prevailing model of inflammation as an important link between obesity and insulin resistance.

The effects of chronic GC exposure due to Cushing syndrome on proinflammatory mediators have not been well studied. IL-1β, IL-6, and TNF-α levels in female patients with Cushing syndrome were not different compared with those in controls,[213] although acute elevations in these cytokines were observed in the immediate postoperative hypocortisolemic period. Whether the latter observation is due to the hypocortisolism rather than the preceding stress of surgery is unclear. Other studies have shown elevated circulating cytokines in both active[214] and treated[42] patients with Cushing syndrome in comparison with controls, including elevated CRP, IL-6, and TNF-α concentrations, with increased endothelin-1 after insulin bolus and reduced basal and stimulated nitric oxide release, suggesting an increased proatherogenic risk profile in addition to increased inflammatory markers in Cushing syndrome.[214] Furthermore, IL-1 receptor antagonist was found to be high in active Cushing syndrome and decreased after surgery, in association with decreased fat, particularly trunk fat (quantified by dual-energy x-ray absorptiometry).[215] Whether this represents a relationship between body composition and markers of inflammation in Cushing syndrome requires further supportive data. Future studies will need to clarify the chronic effects of hypercortisolemia on serum and adipose tissue inflammatory cytokines, and correlate this inflammatory profile with measures of insulin action and cardiovascular risk. Whether the anti-inflammatory actions of GCs are duration or tissue dependent will be an important area of future investigations.

SUMMARY AND FUTURE DIRECTIONS

GCs are critical in the regulation of energy homeostasis, in large part owing to their control of lipid metabolism and adipose tissue function. Although physiologic exposure to GCs and a dynamic HPA axis that is responsive to metabolic and environmental cues are essential for the survival of any organism, chronic exposure to even subtle GC excess cause adverse sequelae, including the development of excess abdominal and ectopic adipose tissue, dyslipidemia, cardiovascular disease, and, ultimately, decreased survival. Prevalent forms of subtle GC excess include exogenous exposure, which is widely used in the treatment of autoimmune and rheumatologic diseases, and chronic stress with resultant activation of the HPA axis. Even common obesity and the metabolic syndrome have been proposed as models of excess endogenous GCs, through enhanced HPA-axis activation, altered metabolism, and/ or a flattened cortisol circadian rhythm.

Thus, the study of GC regulation of insulin action and lipid metabolism in target organs is of critical importance. Further investigation is needed to address critical gaps in our understanding of the regulation of GCs on adipose tissue function. First, the effects of prolonged versus acute in vivo GC exposure on insulin action in adipose tissue need further exploration, including investigation of the effects of GC-induced systemic hyperinsulinemia and insulin resistance on adipose tissue function. Second, while some studies have suggested that the post-hypercortisolemic state is associated with persistent adverse metabolic and cardiovascular risk, the extent and precise mechanisms of these abnormal patterns, at both the systemic and tissue levels, have not been delineated. Third, the paradox of GC anti-inflammatory yet diabetogenic effects, and the investigation of serum and tissue markers of inflammation in the context of obesity and insulin resistance need clarification. Finally, further knowledge of the underpinnings of GC effects on adipose tissue and metabolic function will provide a rationale for new GC therapeutic agents with enhanced beneficial (eg, anti-inflammatory) but reduced adverse (eg, diabetogenic and adipogenic) effects.

REFERENCES

1. Geer EB, Shen W, Gallagher D, et al. MRI assessment of lean and adipose tissue distribution in female patients with Cushing's disease. Clin Endocrinol (Oxf) 2010;73(4):469–75.
2. Geer EB, Shen W, Strohmayer E, et al. Body composition and cardiovascular risk markers after remission of Cushing's disease: a prospective study using whole-body MRI. J Clin Endocrinol Metab 2012;97(5):1702–11.
3. van Staa TP, Leufkens HG, Abenhaim L, et al. Use of oral corticosteroids in the United Kingdom. QJM 2000;93(2):105–11.
4. Kershaw EE, Flier JS. Adipose tissue as an endocrine organ. J Clin Endocrinol Metab 2004;89(6):2548–56.
5. Eckel RH, Kahn R, Robertson RM, et al. Preventing cardiovascular disease and diabetes: a call to action from the American Diabetes Association and the American Heart Association. Circulation 2006;113(25):2943–6.
6. Ridker PM, Buring JE, Cook NR, et al. C-reactive protein, the metabolic syndrome, and risk of incident cardiovascular events: an 8-year follow-up of 14 719 initially healthy American women. Circulation 2003;107(3):391–7.
7. Girman CJ, Rhodes T, Mercuri M, et al. The metabolic syndrome and risk of major coronary events in the Scandinavian Simvastatin Survival Study (4S) and the Air Force/Texas Coronary Atherosclerosis Prevention Study (AFCAPS/Tex-CAPS). Am J Cardiol 2004;93(2):136–41.
8. Solymoss BC, Bourassa MG, Campeau L, et al. Effect of increasing metabolic syndrome score on atherosclerotic risk profile and coronary artery disease angiographic severity. Am J Cardiol 2004;93(2):159–64.

9. Etxabe J, Vazquez JA. Morbidity and mortality in Cushing's disease: an epidemiological approach. Clin Endocrinol (Oxf) 1994;40(4):479–84.

10. Hauner H, Schmid P, Pfeiffer EF. Glucocorticoids and insulin promote the differentiation of human adipocyte precursor cells into fat cells. J Clin Endocrinol Metab 1987;64(4):832–5.

11. Campbell JE, Peckett AJ, D'Souza AM, et al. Adipogenic and lipolytic effects of chronic glucocorticoid exposure. Am J Physiol Cell Physiol 2011;300(1): C198–209.

12. Slavin BG, Ong JM, Kern PA. Hormonal regulation of hormone-sensitive lipase activity and mRNA levels in isolated rat adipocytes. J Lipid Res 1994;35(9): 1535–41.

13. Samra JS, Clark ML, Humphreys SM, et al. Effects of physiological hypercortisolemia on the regulation of lipolysis in subcutaneous adipose tissue. J Clin Endocrinol Metab 1998;83(2):626–31.

14. Djurhuus CB, Gravholt CH, Nielsen S, et al. Additive effects of cortisol and growth hormone on regional and systemic lipolysis in humans. Am J Physiol Endocrinol Metab 2004;286(3):E488–94.

15. Lee MJ, Fried SK. Glucocorticoids antagonize tumor necrosis factor-alpha-stimulated lipolysis and resistance to the antilipolytic effect of insulin in human adipocytes. Am J Physiol Endocrinol Metab 2012;303(9):E1126–33.

16. Villena JA, Roy S, Sarkadi-Nagy E, et al. Desnutrin, an adipocyte gene encoding a novel patatin domain-containing protein, is induced by fasting and glucocorticoids: ectopic expression of desnutrin increases triglyceride hydrolysis. J Biol Chem 2004;279(45):47066–75.

17. Gao Z, Zhang X, Zuberi A, et al. Inhibition of insulin sensitivity by free fatty acids requires activation of multiple serine kinases in 3T3-L1 adipocytes. Mol Endocrinol 2004;18(8):2024–34.

18. Lee MJ, Fried SK, Mundt SS, et al. Depot-specific regulation of the conversion of cortisone to cortisol in human adipose tissue. Obesity (Silver Spring) 2008; 16(6):1178–85.

19. Rebuffe-Scrive M, Krotkiewski M, Elfverson J, et al. Muscle and adipose tissue morphology and metabolism in Cushing's syndrome. J Clin Endocrinol Metab 1988;67(6):1122–8.

20. Krsek M, Rosicka M, Nedvidkova J, et al. Increased lipolysis of subcutaneous abdominal adipose tissue and altered noradrenergic activity in patients with Cushing's syndrome: an in-vivo microdialysis study. Physiol Res 2006;55(4): 421–8.

21. Diraison F, Dusserre E, Vidal H, et al. Increased hepatic lipogenesis but decreased expression of lipogenic gene in adipose tissue in human obesity. Am J Physiol Endocrinol Metab 2002;282(1):E46–51.

22. Roberts R, Hodson L, Dennis AL, et al. Markers of de novo lipogenesis in adipose tissue: associations with small adipocytes and insulin sensitivity in humans. Diabetologia 2009;52(5):882–90.

23. Mayas MD, Ortega FJ, Macias-Gonzalez M, et al. Inverse relation between FASN expression in human adipose tissue and the insulin resistance level. Nutr Metab (Lond) 2010;7:3.

24. Eissing L, Scherer T, Todter K, et al. De novo lipogenesis in human fat and liver is linked to ChREBP-beta and metabolic health. Nat Commun 2013;4:1528.

25. Gathercole LL, Morgan SA, Bujalska IJ, et al. Regulation of lipogenesis by glucocorticoids and insulin in human adipose tissue. PLoS One 2011;6(10): e26223.

26. Postic C, Girard J. Contribution of de novo fatty acid synthesis to hepatic steatosis and insulin resistance: lessons from genetically engineered mice. J Clin Invest 2008;118(3):829–38.

27. Gathercole LL, Bujalska IJ, Stewart PM, et al. Glucocorticoid modulation of insulin signaling in human subcutaneous adipose tissue. J Clin Endocrinol Metab 2007;92(11):4332–9.

28. Tomlinson JJ, Boudreau A, Wu D, et al. Insulin sensitization of human preadipocytes through glucocorticoid hormone induction of forkhead transcription factors. Mol Endocrinol 2010;24(1):104–13.

29. Gathercole LL, Morgan SA, Bujalska IJ, et al. Short- and long-term glucocorticoid treatment enhances insulin signalling in human subcutaneous adipose tissue. Nutr Diabetes 2011;1:e3.

30. Hazlehurst JM, Gathercole LL, Nasiri M, et al. Glucocorticoids fail to cause insulin resistance in human subcutaneous adipose tissue in vivo. J Clin Endocrinol Metab 2013;98(4):1631–40.

31. Buren J, Liu HX, Jensen J, et al. Dexamethasone impairs insulin signalling and glucose transport by depletion of insulin receptor substrate-1, phosphatidylinositol 3-kinase and protein kinase B in primary cultured rat adipocytes. Eur J Endocrinol 2002;146(3):419–29.

32. Lundgren M, Buren J, Ruge T, et al. Glucocorticoids down-regulate glucose uptake capacity and insulin-signaling proteins in omental but not subcutaneous human adipocytes. J Clin Endocrinol Metab 2004;89(6):2989–97.

33. Sakoda H, Ogihara T, Anai M, et al. Dexamethasone-induced insulin resistance in 3T3-L1 adipocytes is due to inhibition of glucose transport rather than insulin signal transduction. Diabetes 2000;49(10):1700–8.

34. Baxter JD, Forsham PH. Tissue effects of glucocorticoids. Am J Med 1972; 53(5):573–89.

35. Donahue RP, Abbott RD. Central obesity and coronary heart disease in men. Lancet 1987;2(8569):1215.

36. Despres JP, Lemieux I, Bergeron J, et al. Abdominal obesity and the metabolic syndrome: contribution to global cardiometabolic risk. Arterioscler Thromb Vasc Biol 2008;28(6):1039–49.

37. Lean ME, Han TS, Seidell JC. Impairment of health and quality of life in people with large waist circumference. Lancet 1998;351(9106):853–6.

38. Chan JM, Rimm EB, Colditz GA, et al. Obesity, fat distribution, and weight gain as risk factors for clinical diabetes in men. Diabetes Care 1994;17(9):961–9.

39. Carey DG, Jenkins AB, Campbell LV, et al. Abdominal fat and insulin resistance in normal and overweight women: direct measurements reveal a strong relationship in subjects at both low and high risk of NIDDM. Diabetes 1996;45(5): 633–8.

40. Kissebah AH, Krakower GR. Regional adiposity and morbidity. Physiol Rev 1994;74(4):761–811.

41. Ducluzeau PH, Manchec-Poilblanc P, Roullier V, et al. Distribution of abdominal adipose tissue as a predictor of hepatic steatosis assessed by MRI. Clin Radiol 2010;65(9):695–700.

42. Barahona MJ, Sucunza N, Resmini E, et al. Persistent body fat mass and inflammatory marker increases after long-term cure of Cushing's syndrome. J Clin Endocrinol Metab 2009;94(9):3365–71.

43. Mayo-Smith W, Hayes CW, Biller BM, et al. Body fat distribution measured with CT: correlations in healthy subjects, patients with anorexia nervosa, and patients with Cushing syndrome. Radiology 1989;170(2):515–8.

44. Garrapa GG, Pantanetti P, Arnaldi G, et al. Body composition and metabolic features in women with adrenal incidentaloma or Cushing's syndrome. J Clin Endocrinol Metab 2001;86(11):5301–6.

45. Schafroth U, Godang K, Ueland T, et al. Leptin levels in relation to body composition and insulin concentration in patients with endogenous Cushing's syndrome compared to controls matched for body mass index. J Endocrinol Invest 2000;23(6):349–55.

46. Wajchenberg BL, Bosco A, Marone MM, et al. Estimation of body fat and lean tissue distribution by dual energy X-ray absorptiometry and abdominal body fat evaluation by computed tomography in Cushing's disease. J Clin Endocrinol Metab 1995;80(9):2791–4.

47. Burt MG, Gibney J, Ho KK. Characterization of the metabolic phenotypes of Cushing's syndrome and growth hormone deficiency: a study of body composition and energy metabolism. Clin Endocrinol (Oxf) 2006;64(4):436–43.

48. Burt MG, Gibney J, Ho KK. Protein metabolism in glucocorticoid excess: study in Cushing's syndrome and the effect of treatment. Am J Physiol Endocrinol Metab 2007;292(5):E1426–32.

49. Rockall AG, Sohaib SA, Evans D, et al. Computed tomography assessment of fat distribution in male and female patients with Cushing's syndrome. Eur J Endocrinol 2003;149(6):561–7.

50. Calao A, Pivonello R, Spiezia S, et al. Persistence of increased cardiovascular risk in patients with Cushing's disease after five years of successful cure. J Clin Endocrinol Metab 1999;84:2664–72.

51. Faggiano A, Pivonello R, Spiezia S, et al. Cardiovascular risk factors and common carotid artery caliber and stiffness in patients with Cushing's disease during active disease and 1 year after disease remission. J Clin Endocrinol Metab 2003;88:2527–33.

52. Pivonello R, Faggiano A, Lombardi G, et al. The metabolic syndrome and cardiovascular risk in Cushing's syndrome. Endocrinol Metab Clin North Am 2005;34(2):327–39, viii.

53. Lambert JK, Goldberg L, Fayngold S, et al. Predictors of mortality and long-term outcomes in treated Cushing's disease: a study of 346 patients. J Clin Endocrinol Metab 2013;98(3):1022–30.

54. Masuzaki H, Paterson J, Shinyama H, et al. A transgenic model of visceral obesity and the metabolic syndrome. Science 2001;294(5549):2166–70.

55. Veilleux A, Rheaume C, Daris M, et al. Omental adipose tissue type 1 11 beta-hydroxysteroid dehydrogenase oxoreductase activity, body fat distribution, and metabolic alterations in women. J Clin Endocrinol Metab 2009;94(9):3550–7.

56. Varma V, Yao-Borengasser A, Bodles AM, et al. Thrombospondin-1 is an adipokine associated with obesity, adipose inflammation, and insulin resistance. Diabetes 2008;57(2):432–9.

57. Spencer M, Yao-Borengasser A, Unal R, et al. Adipose tissue macrophages in insulin-resistant subjects are associated with collagen VI and fibrosis and demonstrate alternative activation. Am J Physiol Endocrinol Metab 2010; 299(6):E1016–27.

58. Pasarica M, Gowronska-Kozak B, Burk D, et al. Adipose tissue collagen VI in obesity. J Clin Endocrinol Metab 2009;94(12):5155–62.

59. Spencer M, Unal R, Zhu B, et al. Adipose tissue extracellular matrix and vascular abnormalities in obesity and insulin resistance. J Clin Endocrinol Metab 2011;96(12):E1990–8.

60. Papaspyrou-Rao S, Schneider SH, Petersen RN, et al. Dexamethasone increases leptin expression in humans in vivo. J Clin Endocrinol Metab 1997; 82(5):1635–7.
61. Masuzaki H, Ogawa Y, Hosoda K, et al. Glucocorticoid regulation of leptin synthesis and secretion in humans: elevated plasma leptin levels in Cushing's syndrome. J Clin Endocrinol Metab 1997;82(8):2542–7.
62. Hube F, Lietz U, Igel M, et al. Difference in leptin mRNA levels between omental and subcutaneous abdominal adipose tissue from obese humans. Horm Metab Res 1996;28(12):690–3.
63. Aso Y, Yamamoto R, Wakabayashi S, et al. Comparison of serum high-molecular weight (HMW) adiponectin with total adiponectin concentrations in type 2 diabetic patients with coronary artery disease using a novel enzyme-linked immunosorbent assay to detect HMW adiponectin. Diabetes 2006;55(7):1954–60.
64. Heidemann C, Sun Q, van Dam RM, et al. Total and high-molecular-weight adiponectin and resistin in relation to the risk for type 2 diabetes in women. Ann Intern Med 2008;149(5):307–16.
65. Fasshauer M, Klein J, Neumann S, et al. Hormonal regulation of adiponectin gene expression in 3T3-L1 adipocytes. Biochem Biophys Res Commun 2002; 290(3):1084–9.
66. Paschke L, Zemleduch T, Rucinski M, et al. Adiponectin and adiponectin receptor system in the rat adrenal gland: ontogenetic and physiologic regulation, and its involvement in regulating adrenocortical growth and steroidogenesis. Peptides 2010;31(9):1715–24.
67. Bruun JM, Lihn AS, Madan AK, et al. Higher production of IL-8 in visceral vs. subcutaneous adipose tissue. Implication of nonadipose cells in adipose tissue. Am J Physiol Endocrinol Metab 2004;286(1):E8–13.
68. Fried SK, Bunkin DA, Greenberg AS. Omental and subcutaneous adipose tissues of obese subjects release interleukin-6: depot difference and regulation by glucocorticoid. J Clin Endocrinol Metab 1998;83(3):847–50.
69. Trujillo ME, Scherer PE. Adipose tissue-derived factors: impact on health and disease. Endocr Rev 2006;27(7):762–78.
70. Weisberg SP, McCann D, Desai M, et al. Obesity is associated with macrophage accumulation in adipose tissue. J Clin Invest 2003;112(12):1796–808.
71. Wang L, Liu J, Zhang A, et al. BVT.2733, a selective 11beta-hydroxysteroid dehydrogenase type 1 inhibitor, attenuates obesity and inflammation in diet-induced obese mice. PLoS One 2012;7(7):e40056.
72. Cannon B, Nedergaard J. Developmental biology: neither fat nor flesh. Nature 2008;454(7207):947–8.
73. Almind K, Manieri M, Sivitz WI, et al. Ectopic brown adipose tissue in muscle provides a mechanism for differences in risk of metabolic syndrome in mice. Proc Natl Acad Sci U S A 2007;104(7):2366–71.
74. Tateishi K, Okada Y, Kallin EM, et al. Role of Jhdm2a in regulating metabolic gene expression and obesity resistance. Nature 2009;458(7239):757–61.
75. Cypess AM, Lehman S, Williams G, et al. Identification and importance of brown adipose tissue in adult humans. N Engl J Med 2009;360(15):1509–17.
76. van Marken Lichtenbelt WD, Vanhommerig JW, Smulders NM, et al. Cold-activated brown adipose tissue in healthy men. N Engl J Med 2009;360(15): 1500–8.
77. Virtanen KA, Lidell ME, Orava J, et al. Functional brown adipose tissue in healthy adults. N Engl J Med 2009;360(15):1518–25.

78. Liu J, Kong X, Wang L, et al. Essential roles of 11beta-HSD1 in regulating brown adipocyte function. J Mol Endocrinol 2013;50(1):103–13.

79. Morgan SA, Sherlock M, Gathercole LL, et al. 11beta-hydroxysteroid dehydrogenase type 1 regulates glucocorticoid-induced insulin resistance in skeletal muscle. Diabetes 2009;58(11):2506–15.

80. Lim S, Son KR, Song IC, et al. Fat in liver/muscle correlates more strongly with insulin sensitivity in rats than abdominal fat. Obesity (Silver Spring) 2009;17(1): 188–95.

81. Greco AV, Mingrone G, Giancaterini A, et al. Insulin resistance in morbid obesity: reversal with intramyocellular fat depletion. Diabetes 2002;51(1):144–51.

82. Jacob S, Machann J, Rett K, et al. Association of increased intramyocellular lipid content with insulin resistance in lean nondiabetic offspring of type 2 diabetic subjects. Diabetes 1999;48(5):1113–9.

83. Misra A, Sinha S, Kumar M, et al. Proton magnetic resonance spectroscopy study of soleus muscle in non-obese healthy and Type 2 diabetic Asian Northern Indian males: high intramyocellular lipid content correlates with excess body fat and abdominal obesity. Diabet Med 2003;20(5):361–7.

84. Perseghin G, Scifo P, De Cobelli F, et al. Intramyocellular triglyceride content is a determinant of in vivo insulin resistance in humans: a ^{1}H-^{13}C nuclear magnetic resonance spectroscopy assessment in offspring of type 2 diabetic parents. Diabetes 1999;48(8):1600–6.

85. Morino K, Petersen KF, Shulman GI. Molecular mechanisms of insulin resistance in humans and their potential links with mitochondrial dysfunction. Diabetes 2006;55(Suppl 2):S9–15.

86. Morgan SA, Gathercole LL, Simonet C, et al. Regulation of lipid metabolism by glucocorticoids and 11beta-HSD1 in skeletal muscle. Endocrinology 2013; 154(7):2374–84.

87. Goodpaster BH, Thaete FL, Kelley DE. Thigh adipose tissue distribution is associated with insulin resistance in obesity and in type 2 diabetes mellitus. Am J Clin Nutr 2000;71(4):885–92.

88. Fabbrini E, Magkos F, Mohammed BS, et al. Intrahepatic fat, not visceral fat, is linked with metabolic complications of obesity. Proc Natl Acad Sci U S A 2009; 106(36):15430–5.

89. Amatruda JM, Danahy SA, Chang CL. The effects of glucocorticoids on insulin-stimulated lipogenesis in primary cultures of rat hepatocytes. Biochem J 1983; 212(1):135–41.

90. Zhao LF, Iwasaki Y, Zhe W, et al. Hormonal regulation of acetyl-CoA carboxylase isoenzyme gene transcription. Endocr J 2010;57(4):317–24.

91. Dolinsky VW, Douglas DN, Lehner R, et al. Regulation of the enzymes of hepatic microsomal triacylglycerol lipolysis and re-esterification by the glucocorticoid dexamethasone. Biochem J 2004;378(Pt 3):967–74.

92. Schwarz JM, Linfoot P, Dare D, et al. Hepatic de novo lipogenesis in normoinsulinemic and hyperinsulinemic subjects consuming high-fat, low-carbohydrate and low-fat, high-carbohydrate isoenergetic diets. Am J Clin Nutr 2003;77(1): 43–50.

93. Lemke U, Krones-Herzig A, Berriel Diaz M, et al. The glucocorticoid receptor controls hepatic dyslipidemia through Hes1. Cell Metab 2008;8(3):212–23.

94. Zoppini G, Targher G, Venturi C, et al. Relationship of nonalcoholic hepatic steatosis to overnight low-dose dexamethasone suppression test in obese individuals. Clin Endocrinol (Oxf) 2004;61(6):711–5.

95. Ahmed A, Rabbitt E, Brady T, et al. A switch in hepatic cortisol metabolism across the spectrum of non alcoholic fatty liver disease. PLoS One 2012;7(2): e29531.

96. Westerbacka J, Yki-Jarvinen H, Vehkavaara S, et al. Body fat distribution and cortisol metabolism in healthy men: enhanced 5beta-reductase and lower cortisol/cortisone metabolite ratios in men with fatty liver. J Clin Endocrinol Metab 2003;88(10):4924–31.

97. Targher G, Bertolini L, Zoppini G, et al. Relationship of non-alcoholic hepatic steatosis to cortisol secretion in diet-controlled Type 2 diabetic patients. Diabet Med 2005;22(9):1146–50.

98. Rockall AG, Sohaib SA, Evans D, et al. Hepatic steatosis in Cushing's syndrome: a radiological assessment using computed tomography. Eur J Endocrinol 2003; 149(6):543–8.

99. Dourakis SP, Sevastianos VA, Kaliopi P. Acute severe steatohepatitis related to prednisolone therapy. Am J Gastroenterol 2002;97(4):1074–5.

100. Nanki T, Koike R, Miyasaka N. Subacute severe steatohepatitis during prednisolone therapy for systemic lupus erythematosus. Am J Gastroenterol 1999; 94(11):3379.

101. Choi HK, Seeger JD. Glucocorticoid use and serum lipid levels in US adults: the Third National Health and Nutrition Examination Survey. Arthritis Rheum 2005; 53(4):528–35.

102. Wang X, Magkos F, Patterson BW, et al. Low-dose dexamethasone administration for 3 weeks favorably affects plasma HDL concentration and composition but does not affect very low-density lipoprotein kinetics. Eur J Endocrinol 2012;167(2):217–23.

103. Filipsson H, Monson JP, Koltowska-Haggstrom M, et al. The impact of glucocorticoid replacement regimens on metabolic outcome and comorbidity in hypopituitary patients. J Clin Endocrinol Metab 2006;91(10):3954–61.

104. Berg AL, Nilsson-Ehle P. ACTH lowers serum lipids in steroid-treated hyperlipemic patients with kidney disease. Kidney Int 1996;50(2):538–42.

105. Berg AL, Hansson P, Nilsson-Ehle P. ACTH 1-24 decreases hepatic lipase activities and low density lipoprotein concentrations in healthy men. J Intern Med 1991;229(2):201–3.

106. Berg AL, Nilsson-Ehle P. Direct effects of corticotropin on plasma lipoprotein metabolism in man—studies in vivo and in vitro. Metabolism 1994;43(1):90–7.

107. Arnaldi G, Angeli A, Atkinson AB, et al. Diagnosis and complications of Cushing's syndrome: a consensus statement. J Clin Endocrinol Metab 2003;88(12): 5593–602.

108. Giordano R, Picu A, Marinazzo E, et al. Metabolic and cardiovascular outcomes in patients with Cushing's syndrome of different aetiologies during active disease and 1 year after remission. Clin Endocrinol 2011;75(3):354–60.

109. Mancini T, Kola B, Mantero F, et al. High cardiovascular risk in patients with Cushing's syndrome according to 1999 WHO/ISH guidelines. Clin Endocrinol (Oxf) 2004;61(6):768–77.

110. Moisan MP, Seckl JR, Edwards CR. 11 beta-hydroxysteroid dehydrogenase bioactivity and messenger RNA expression in rat forebrain: localization in hypothalamus, hippocampus, and cortex. Endocrinology 1990;127(3):1450–5.

111. Lakshmi V, Sakai RR, McEwen BS, et al. Regional distribution of 11 beta-hydroxysteroid dehydrogenase in rat brain. Endocrinology 1991;128(4): 1741–8.

112. Seckl JR, Dow RC, Low SC, et al. The 11 beta-hydroxysteroid dehydrogenase inhibitor glycyrrhetinic acid affects corticosteroid feedback regulation of hypothalamic corticotrophin-releasing peptides in rats. J Endocrinol 1993;136(3):471–7.

113. Bisschop PH, Dekker MJ, Osterthun W, et al. Expression of 11beta-hydroxysteroid dehydrogenase type 1 in the human hypothalamus. J Neuroendocrinol 2013;25(5):425–32.

114. Zakrzewska KE, Cusin I, Stricker-Krongrad A, et al. Induction of obesity and hyperleptinemia by central glucocorticoid infusion in the rat. Diabetes 1999;48(2): 365–70.

115. Asensio C, Muzzin P, Rohner-Jeanrenaud F. Role of glucocorticoids in the physiopathology of excessive fat deposition and insulin resistance. Int J Obes Relat Metab Disord 2004;28(Suppl 4):S45–52.

116. Cusin I, Rouru J, Rohner-Jeanrenaud F. Intracerebroventricular glucocorticoid infusion in normal rats: induction of parasympathetic-mediated obesity and insulin resistance. Obes Res 2001;9(7):401–6.

117. Yi CX, Foppen E, Abplanalp W, et al. Glucocorticoid signaling in the arcuate nucleus modulates hepatic insulin sensitivity. Diabetes 2012;61(2):339–45.

118. Kuo LE, Kitlinska JB, Tilan JU, et al. Neuropeptide Y acts directly in the periphery on fat tissue and mediates stress-induced obesity and metabolic syndrome. Nat Med 2007;13(7):803–11.

119. Kola B, Christ-Crain M, Lolli F, et al. Changes in adenosine 5'-monophosphate-activated protein kinase as a mechanism of visceral obesity in Cushing's syndrome. J Clin Endocrinol Metab 2008;93(12):4969–73.

120. Kola B, Boscaro M, Rutter GA, et al. Expanding role of AMPK in endocrinology. Trends Endocrinol Metab 2006;17(5):205–15.

121. Gauthier MS, O'Brien EL, Bigornia S, et al. Decreased AMP-activated protein kinase activity is associated with increased inflammation in visceral adipose tissue and with whole-body insulin resistance in morbidly obese humans. Biochem Biophys Res Commun 2011;404(1):382–7.

122. Christ-Crain M, Kola B, Lolli F, et al. AMP-activated protein kinase mediates glucocorticoid-induced metabolic changes: a novel mechanism in Cushing's syndrome. FASEB J 2008;22(6):1672–83.

123. Butler H, Korbonits M. Cannabinoids for clinicians: the rise and fall of the cannabinoid antagonists. Eur J Endocrinol 2009;161(5):655–62.

124. Cota D, Marsicano G, Tschop M, et al. The endogenous cannabinoid system affects energy balance via central orexigenic drive and peripheral lipogenesis. J Clin Invest 2003;112(3):423–31.

125. Di S, Malcher-Lopes R, Halmos KC, et al. Nongenomic glucocorticoid inhibition via endocannabinoid release in the hypothalamus: a fast feedback mechanism. J Neurosci 2003;23(12):4850–7.

126. Di S, Malcher-Lopes R, Marcheselli VL, et al. Rapid glucocorticoid-mediated endocannabinoid release and opposing regulation of glutamate and gamma-aminobutyric acid inputs to hypothalamic magnocellular neurons. Endocrinology 2005;146(10):4292–301.

127. Scerif M, Fuzesi T, Thomas JD, et al. CB1 receptor mediates the effects of glucocorticoids on AMPK activity in the hypothalamus. J Endocrinol 2013;219(1):79–88.

128. Scherer T, Buettner C. The dysregulation of the endocannabinoid system in diabesity—a tricky problem. J Mol Med (Berl) 2009;87(7):663–8.

129. Tomlinson JW, Walker EA, Bujalska IJ, et al. 11beta-hydroxysteroid dehydrogenase type 1: a tissue-specific regulator of glucocorticoid response. Endocr Rev 2004;25(5):831–66.

130. Rask E, Olsson T, Soderberg S, et al. Tissue-specific dysregulation of cortisol metabolism in human obesity. J Clin Endocrinol Metab 2001;86(3):1418–21.
131. Engeli S, Bohnke J, Feldpausch M, et al. Regulation of 11beta-HSD genes in human adipose tissue: influence of central obesity and weight loss. Obes Res 2004;12(1):9–17.
132. Paulsen SK, Pedersen SB, Fisker S, et al. 11Beta-HSD type 1 expression in human adipose tissue: impact of gender, obesity, and fat localization. Obesity (Silver Spring) 2007;15(8):1954–60.
133. Anagnostis P, Athyros VG, Tziomalos K, et al. Clinical review: the pathogenetic role of cortisol in the metabolic syndrome: a hypothesis. J Clin Endocrinol Metab 2009;94(8):2692–701.
134. Bujalska IJ, Kumar S, Stewart PM. Does central obesity reflect "Cushing's disease of the omentum"? Lancet 1997;349(9060):1210–3.
135. Stimson RH, Andersson J, Andrew R, et al. Cortisol release from adipose tissue by 11beta-hydroxysteroid dehydrogenase type 1 in humans. Diabetes 2009; 58(1):46–53.
136. Morton NM, Seckl JR. 11beta-hydroxysteroid dehydrogenase type 1 and obesity. Front Horm Res 2008;36:146–64.
137. Bujalska IJ, Gathercole LL, Tomlinson JW, et al. A novel selective 11beta-hydroxysteroid dehydrogenase type 1 inhibitor prevents human adipogenesis. J Endocrinol 2008;197(2):297–307.
138. Kotelevtsev Y, Holmes MC, Burchell A, et al. 11beta-hydroxysteroid dehydrogenase type 1 knockout mice show attenuated glucocorticoid-inducible responses and resist hyperglycemia on obesity or stress. Proc Natl Acad Sci U S A 1997; 94(26):14924–9.
139. Holmes MC, Kotelevtsev Y, Mullins JJ, et al. Phenotypic analysis of mice bearing targeted deletions of 11beta-hydroxysteroid dehydrogenases 1 and 2 genes. Mol Cell Endocrinol 2001;171(1–2):15–20.
140. Alberts P, Engblom L, Edling N, et al. Selective inhibition of 11beta-hydroxysteroid dehydrogenase type 1 decreases blood glucose concentrations in hyperglycaemic mice. Diabetologia 2002;45(11):1528–32.
141. Morton NM, Paterson JM, Masuzaki H, et al. Novel adipose tissue-mediated resistance to diet-induced visceral obesity in 11 beta-hydroxysteroid dehydrogenase type 1-deficient mice. Diabetes 2004;53(4):931–8.
142. Bujalska IJ, Kumar S, Hewison M, et al. Differentiation of adipose stromal cells: the roles of glucocorticoids and 11beta-hydroxysteroid dehydrogenase. Endocrinology 1999;140(7):3188–96.
143. Basu R, Basu A, Grudzien M, et al. Liver is the site of splanchnic cortisol production in obese nondiabetic humans. Diabetes 2009;58(1):39–45.
144. Lavery GG, Zielinska AE, Gathercole LL, et al. Lack of significant metabolic abnormalities in mice with liver-specific disruption of 11beta-hydroxysteroid dehydrogenase type 1. Endocrinology 2012;153(7):3236–48.
145. Masuzaki H, Yamamoto H, Kenyon CJ, et al. Transgenic amplification of glucocorticoid action in adipose tissue causes high blood pressure in mice. J Clin Invest 2003;112(1):83–90.
146. Paterson JM, Morton NM, Fievet C, et al. Metabolic syndrome without obesity: hepatic overexpression of 11beta-hydroxysteroid dehydrogenase type 1 in transgenic mice. Proc Natl Acad Sci U S A 2004;101(18):7088–93.
147. Morton NM, Densmore V, Wamil M, et al. A polygenic model of the metabolic syndrome with reduced circulating and intra-adipose glucocorticoid action. Diabetes 2005;54(12):3371–8.

148. Stewart PM, Tomlinson JW. Selective inhibitors of 11beta-hydroxysteroid dehydrogenase type 1 for patients with metabolic syndrome: is the target liver, fat, or both? Diabetes 2009;58(1):14–5.

149. Harno E, Cottrell EC, Keevil BG, et al. 11-Dehydrocorticosterone causes metabolic syndrome, which is prevented when 11beta-HSD1 is knocked out in livers of male mice. Endocrinology 2013;154(10):3599–609.

150. Rask E, Walker BR, Soderberg S, et al. Tissue-specific changes in peripheral cortisol metabolism in obese women: increased adipose 11beta-hydroxysteroid dehydrogenase type 1 activity. J Clin Endocrinol Metab 2002;87(7):3330–6.

151. Mariniello B, Ronconi V, Rilli S, et al. Adipose tissue 11beta-hydroxysteroid dehydrogenase type 1 expression in obesity and Cushing's syndrome. Eur J Endocrinol 2006;155(3):435–41.

152. Paulmyer-Lacroix O, Boullu S, Oliver C, et al. Expression of the mRNA coding for 11beta-hydroxysteroid dehydrogenase type 1 in adipose tissue from obese patients: an in situ hybridization study. J Clin Endocrinol Metab 2002;87(6):2701–5.

153. Tomlinson JW, Moore JS, Clark PM, et al. Weight loss increases 11beta-hydroxysteroid dehydrogenase type 1 expression in human adipose tissue. J Clin Endocrinol Metab 2004;89(6):2711–6.

154. Basu R, Singh RJ, Basu A, et al. Obesity and type 2 diabetes do not alter splanchnic cortisol production in humans. J Clin Endocrinol Metab 2005; 90(7):3919–26.

155. Tomlinson JW, Sinha B, Bujalska I, et al. Expression of 11beta-hydroxysteroid dehydrogenase type 1 in adipose tissue is not increased in human obesity. J Clin Endocrinol Metab 2002;87(12):5630–5.

156. Valsamakis G, Anwar A, Tomlinson JW, et al. 11beta-hydroxysteroid dehydrogenase type 1 activity in lean and obese males with type 2 diabetes mellitus. J Clin Endocrinol Metab 2004;89(9):4755–61.

157. Kerstens MN, Riemens SC, Sluiter WJ, et al. Lack of relationship between 11beta-hydroxysteroid dehydrogenase setpoint and insulin sensitivity in the basal state and after 24h of insulin infusion in healthy subjects and type 2 diabetic patients. Clin Endocrinol (Oxf) 2000;52(4):403–11.

158. Purnell JQ, Kahn SE, Samuels MH, et al. Enhanced cortisol production rates, free cortisol, and 11beta-HSD-1 expression correlate with visceral fat and insulin resistance in men: effect of weight loss. Am J Physiol Endocrinol Metab 2009; 296(2):E351–7.

159. Alberti L, Girola A, Gilardini L, et al. Type 2 diabetes and metabolic syndrome are associated with increased expression of 11beta-hydroxysteroid dehydrogenase 1 in obese subjects. Int J Obes (Lond) 2007;31(12):1826–31.

160. Uckaya G, Karadurmus N, Kutlu O, et al. Adipose tissue 11-beta-hydroxysteroid dehydrogenase type 1 and hexose-6-phosphate dehydrogenase gene expressions are increased in patients with type 2 diabetes mellitus. Diabetes Res Clin Pract 2008;82(Suppl 2):S135–40.

161. Tomlinson JW, Finney J, Gay C, et al. Impaired glucose tolerance and insulin resistance are associated with increased adipose 11beta-hydroxysteroid dehydrogenase type 1 expression and elevated hepatic 5alpha-reductase activity. Diabetes 2008;57(10):2652–60.

162. Stewart PM, Boulton A, Kumar S, et al. Cortisol metabolism in human obesity: impaired cortisone–>cortisol conversion in subjects with central adiposity. J Clin Endocrinol Metab 1999;84(3):1022–7.

163. Lindsay RS, Wake DJ, Nair S, et al. Subcutaneous adipose 11 beta-hydroxysteroid dehydrogenase type 1 activity and messenger ribonucleic

acid levels are associated with adiposity and insulinemia in Pima Indians and Caucasians. J Clin Endocrinol Metab 2003;88(6):2738–44.

164. Tomlinson JW, Moore J, Cooper MS, et al. Regulation of expression of 11beta-hydroxysteroid dehydrogenase type 1 in adipose tissue: tissue-specific induction by cytokines. Endocrinology 2001;142(5):1982–9.

165. Espindola-Antunes D, Kater CE. Adipose tissue expression of 11beta-hydroxysteroid dehydrogenase type 1 in Cushing's syndrome and in obesity. Arq Bras Endocrinol Metabol 2007;51(8):1397–403.

166. Walker BR, Connacher AA, Lindsay RM, et al. Carbenoxolone increases hepatic insulin sensitivity in man: a novel role for 11-oxosteroid reductase in enhancing glucocorticoid receptor activation. J Clin Endocrinol Metab 1995;80(11):3155–9.

167. Andrews RC, Rooyackers O, Walker BR. Effects of the 11 beta-hydroxysteroid dehydrogenase inhibitor carbenoxolone on insulin sensitivity in men with type 2 diabetes. J Clin Endocrinol Metab 2003;88(1):285–91.

168. Tomlinson JW, Sherlock M, Hughes B, et al. Inhibition of 11beta-hydroxysteroid dehydrogenase type 1 activity in vivo limits glucocorticoid exposure to human adipose tissue and decreases lipolysis. J Clin Endocrinol Metab 2007;92(3): 857–64.

169. Barf T, Vallgarda J, Emond R, et al. Arylsulfonamidothiazoles as a new class of potential antidiabetic drugs. Discovery of potent and selective inhibitors of the 11beta-hydroxysteroid dehydrogenase type 1. J Med Chem 2002;45(18): 3813–5.

170. Hermanowski-Vosatka A, Balkovec JM, Cheng K, et al. 11beta-HSD1 inhibition ameliorates metabolic syndrome and prevents progression of atherosclerosis in mice. J Exp Med 2005;202(4):517–27.

171. Sundbom M, Kaiser C, Bjorkstrand E, et al. Inhibition of 11betaHSD1 with the S-phenylethylaminothiazolone BVT116429 increases adiponectin concentrations and improves glucose homeostasis in diabetic KKAy mice. BMC Pharmacol 2008;8:3.

172. Berthiaume M, Laplante M, Festuccia W, et al. Depot-specific modulation of rat intraabdominal adipose tissue lipid metabolism by pharmacological inhibition of 11beta-hydroxysteroid dehydrogenase type 1. Endocrinology 2007;148(5): 2391–7.

173. Berthiaume M, Laplante M, Festuccia WT, et al. 11beta-HSD1 inhibition improves triglyceridemia through reduced liver VLDL secretion and partitions lipids toward oxidative tissues. Am J Physiol Endocrinol Metab 2007;293(4): E1045–52.

174. Berthiaume M, Laplante M, Festuccia WT, et al. Additive action of 11beta-HSD1 inhibition and PPAR-gamma agonism on hepatic steatosis and triglyceridemia in diet-induced obese rats. Int J Obes (Lond) 2009;33(5):601–4.

175. Edgerton DS, Basu R, Ramnanan CJ, et al. Effect of 11 beta-hydroxysteroid dehydrogenase-1 inhibition on hepatic glucose metabolism in the conscious dog. Am J Physiol Endocrinol Metab 2010;298(5):E1019–26.

176. Rosenstock J, Banarer S, Fonseca VA, et al. The 11-beta-hydroxysteroid dehydrogenase type 1 inhibitor INCB13739 improves hyperglycemia in patients with type 2 diabetes inadequately controlled by metformin monotherapy. Diabetes Care 2010;33(7):1516–22.

177. Feig PU, Shah S, Hermanowski-Vosatka A, et al. Effects of an 11beta-hydroxysteroid dehydrogenase type 1 inhibitor, MK-0916, in patients with type 2 diabetes mellitus and metabolic syndrome. Diabetes Obes Metab 2011;13(6): 498–504.

178. Shah S, Hermanowski-Vosatka A, Gibson K, et al. Efficacy and safety of the selective 11beta-HSD-1 inhibitors MK-0736 and MK-0916 in overweight and obese patients with hypertension. J Am Soc Hypertens 2011;5(3):166–76.

179. Abrahams L, Semjonous NM, Guest P, et al. Biomarkers of hypothalamic-pituitary-adrenal axis activity in mice lacking 11beta-HSD1 and H6PDH. J Endocrinol 2012;214(3):367–72.

180. Pasquali R, Ambrosi B, Armanini D, et al. Cortisol and ACTH response to oral dexamethasone in obesity and effects of sex, body fat distribution, and dexamethasone concentrations: a dose-response study. J Clin Endocrinol Metab 2002;87(1):166–75.

181. Mattsson C, Reynolds RM, Simonyte K, et al. Combined receptor antagonist stimulation of the hypothalamic-pituitary-adrenal axis test identifies impaired negative feedback sensitivity to cortisol in obese men. J Clin Endocrinol Metab 2009;94(4):1347–52.

182. Vicennati V, Pasquali R. Abnormalities of the hypothalamic-pituitary-adrenal axis in nondepressed women with abdominal obesity and relations with insulin resistance: evidence for a central and a peripheral alteration. J Clin Endocrinol Metab 2000;85(11):4093–8.

183. Lottenberg SA, Giannella-Neto D, Derendorf H, et al. Effect of fat distribution on the pharmacokinetics of cortisol in obesity. Int J Clin Pharmacol Ther 1998;36(9):501–5.

184. Korbonits M, Trainer PJ, Nelson ML, et al. Differential stimulation of cortisol and dehydroepiandrosterone levels by food in obese and normal subjects: relation to body fat distribution. Clin Endocrinol 1996;45(6):699–706.

185. Pasquali R, Anconetani B, Chattat R, et al. Hypothalamic-pituitary-adrenal axis activity and its relationship to the autonomic nervous system in women with visceral and subcutaneous obesity: effects of the corticotropin-releasing factor/arginine-vasopressin test and of stress. Metabolism 1996;45(3):351–6.

186. Fraser R, Ingram MC, Anderson NH, et al. Cortisol effects on body mass, blood pressure, and cholesterol in the general population. Hypertension 1999;33(6):1364–8.

187. Marin P, Darin N, Amemiya T, et al. Cortisol secretion in relation to body fat distribution in obese premenopausal women. Metabolism 1992;41(8):882–6.

188. Pasquali R, Biscotti D, Spinucci G, et al. Pulsatile secretion of ACTH and cortisol in premenopausal women: effect of obesity and body fat distribution. Clin Endocrinol (Oxf) 1998;48(5):603–12.

189. Adam EK, Doane LD, Zinbarg RE, et al. Prospective prediction of major depressive disorder from cortisol awakening responses in adolescence. Psychoneuroendocrinology 2010;35(6):921–31.

190. Adam TC, Hasson RE, Ventura EE, et al. Cortisol is negatively associated with insulin sensitivity in overweight Latino youth. J Clin Endocrinol Metab 2010;95(10):4729–35.

191. Otte C, Wust S, Zhao S, et al. Glucocorticoid receptor gene, low-grade inflammation, and heart failure: the Heart and Soul study. J Clin Endocrinol Metab 2010;95(6):2885–91.

192. Manenschijn L, van den Akker EL, Lamberts SW, et al. Clinical features associated with glucocorticoid receptor polymorphisms. An overview. Ann N Y Acad Sci 2009;1179:179–98.

193. Geelen CC, van Greevenbroek MM, van Rossum EF, et al. Bcll glucocorticoid receptor polymorphism is associated with greater body fatness: the Hoorn and CODAM studies. J Clin Endocrinol Metab 2013;98(3):E595–9.

194. Epel ES, McEwen B, Seeman T, et al. Stress and body shape: stress-induced cortisol secretion is consistently greater among women with central fat. Psychosom Med 2000;62(5):623–32.
195. Pasquali R, Vicennati V. Activity of the hypothalamic-pituitary-adrenal axis in different obesity phenotypes. Int J Obes Relat Metab Disord 2000;24(Suppl 2):S47–9.
196. Manenschijn L, Schaap L, van Schoor NM, et al. High long-term cortisol levels, measured in scalp hair, are associated with a history of cardiovascular disease. J Clin Endocrinol Metab 2013;98(5):2078–83.
197. Stalder T, Kirschbaum C, Alexander N, et al. Cortisol in hair and the metabolic syndrome. J Clin Endocrinol Metab 2013;98(6):2573–80.
198. Huizenga NA, Koper JW, de Lange P, et al. Interperson variability but intraperson stability of baseline plasma cortisol concentrations, and its relation to feedback sensitivity of the hypothalamo-pituitary-adrenal axis to a low dose of dexamethasone in elderly individuals. J Clin Endocrinol Metab 1998;83(1): 47–54.
199. Xu H, Barnes GT, Yang Q, et al. Chronic inflammation in fat plays a crucial role in the development of obesity-related insulin resistance. J Clin Invest 2003; 112(12):1821–30.
200. Large V, Reynisdottir S, Langin D, et al. Decreased expression and function of adipocyte hormone-sensitive lipase in subcutaneous fat cells of obese subjects. J Lipid Res 1999;40(11):2059–66.
201. Cawthorn WP, Sethi JK. TNF-alpha and adipocyte biology. FEBS Lett 2008; 582(1):117–31.
202. Borst SE. The role of TNF-alpha in insulin resistance. Endocrine 2004;23(2–3): 177–82.
203. Kosteli A, Sugaru E, Haemmerle G, et al. Weight loss and lipolysis promote a dynamic immune response in murine adipose tissue. J Clin Invest 2010; 120(10):3466–79.
204. Capel F, Klimcakova E, Viguerie N, et al. Macrophages and adipocytes in human obesity: adipose tissue gene expression and insulin sensitivity during calorie restriction and weight stabilization. Diabetes 2009;58(7):1558–67.
205. Waage A, Bakke O. Glucocorticoids suppress the production of tumour necrosis factor by lipopolysaccharide-stimulated human monocytes. Immunology 1988; 63(2):299–302.
206. Udono-Fujimori R, Totsune K, Murakami O, et al. Suppression of cytokine-induced expression of endothelin-1 by dexamethasone in human retinal pigment epithelial cells. J Cardiovasc Pharmacol 2004;44:S471–3.
207. Pereda MP, Lohrer P, Kovalovsky D, et al. Interleukin-6 is inhibited by glucocorticoids and stimulates ACTH secretion and POMC expression in human corticotroph pituitary adenomas. Exp Clin Endocrinol Diabetes 2000;108:202–7.
208. Barber AE, Coyle SM, Marano MA, et al. Glucocorticoid therapy alters hormonal and cytokine responses to endotoxin in man. J Immunol 1993;150(5): 1999–2006.
209. DeRijk R, Michelson D, Karp B, et al. Exercise and circadian rhythm-induced variations in plasma cortisol differentially regulate interleukin-1 beta (IL-1 beta), IL-6, and tumor necrosis factor-alpha (TNF alpha) production in humans: high sensitivity of TNF alpha and resistance of IL-6. J Clin Endocrinol Metab 1997;82(7):2182–91.
210. Lionakis MS, Kontoyiannis DP. Glucocorticoids and invasive fungal infections. Lancet 2003;362(9398):1828–38.

211. Rajala MW, Scherer PE. Minireview: the adipocyte—at the crossroads of energy homeostasis, inflammation, and atherosclerosis. Endocrinology 2003;144(9):3765–73.
212. Trayhurn P, Wood IS. Adipokines: inflammation and the pleiotropic role of white adipose tissue. Br J Nutr 2004;92(3):347–55.
213. Papanicolaou DA, Tsigos C, Oldfield EH, et al. Acute glucocorticoid deficiency is associated with plasma elevations of interleukin-6: does the latter participate in the symptomatology of steroid withdrawal syndrome and adrenal insufficiency? J Clin Endocrinol Metab 1996;81:2303–6.
214. Setola E, Losa M, Lanzi R, et al. Increased insulin-stimulated endothelin-1 release is a distinct vascular phenotype distinguishing Cushing's disease from metabolic syndrome. Clin Endocrinol 2007;66:586–92.
215. Ueland T, Kristo C, Godang K, et al. Interleukin-1 receptor antagonist is associated with fat distribution in endogenous Cushing's syndrome: a longitudinal study. J Clin Endocrinol Metab 2003;88:1492–6.

Type 2 Diabetes Mellitus and Hypertension: An Update

Guido Lastra, MD[a,b,c], Sofia Syed, MD[a,b],
L. Romayne Kurukulasuriya, MD[a], Camila Manrique, MD[a,b,c],
James R. Sowers, MD[a,b,c,d],*

KEYWORDS

- Diabetes • Hypertension • Cardiovascular disease • Chronic kidney disease
- Renin-angiotensin-aldosterone system • Sympathetic nervous system

KEY POINTS

- Patients with hypertension and type 2 diabetes are at increased risk of cardiovascular and chronic renal disease.
- Factors involved in the pathogenesis of both hypertension and type 2 diabetes include inappropriate activation of the renin-angiotensin-aldosterone system, oxidative stress, inflammation, impaired insulin-mediated vasodilatation, augmented sympathetic nervous system activation, altered innate and adaptive immunity, and abnormal sodium processing by the kidney.
- The renin-angiotensin-aldosterone system blockade is a key therapeutic strategy in the treatment of hypertension in type 2 diabetes.
- Emerging therapies include renal denervation and carotid body denervation.

INTRODUCTION

Hypertension (HTN) is present in more than 50% of patients with diabetes mellitus (DM) and contributes significantly to both microvascular and macrovascular disease in DM (**Fig. 1**).[1–4] The risk for cardiovascular disease (CVD) is 4-fold higher in patients

Disclosures: The authors have nothing to disclose.
Funding Sources: Dr J.R. Sowers, NIH (R01 HL73101-01A1 and R01 HL107910-01), Veterans Affairs Merit System 0018.
Conflict of Interest: Dr J.R. Sowers is on the Merck Pharmaceuticals Advisory Board.
[a] Division of Endocrinology, Diabetes & Metabolism, Department of Internal Medicine, University of Missouri Columbia School of Medicine, D109 Diabetes Center HSC, One Hospital Drive, Columbia, MO 65212, USA; [b] Diabetes and Cardiovascular Research Center, University of Missouri, One Hospital Drive, Columbia, MO 65212, USA; [c] Harry S Truman Memorial Veterans Hospital, 800 Hospital Drive, Columbia, MO 65201, USA; [d] Department of Medical Physiology and Pharmacology, University of Missouri, One Hospital Drive, Columbia, MO 65212, USA
* Corresponding author. University of Missouri, D109 Diabetes Center HSC, One Hospital Drive, Columbia, MO 65212.
E-mail address: sowersj@health.missouri.edu

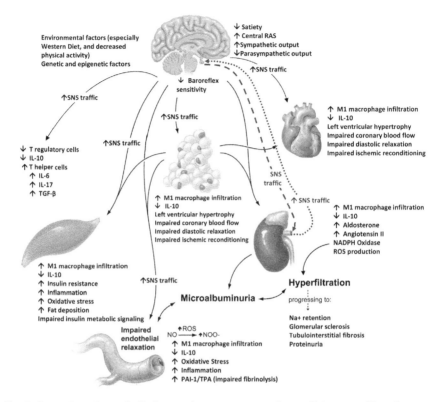

Fig. 1. Systemic and metabolic factors that promote coexistent diabetes mellitus, hypertension, cardiovascular, and chronic kidney disease. IL-10, interleukin 10; NADPH, nicotinamide adenine dinucleotide phosphate oxidase; PAI-1, plasminogen activator inhibitor 1; RAS, renin-angiotensin system; ROS, reactive oxygen species; SNS, sympathetic nervous system; TGF, tumor growth factor; TPA, tissue plasminogen activator. (*Adapted from* Sowers JR. Recent advances in hypertension. Diabetes Mellitus and Vascular Disease. Hypertension 2013;61:94; with permission.)

with both DM and HTN compared with the normotensive nondiabetic controls.[4,5] To this point, a meta-analysis of 102 prospective studies involving 698,782 individuals found that DM is responsible for approximately a 2-fold increased risk for coronary heart disease, stroke, and deaths from cardiovascular cause, including heart failure, cardiac arrhythmia, sudden death, hypertensive disease, and aortic aneurysms.[6] These data suggest that about 10% of vascular deaths in industrialized countries can be attributed to DM, and this burden will further increase as the incidence of diabetes continues to increase.[6] In the Framingham Heart Study, DM was associated with a 2-fold to 4-fold increased risk of myocardial infarction (MI), congestive heart failure, peripheral arterial disease, stroke, and death.[7] Furthermore, a more recent analysis of the Framingham data showed that the population with HTN at the time of DM diagnosis had higher rates of mortality for all causes (32 vs 20 per 1000 person-years; *P*<.001) and cardiovascular events (52 vs 31 per 1000 person-years; *P*<.001) compared with normotensive subjects with DM, thus suggesting that much of this excess risk is attributable to coexistent HTN.[8]

THE BURDEN

The National Health and Nutrition Examination Survey (NHANES) conducted from 2005 through 2008 estimated that HTN affects up to 65 million adults in the United States.[9] Only 50% of hypertensive individuals have their blood pressure (BP) under control.[10] The incidence of HTN is expected to increase further as the population ages and the frequency of obesity increases.[10,11] In a cross-sectional analysis of data from the Study to Help Improve Early Evaluation and Management of Risk Factors Leading to Diabetes (SHIELD) comparing health outcomes between patients with DM, HTN, and obesity relative to those with DM alone, obese patients with both DM and HTN had greater health care resource use, higher incidence of depression, and lower quality of life.[12] Another retrospective study assessed economic trends in patients with newly treated HTN only, DM only, and both newly treated HTN and DM for a period of time up to 24 months. Coexistent HTN and DM were associated with higher costs and resource use.[13] Furthermore, the post hoc analysis of CVD events found that the comorbid cohort had significantly more MIs and acute ischemic events, further increasing the cost of care.[13]

EPIDEMIOLOGY

In nondiabetic individuals, the prevalence of HTN is higher in men than in women until the age of 64 years when the gap closes and prevalence in women reaches that of men.[8] Women with impaired glucose tolerance (IGT) and DM have a higher incidence of HTN than men with equivalent impairment in glucose homeostasis.[14] Diabetic women also have higher relative risk for death from CVD than diabetic men.[15] The reason underlying the excess risk in diabetic women is still unclear. However, the increased risk of HTN in women with abnormal glucose tolerance may partially explain the high risk of CVD in this population.

The prevalence of HTN is different within various ethnic groups. In African Americans, the incidence of HTN is higher compared with white people between the ages of 45 and 75 years, after which it is same in both ethnicities.[16] Several mechanisms have been proposed to explain this finding, including higher rate of obesity, genetic predisposition, and environmental factors.[17] Defects in renal sodium processing have also been observed more frequently in the African American hypertensive populations, who have a greater prevalence of HTN and DM than other ethnic groups, further contributing to increased incidence of HTN.[18] In contrast, a recent analysis of the NHANES 1999 to 2008 data revealed that the Mexican-American populations, who have a high prevalence of DM, have a lower risk of coexistent uncontrolled HTN and DM compared with African Americans and white participants.[19] At present, limited data are available on the incidence of coexistent HTN and DM among Asian people in the United States.

There are several factors that contribute to increased coexistence of DM and HTN. The frequency of obesity in children and adolescents in industrialized countries has increased greatly over the last several decades, with an ominous parallel increment in the incidence of HTN and DM.[2,20] The multicenter Treatment Options for DM in Adolescents and Youth (TODAY) trial, which included 699 adolescents with DM aged 10 to 17 years, revealed that the prevalence of HTN increased from 11.6% at baseline to 33.8% by the end of study. Contrary to the adult data, the incidence of HTN was significantly increased in men versus women during the same period of time.[21]

PATHOPHYSIOLOGY: CONVERGING PATHWAYS IN COEXISTING DM AND HTN

DM and HTN share several pathophysiologic mechanisms including inappropriate activation of the renin-angiotensin-aldosterone system (RAAS), oxidative stress secondary to excessive production of reactive oxygen species (ROS), inflammation, impaired insulin-mediated vasodilatation, increased sympathetic nervous system (SNS) activation, dysfunctional innate and adaptive immune responses, and abnormal renal processing of sodium.[2,3] Obesity and increased visceral adiposity are key pathogenic factors behind the coexistence of both DM and HTN.[3] Chronic low-grade inflammation and oxidative stress in the adipose tissue lead to increased production of angiotensinogen (AGT) and angiotensin II (Ang II) with consequent tissue RAAS activation.[22,23] Further, overexpression of AGT in the white adipose tissue results in increased BP.[22] Hence, AGT and Ang II have local as well as systemic effects on BP regulation.[22,23] Ang II exerts many of its detrimental effects via activation of the Ang II type 1 receptor (AT1R).[24] The activation of AT1R in nonadrenal tissues results in multiple intracellular events, including production of ROS, reduced insulin metabolic signaling, and proliferative and inflammatory vascular responses resulting in endothelial dysfunction, insulin resistance and HTN.[24] Thus, there is often an activated RAAS in coexistent DM and HTN.

Increased aldosterone production and augmented signaling through the mineralocorticoid receptor (MR) are also key events in the pathogenesis of HTN.[25] Corticosteroids may also contribute to CVD in patients with DM via actions mediated in part through activation of the MR.[3] Adipose tissue is known to produce a lipid-soluble factor that stimulates aldosterone production from the adrenal zona glomerulosa.[26,27] Complement-C1q tumor necrosis factor (TNF)–related protein 1 (CTRP1) is a novel adipokine that promotes aldosterone production in a rodent model of obesity and insulin resistance.[28] Aldosterone activation of the MR in the renal distal tubule and collecting duct increases sodium retention leading to expansion of plasma volume and increased BP. In addition, aldosterone exerts nongenomic actions also likely through MR activation, which contribute to HTN by altering cellular redox state, signaling, and endothelial-mediated vascular relaxation.[25,27] Thus, adipose tissue contributes to systemic increases in BP, in part through local production of components of the RAAS.

ROLE OF OXIDATIVE STRESS

Increased oxidative stress is a key pathogenic factor in the development of insulin resistance, DM, and HTN.[29] ROS can be produced in different vascular cell types, including endothelial cells (ECs) and vascular smooth muscle cells (VSMCs) through activation of xanthine oxidase (XO), nitric oxide (NO) synthase, and the mitochondrial respiratory chain.[30–33] In turn, ROS can lead to impaired endothelial function by direct tissue injury, reduction of bioavailable NO, and impaired NO-mediated vasodilation.[30] One important additional source of ROS and endothelial dysfunction is endothelial NO synthase (eNOS) uncoupling. Under conditions of decreased availability of tetrahydrobiopterin (BH4, a cofactor in NO production) or the substrate L-arginine, eNOS switches from this coupled state to an uncoupled state, resulting in production of superoxide (O_{2-}).[31] Mitochondrial and XO-mediated oxidative stress also contribute to this excess generation of ROS in coexistent DM and HTN.[3] XO is also expressed in vascular endothelial cells and VSMC, and is another source of vascular oxidative stress, which generates O_{2-} by catalyzing hypoxanthine and xanthine to uric acid.[32] A major source of ROS is the membrane-bound vascular-derived nicotinamide adenine dinucleotide phosphate oxidase (NADPH), a protein enzyme composed of several subunits, including the membrane-bound subunits $p22^{phox}$ and Nox2; the cytosolic regulatory subunits $p47^{phox}$, $p67^{phox}$, $p40^{phox}$; and the small GTP-binding protein Rac1/Rac2.[34] Increased ROS production in turn results in cell as well as tissue damage by activating inflammatory pathways such as nuclear factor kappa B.

Inflammation is characterized by increased activity of adhesion molecules; proinflammatory cytokines, including TNF-α, interleukin (IL)-1 and IL-6, as well as acute-phase reactants such as C-reactive protein and molecules that promote fibrosis and remodeling, such as transforming growth factor beta (TGF-β) and plasminogen activator inhibitor 1 (PAI-1).[35] Mechanical stretch (a characteristic phenomenon in HTN) can lead to membrane translocation and activation of p47[phox] and Rac1, thus leading to NADPH oxidase activation.[32] Ang II and aldosterone can also directly activate NADPH oxidase and trigger oxidative stress.[33]

INSULIN RESISTANCE AND HYPERINSULINEMIA

Insulin resistance plays an important role in the development of both DM and HTN, as shown by approximately 50% of hypertensive patients manifesting systemic insulin resistance.[3,36,37] Binding of insulin to the insulin receptor (IR) triggers 2 major pathways. A metabolic signaling pathway mediated by phosphatidylinositol 3-kinase (PI3K), downstream protein kinase B signaling, results in translocation of glucose transporter 4 (GLUT-4) to plasma membrane, thus resulting in increased insulin-mediated glucose transport in insulin-sensitive tissues such as skeletal muscle.[38] In addition, signaling through the PI3K/Akt pathway results in phosphorylation/activation of eNOS and consequent NO production promotes endothelium-mediated vasodilation.[39] Insulin also signals through the growth/proliferative signaling pathway, which is mediated by mitogen-activated protein kinase (MAPK).[38,40] By activating MAPK-dependent signaling pathways, insulin stimulates secretion of vasoconstrictor mediators, such as endothelin-1,[41,42] as well as increased expression of PAI-1, and vascular cell adhesion molecule-1.[43] In conditions of normal insulin sensitivity, the balance between these vasoconstrictor and vasodilatory actions favors vasodilation. In insulin-resistant states there is often deficient insulin metabolic signaling in concert with unchecked signaling through the growth pathway.[1–3]

Maladaptive hyperinsulinemia/insulin resistance leads to abnormalities in vascular function, vascular stiffness, hypertrophy, fibrosis, and remodeling.[44] Hyperinsulinemia also results in enhanced sympathetic output in humans through ventromedial hypothalamus mechanisms.[45,46] In addition, leptin, which is an adipokine produced in adipose tissue and is increased in obese individuals, also increases sympathetic nerve activation likely through a central nervous system effect involving leptin receptor activation.[47,48] There is increasing evidence that increased afferent traffic from, and efferent activity to, the kidney plays an important role in development of HTN associated with obesity and insulin resistance.[3]

Insulin enhances sodium reabsorption in the diluting segment of the distal nephron, in part through increased expression of sodium transporters like the epithelial sodium channel (ENaC), with consequent decreases in sodium excretion.[49] Hyperinsulinemia-mediated sodium retention could potentially contribute to the genesis of HTN via increased activation of sodium-hydrogen exchanger activity in the proximal tubule as well as through the effects on ENaC more distally. Although this is an attractive hypothesis, in an animal model of knockout of IR in the renal tubule epithelial cells, the absence of insulin action resulted in impaired natriuretic responses and HTN, likely because of reduce NO production.[50] Because of these contradictory results, further studies are needed to clarify the physiologic role of insulin on renal sodium processing.

In addition, sodium and uric acid are generally handled together; hence excess uric acid can increase along with sodium retention, thereby contributing to hyperuricemia, which is frequently seen in hypertensive patients.[51] The propensity for increased uric acid levels is increased with westernized diets that are high in fructose (see **Fig. 1**).[3]

TREATMENT OF HTN: RATIONALE, STRATEGIES, AND CHALLENGES IN HTN
Impact of BP Control

High BP is a strong independent risk factor for CVD and chronic kidney disease (CKD), and, when HTN is associated with DM, the risk is increased even further.[4,52] Although controversy exists regarding the optimal target for BP reduction,[3,52,53] consistent control of BP in patients with DM is important for preventing and delaying both microvascular and macrovascular complications.[54,55] Early data from landmark trials such as the United Kingdom Prospective Diabetes Study (UKPDS), Hypertension Optimal Treatment (HOT), Systolic Hypertension in the Elderly (SHEP), and Systolic Hypertension in Europe (Syst-Eur) showed that strict BP control was beneficial in hypertensive patients with diabetes. In a 9-year follow-up of the UKPDS cohort, patients with both HTN and DM assigned to strict BP control (mean BP, 144/82 mm Hg) achieved a significant reduction in risk for all of the end points related to DM, including death related to DM and microvascular disease, relative to patients who were treated conventionally (mean BP, 154/87 mm Hg).[55] The group allocated to tight BP control had a significant reduction in the risk of heart failure, with an additional nonsignificant reduction in the risk of MI. However, when all macrovascular diseases were combined, including MI, sudden death, stroke, and peripheral vascular disease, the group assigned to tight BP control still had a significant reduction in risk compared with the group assigned to less tight control.[55]

The HOT study revealed that, among the 1501 patients with DM at baseline, a stricter BP control (mean BP, 140/81 mm Hg) halved the risk of major cardiovascular events compared with the control group (mean BP, 144/85 mm Hg).[56] The risk for stroke decreased significantly in individuals who reached the lower target BP. In participants reaching diastolic BP less than 80 mm Hg the risk was reduced roughly 30% relative to individuals who only reached a diastolic BP less than 90 mm Hg. In addition, cardiovascular mortality was also significantly lower in this group (diastolic BP less than 80 mm Hg) than in each of the other target groups. In addition, a nonsignificant decline was seen in the risk for all (MI) in the group with stricter BP control.[56]

In the Syst-Eur trial, 492 patients (10.5%) had DM; after a 2-year follow-up, the active treatment with antihypertensive drugs reduced overall mortality by 55%, mortality from cardiovascular causes by 76%, all cardiovascular events by 69%, fatal and nonfatal stroke by 73%, as well as all cardiac events by 63%.[57] In the SHEP trial, patients with DM randomized to active treatment with antihypertensive medications had lower frequency of stroke, nonfatal MI and fatal coronary heart disease (CHD), major coronary events, and all-cause mortality relative to patients treated with placebo.[58] The Appropriate Blood Pressure Control in Diabetes (ABCD) trial showed a significant decrease in all-cause stroke with intensive (mean BP, 133/78 mm Hg) versus moderate antihypertensive therapy (mean BP, 139/86 mm Hg) in patients with DM.[59] This finding is important because of the increased risk of both fatal and nonfatal stroke in patients with coexistent DM and HTN. In summary, although specific targets are still controversial, control of HTN in the setting of DM is strongly supported by current evidence showing the critical impact that BP has on CVD in diabetic individuals.[52,55,59]

BP Targets

Clinical management guidelines derived from the widely accepted Seventh Report of the Joint National Committee on Prevention, Detection, Evaluation, and Treatment of High Blood Pressure (JNC 7) and the American Diabetes Association (ADA) have recommended strict treatment of HTN in the setting of DM, aiming at values less than 130 mm Hg for systolic BP and less than 80 mm Hg for diastolic BP.[54] Nonetheless, the additional beneficial effects of such lower BP targets remain unproved.[53,60] Hence, the recently revised ADA guidelines suggest that the BP goal for people with DM and HTN should be less than 140/80 mm Hg.[61]

Most guidelines for management of HTN are based on the landmark UKPDS and HOT trials. However, the systolic BP achieved in the tight control arm in these trials was between 140 and 150 mm Hg. Only the intensive BP control groups in the hypertensive and normotensive ABCD studies reached the consensus JNC 7 goal of less than 130/80 mm Hg. The results of the Action to Control Cardiovascular Risk in Diabetes (ACCORD) BP study,[53] recently showed that, in patients with DM, targeting systolic BP to less than 120 mm Hg did not reduce the rate of CV events (nonfatal MI and death from cardiovascular causes), compared with subjects in whom the target was less than 140 mm Hg, except for fatal and nonfatal strokes. As expected, adverse events that were attributed to BP medication were more frequent in the intensive therapy group.[53] Likewise, a post hoc analysis of the International Verapamil SR-Trandolapril (INVEST) study concluded that reducing systolic BP to less than 130 mm Hg in patients with DM and coronary artery disease was not associated with improved CVD outcomes compared with conventional BP control (systolic BP of 130–139 mm Hg).[60]

In another post hoc analysis of the Ongoing Telmisartan Alone and in Combination with Ramipril Global Endpoint Trial (ONTARGET), the relationship between BP and overall cardiovascular risk followed a similar pattern in diabetic and nondiabetic patients. With the exception of stroke, reducing systolic BP to less than 130 mm Hg did not result in improvements in either fatal or nonfatal CVD outcomes.[62] Furthermore, a recent meta-analysis of 13 major trials done in patients with DM or IGT showed that at a systolic BP of less than 130 mm Hg there was only significant reduction in the rate of stroke, with no further reduction in cardiac, renal, or retinal outcomes; however, there was an increased incidence of major adverse events such as hyperkalemia, symptomatic hypotension, bradycardia, and cardiac arrhythmias.[63] An additional concern about strict BP targets is the possible deficiency in blood perfusion to the central nervous system in diabetic patients, who already have microvascular disease and impaired cerebrovascular autoregulation.[64]

The optimal BP goal for diabetic patients should be individualized. Nevertheless, available literature suggests that a maximal benefit of BP control in patients with DM is attained with systolic BP between 130 and 135 mm Hg and diastolic BP from 80 to 85 mm Hg, except in stoke prevention, for which data suggest that further lowering BP may be beneficial.

NONPHARMACOLOGIC TREATMENT: THE ROLE OF THERAPEUTIC LIFESTYLE INTERVENTION

Despite significant advances over the last several decades, the management of HTN is still not ideal, and about 50% of hypertensive patients are still not optimally controlled. The reasons underlying these results seem to be multiple and include deficiencies in current nonpharmacologic and pharmacologic management strategies. One of these issues, access to antihypertensive medications and BP control, was studied in the cross-sectional Reasons for Geographic And Racial Differences in Stroke (REGARDS) cohort study.[65] Although access to antihypertensive medications increased significantly from 66% in 2003 to 81% in 2007, this was not independently associated with improved BP control. African American ethnicity, male sex, low income, and medication nonadherence were significant predictors of inadequate BP control, suggesting that poor BP control is multifactorial.[65]

Nonpharmacologic lifestyle interventions, which include dietary changes, low-salt diet, weight loss, increased physical activity on a regular basis, and alcohol restriction, have been shown to reduce BP in several controlled studies. Lifestyle changes including individualized counseling designed to reduce total intake of fat and intake of saturated fat, and increasing intake of fiber and physical activity, result in significant improvements in BP and reduction in the incidence of DM.[66]

The Dietary Approach to Stop Hypertension (DASH) is a nutritional strategy promoted by the United States National Heart, Lungs and Blood Institute (NHLBI) as a nonpharmacologic intervention to prevent and control HTN. The DASH diet includes foods rich in fruits, vegetables, whole grains, and low-fat dairy products, and low in total fat and saturated fat, cholesterol, refined grains, and sweets, and has been shown to provide beneficial metabolic and cardiovascular effects in DM. Adherence to the DASH diet results in lower systolic as well as diastolic BP, body weight, waist circumference, blood glucose levels, and hemoglobin A1C. It also has beneficial actions on lipid profile, and has been shown to improve high-density lipoprotein cholesterol levels and reduce low-density lipoprotein cholesterol.[67,68]

The beneficial effects of the DASH diet are probably caused by its effect on some cardiovascular risk factors. After following the DASH diet for 8 weeks, liver aminotransferase enzymes, plasma fibrinogen levels, and high-sensitivity C-reactive protein (hs-CRP) were all reduced, suggesting that this type of diet can play an important role in reducing inflammation in DM.[69] In the Lifestyle Changes Through the Use of Delivered Meals and Dietary Counseling in a Single-blind Study (STYLIST), the combination of dietary counseling by dietitians and delivery of calorie-controlled meals was effective in reducing body weight, BP, and hemoglobin A1C in patients with HTN and/or DM.[70]

In addition, sodium intake has also been associated with CVD. Results from multiple trials have shown that reduction of dietary sodium (from a daily intake of 200 mmol [4600 mg] to 100 mmol [2300 mg] of sodium per day) reduces BP and may also reduce long-term risk of cardiovascular events.[71,72] However, results from a recent meta-analysis of 7 randomized controlled trials failed to provide strong evidence that salt reduction reduced all-cause mortality or CVD morbidity in normotensive or hypertensive individuals.[73] The interventions used in this meta-analysis were capable of reducing urinary sodium excretion. Systolic and diastolic BPs were also reduced by an average of 1 mm Hg in normotensives and by an average of 2 to 4 mm Hg in persons with HTN and those with heart failure.[73] However, the methods of achieving salt reduction in the trials included in the review were modest in their impacts on sodium excretion and on BP levels, and would not be expected to have major impacts on the burden of CVD. Sodium restriction has not been tested in the diabetic population in controlled clinical trials. However, in a recent animal study, the results are in favor of oxidative stress normalization as the beneficial influence of dietary sodium deprivation on cardiovascular remodeling in the model of insulin resistance in rats. Withdrawal of sodium from the fructose diet in these rats showed prevention of CVD effects of high fructose consumption, including production of superoxide anions/oxidative stress.[74] In summary, the available literature suggests that reduction of dietary salt reduces BP and may also reduce long-term risk of CVD events in hypertensive patients; however, the data in diabetic individuals are limited. Further, more studies are need to determine whether increasing dietary potassium, calcium, and magnesium may have beneficial effects on BP, CVD, and metabolic control in patients with coexistent DM and HTN.

In addition, physical inactivity is a major underlying risk for CVD. In addition to changing the dietary patterns, increased aerobic physical activity on a regular basis (such as brisk walking) is important in this population. Between 30 and 45 minutes of brisk walking 3 to 5 days a week has been shown to improve lipid profiles, BP, and insulin resistance,[75] and is currently recommended in most management guidelines.[61] Increased physical activity may decrease the rapidity of development of both CVD and CKD events in persons with DM and HTN.

PHARMACOLOGIC THERAPY
RAAS Blockade

Use of Ang II–converting enzyme inhibitors (ACEI) reduces the activity of Ang II, which results in vasodilatation, decreased BP, and improvement in the deleterious effects of Ang II on cardiac, vascular, and renal tissues.[76,77] The Heart Outcomes Prevention Evaluation (HOPE) study compared the effects of the ACE inhibitor ramipril versus placebo on cardiovascular complications and showed 25% risk reduction in MI, stroke, or cardiovascular death after a median follow-up period of 4.5 years.[78] A subgroup of 3577 diabetic patients was analyzed in the microalbuminuria, cardiovascular, and renal outcomes (MICRO)-HOPE study, and showed similar beneficial effects of ramipril on cardiovascular and all-cause mortality in patients with DM.[79]

In contrast with ACEI, Ang II receptor blockers (ARBs) do not increase the levels of bradykinin, which can cause low patient adherence because of induction of cough. In a subset of the Losartan Intervention For Endpoint Reduction in Hypertension (LIFE) study, including 1195 type 2 diabetic patients, a significant reduction in cardiovascular morbidity and mortality was reported in patients treated with losartan compared with individuals taking a β-blocker (atenolol). A relative risk reduction of 24% for the primary composite end point of cardiovascular morbidity and mortality (cardiovascular death, stroke, or MI) was seen in patients treated with losartan compared with atenolol despite similar BP reduction.[80]

In the Antihypertensive Long-Term Use Evaluation (VALUE) and the Candesartan Antihypertensive Survival Evaluation in Japan (CASE-J) trials, cardiac morbidity and mortality were no different in patients treated with ARBs (valsartan and candesartan respectively) relative to patients treated with the long-acting calcium channel blocker (CCB) amlodipine, although they did significantly reduce the incidence of DM.[81,82] In a subgroup analysis of the ONTARGET trial in 6391 patients with DM, telmisartan (ARB) and rampril (ACEI) had similar effects on cardiovascular morbidity and mortality.[83] However, in this study the patients who received combination therapy with ACEI and ARB had an increased risk of adverse side effects including hypotension, syncope, renal dysfunction, and hyperkalemia. The combination-therapy group had a significant increase in the relative risk of impairment of renal function (1.33, $P<.001$). Also the risk of hypotension was higher in the combination group, with a relative risk of 2.75 ($P<.001$). The numbers of patients who had an increase in potassium level of more than 5.5 mmol per liter were similar in the ramipril group (283 patients) and the telmisartan group (287 patients), but the number was significantly higher in the combination-therapy group (480 patients, $P<.001$). Therefore, current literature does not recommend combined treatment with ARB and ACEI.

In addition to cardiovascular protection, available literature shows that RAAS blockade provides renal protective effects. The Bergamo Nephrologic Diabetic complications Trial (BENEDICT) and the Randomized Olmesartan and Diabetes Microalbuminuria Prevention (ROADMAP) trials found that in patients with DM, HTN, and normoalbuminuria (<30 mg/g of creatinine), RAAS blockade with an ACEI and an ARB, respectively, delayed the onset of microalbuminuria (30–300 mg/g).[84,85] Nevertheless, in the Diabetic Retinopathy Candesartan Trial (DIRECT), RAAS blockade failed to show prevention of microalbuminuria in normotensive patients with type 1 or type 2 DM.[86]

There is significant collective evidence to support RAAS blockade as the first line of therapy for HTN in DM to prevent or delay microalbuminuria; however, evidence to sustain their use in normotensive diabetic patients (type 1 or 2) to prevent or delay the development of microalbuminuria is lacking.

In addition, RAAS blockade also has potential benefits beyond BP-lowering effects, including improvements in insulin resistance, inflammation, oxidative stress, and vascular function.[87] In large clinical trials, the Randomized Aldactone Evaluation Study (RALES) and Eplerenone Post–Acute Myocardial Infarction Heart Failure Efficacy and Survival Study (EPHESUS) trials, MR blockade showed improvement in cardiovascular morbidity and mortality.

Improvement in endothelial dysfunction; decreased activation of matrix metalloproteinases; improved ventricular remodeling; along with improvements in tissue fibrosis, inflammation, oxidative stress, and insulin resistance have been postulated as the possible mechanisms responsible for these actions.[87,88]

CCBs

CCBs are an effective and well-tolerated antihypertensive therapy and have been extensively studied. In the Antihypertensive and Lipid-Lowering Treatment to Prevent Heart Attack Trial (ALLHAT), treatment with amlodipine was associated with similar rates of coronary mortality and nonfatal MI to treatment with ACEI (lisinopril) and the diuretic chlorthalidone.[77] However, the heart failure rate was higher in patients treated with CCBs compared with chlorthalidone, which could be in part caused by lower BP attained in the patients treated with the diuretic, or discontinuation of diuretic therapy in the patients in the CCB group.

In diabetic hypertensive patients, some trials have shown that ACEI significantly reduced the risk of CVD compared with CCB,[89,90] whereas another large-scale trial showed no difference.[91] As described earlier, in the VALUE and the CASE-J trials, no significant difference was seen in cardiac composite end points between ARBs and CCBs.[81,92] In the Irbesartan Diabetic Nephropathy Trial (IDNT), this ARB showed better renal protection compared with CCB, but failed to show any difference in reduction in CVD between the two.[93]

In the large diabetic subgroup (5137 patients) in the BP-lowering arm of the Anglo-Scandinavian Cardiac Outcomes Trial (ASCOT), CCB (amlodipine) showed significant reduction in total cardiovascular events compared with β-blocker.[94]

Diuretics

Thiazide-type diuretics have been the basis of antihypertensive therapy for a long time. In the ALLHAT, the diuretic chlorthalidone was e as effective as CCBs and ACEIs in reducing cardiovascular morbidity and mortality.[77] In the Hypertension in the Very Elderly Trial (HYVET), the thiazidelike diuretic indapamide reduced the rate of stroke, CHD, heart failure, and all-cause mortality in very elderly hypertensive patients.[95]

Thiazide diuretics have some significant negative metabolic effects, in particular impaired glycemic control by impairment of insulin secretion and insulin sensitivity.[96,97] They may also worsen insulin sensitivity and glucose tolerance by activation of the RAAS and the SNS, which can be attenuated by addition of MR blocker.[98]

In high doses, diuretics can result in hypokalemia, hypomagnesemia, and/or hyperuricemia, all of which have been shown to worsen glucose control.[96,97] Most of the adverse effects of thiazides are dose dependent; hence using it in low dose combined with other medications helps to avoid metabolic side effects.

Use of other agents, like β-blockers, remains controversial. There is some emerging evidence that β-blockers may be associated with weight gain, which may further worsen glucose tolerance.[96,99] However, in contrast with conventional β-blockers, nebivolol, a selective blocker of β1-adrenergic receptor with NO-potentiating vasodilatory action, has not been associated with weight gain or with worsened glucose tolerance.[99]

β-Blockers are generally not used as first-line agents for HTN in diabetic individuals; however, they are considered as add-on therapy in patients with coronary artery disease and heart failure.[61]

INCRETIN-BASED THERAPY AND HTN: BEYOND GLYCEMIC CONTROL

A better understanding of the role of gut-derived hormones and their impact on carbohydrate homeostasis has been reached over the last decade, which has led to the development of incretin-based therapy. Glucagonlike peptide 1 (GLP-1) and glucose-dependent insulinotropic peptide have been extensively studied in these regards, and are known to potentiate insulin secretion in a glucose-dependent manner in response to the presence of nutrients in the gut (ie, the incretin effect). In addition, incretin hormones slow gastric emptying, thereby slowing the absorption of nutrients in the digestive tract, and suppressing glucagon production in pancreatic alpha cells.[100]

The incretin effect is typically blunted in the setting of DM, and is restored by GLP-1 analogues such as exenatide or liraglutide, as well as inhibitors of the enzyme dipeptidyl peptidase 4 (DPP-4), which rapidly cleaves and inactivates GLP-1. In turn, reduced degradation of GLP-1 by DPP-4 inhibitors results in an enhanced incretin effect. GLP-1 action derives from activation of a highly specific G protein–coupled receptor (GLP-1R), which is expressed in several tissues, including pancreas, nervous system, kidney, cardiovascular tissue, and immune cells.[101]

In the clinical setting, GLP-1 analogues and DPP-4 inhibitors have proved to be efficacious for DM treatment because they contribute to improved beta cell function and glycemic control. In addition, there is mounting interest in the impact of incretin-based therapy on the cardiovascular and renal systems.[102–110]

Both GLP-1 agonists and DPP-4 inhibitors have been shown to modulate BP, heart rate, and contractility. Knockout of GLP-1R in mice results in impaired myocardial contractility and diastolic function.[102] GLP-1 and DPP-4 inhibitors acutely induce increases in BP and heart rate in rodents.[103,104]

In humans, the actions of GLP-1 on BP and heart rate are less clear and experimental results have been more variable. Chronic treatment with GLP-1 analogues in type 2 diabetic patients results in improvements in both systolic and diastolic BP without affecting heart rate.[103,105] In a study by Mistry and colleagues,[106] treatment with the DPP-4 inhibitor sitagliptin similarly produced a modest reduction in BP. In young Zucker obese rats, treatment with linagliptin for 8 weeks resulted in improved diastolic function, left ventricular hypertrophy, and fibrosis. These changes occurred in concert with significant improvements in BP, eNOS, and calcium processing in cardiomyocytes.[107] In the vasculature, DPP-4 inhibition also seems to affect endothelial function. Two weeks of treatment with sitagliptin improved endothelium-dependent relaxation in renal arteries, restored renal blood flow, and reduced systolic BP in spontaneously hypertensive rats (SHRs).[108] In addition, treatment with GLP-1 reduced the size of MI (23.2%–14.1% of area at risk) in rat hearts.[109]

In addition, the impact of incretin-based therapy on BP seems to be also related to activation of GLP-1R in renal tissue, which results in decreased expression of the sodium-hydrogen transporter type 3 (NH3) and leads to increased diuresis and sodium excretion in renal proximal tubules.[110] DPP-4 inhibition results in lower mean BP in young SHRs treated with sitagliptin for 8 days, in concert with increased urinary flow and decreased NH3 expression and activity.[111]

COMBINED PHARMACOLOGIC THERAPY

Although treatment of HTN is often initiated with a single agent, most diabetic patients typically require combination therapy to control their BP. In a randomized, parallel-group, double-blind international trial comparing the once-daily single-pill combination of telmisartan 80 mg and amlodipine 10 mg (telmisartan/amlodipine; T/A) with once-daily amlodipine 10 mg (A) in patients with DM and HTN, T/A provided prompt and greater BP decreases compared with A monotherapy, with most patients achieving the BP goal (<140/90 mm Hg).[112]

The Avoiding Cardiovascular Events Through Combination Therapy in Patients Living With Systolic Hypertension (ACCOMPLISH) trial, which included 6946 patients with diabetes, compared the outcome effects of the ACEI benazepril (20–40 mg/d) combined with amlodipine (5–10 mg/d) (B + A) or hydrochlorothiazide (12.5–25 mg/d; B + H). B + A was superior to the B + H combination, because there was 20% reduction in the primary end point (CV death, stroke, MI, revascularization, hospitalization for unstable angina, or resuscitated cardiac arrest) in the B + A arm compared with the B + H arm ($P = .0002$) despite a similar reduction in BP in both groups. The mean value of BP after the treatment adjustments were 131.5/72.6 mm Hg in the B + A arm and 132.7/73.7 mm Hg in the B + H arm.[113] The study was stopped early because of a difference in outcomes favoring amlodipine. The data from this study are consistent with the ASCOT study,[114] which also showed the cardiovascular benefits of the ACEI/CCB combination.

Fixed-dose combinations in a single tablet may increase compliance compared with corresponding free-drug components given separately, because they simplify treatment and thereby can improve adherence on the part of the patients.[115]

The escalation of double-drug treatment to triple-drug therapy may improve BP control in clinical practice. A subgroup analysis in African Americans and non–African Americans with HTN compared triple-combination treatment with olmesartan 40 mg, amlodipine 10 mg, and hydrochlorothiazide 25 mg with the component dual-combination treatments. Triple-combination treatment resulted in significant and similar mean reductions in diastolic and systolic BP relative to dual-combination treatment. A greater proportion of participants on triple combination reached the target BP compared with dual-combination treatments at the end of 12 weeks regardless of ethnicity.[116] Because HTN and DM generally require multiple antihypertensive agents to achieve a goal BP, triple-combination therapy may represent an important treatment option to improve BP control in this patient population.

PERSPECTIVES
Telehealth

The treatment of HTN remains challenging and demands constant reshaping. Newer strategies are currently being tried for optimal control of HTN in diabetic patients, including the use of remote services like telehealth. Telehealth encompasses the use of medical information exchange remotely via electronic communications to improve a patient's clinical health status. The use of telehealth for transmission of education and advice to the patient on an ongoing basis with close surveillance by nurses and or physicians improves clinical outcomes.[117] A randomized controlled trial conducted at the Iowa City Veterans Affairs Medical Center, evaluated the efficacy of nurse-managed home telehealth intervention to improve outcomes in veterans with comorbid DM and HTN. Intervention subjects experienced a significant decrease in systolic BP compared with the other groups at 6 months and this pattern was maintained at 12 months.[117]

Renal Denervation

Activation of renal sympathetic nerves plays an important role in the pathogenesis of HTN.[118] Renal denervation (RDN) is a percutaneous catheter-based renal sympathetic denervation procedure to disrupt renal afferent and efferent nerves using radiofrequency ablation.[119–121] In a multicenter, prospective, randomized trial (Symplicity HTN-2) evaluating the role of RDN in patients with resistant HTN, office-based BP measurements in the group assigned to the procedure (n = 52) decreased by 32/12 mm Hg (baseline of 178/96 mm Hg; $P<.0001$). This reduction persisted after 6 months.[119] However, the study did not include ambulatory BP monitoring (ABPM) in the analysis, which has been shown to be more closely related to cardiovascular morbidity and mortality than office BP.[122,123]

Another study of 50 patients investigated the effect of RDN on glucose homeostasis and BP control in patients with resistant HTN. Systolic and diastolic BP, fasting glucose, insulin, C peptide, hemoglobin A1c, and insulin sensitivity were measured before, 1 month after, and 3 months after treatment. At 1 and 3 months, office BP was reduced by 28/10 mm Hg ($P<.001$) and 32/12 mm Hg ($P<.001$) respectively in the treatment groups, without changes in concurrent antihypertensive treatment. There were also significant improvements in fasting glucose, insulin, C-peptide levels, and markers of insulin resistance.[120] In a recent multicenter study, RDN showed significant reductions in systolic and diastolic BP, taken both in the office and through 24-h ABPM.[121] In-office systolic and diastolic BP changes were significantly more pronounced than changes in 24-hour continuous measurements. Furthermore, there was no effect on ABPM in pseudoresistant patients, whereas in-office BP was reduced to a similar extent. Thus, RDN may represent an important and novel approach for selective reduction of renal sympathetic drive that results in improvement in both insulin resistance and resistant HTN. This strategy deserves additional clinical research.

ACKNOWLEDGMENTS

The authors wish to thank Brenda Hunter for editorial assistance.

REFERENCES

1. Sowers JR, Epstein M, Frohlich ED. Diabetes, hypertension, and cardiovascular disease: an update. Hypertension 2001;37:1053–9.
2. Sowers JR, Whaley-Connell A, Hayden M. The role of overweight and obesity in the cardiorenal syndrome. Cardiorenal Med 2011;1:5–12.
3. Sowers JR. Diabetes mellitus and vascular disease. Hypertension 2013;61(5): 943–7.
4. Stamler J, Vaccaro O, Neaton JD, et al. Diabetes, other risk factors, and 12-yr cardiovascular mortality for men screened in the Multiple Risk Factor Intervention Trial. Diabetes Care 1993;16:434–44.
5. Hu G, Jousilahti P, Tuomilehto J. Joint effects of history of hypertension at baseline and type 2 diabetes at baseline and during follow-up on the risk of coronary heart disease. Eur Heart J 2007;28:3059–66.

6. Sarwar N, Gao P, Seshasai SR, et al, Emerging Risk Factors Collaboration. Diabetes mellitus, fasting blood glucose concentration, and risk of vascular disease: a collaborative meta-analysis of 102 prospective studies. Lancet 2010;375:2215–22.
7. Fox CS. Cardiovascular disease risk factors, type 2 diabetes mellitus, and the Framingham Heart Study. Trends Cardiovasc Med 2010;20:90–5.
8. Chen G, McAlister FA, Walker RL, et al. Cardiovascular outcomes in Framingham participants with diabetes: the importance of blood pressure. Hypertension 2011;57:891–7.
9. Egan BM, Zhao Y, Axon RN. US trends in prevalence, awareness, treatment, and control of hypertension, 1988-2008. JAMA 2010;303:2043.
10. Wright JD, Hughes JP, Ostchega Y, et al. Mean systolic and diastolic blood pressure in adults aged 18 and over in the United States, 2001-2008. Natl Health Stat Report 2011;35:1–22, 24.
11. Kaplan NM, Victor RG. Hypertension in the population at large. In: Kaplan NM, Victor RG, editors. Kaplan's clinical hypertension. 10th edition. Philadelphia: Wolter's Kluwer; 2010. p. 1.
12. Green AJ, Bazata DD, Fox KM, et al. Quality of life, depression, and healthcare resource utilization among adults with type 2 diabetes mellitus and concomitant hypertension and obesity: a prospective survey. Cardiol Res Pract 2012. http://dx.doi.org/10.1155/2012/404107.
13. Eaddy MT, Shah M, Lunacsek O, et al. The burden of illness of hypertension and comorbid diabetes. Curr Med Res Opin 2008;24:2501–7.
14. Haffner SM, Valdez R, Morales PA, et al. Greater effect of glycemia on incidence of hypertension in women than in men. Diabetes Care 1992;15:1277–84.
15. Hu G, DECODE Study Group. Gender difference in all-cause and cardiovascular mortality related to hyperglycaemia and newly-diagnosed diabetes. Diabetologia 2003;46:608–17.
16. Carson AP, Howard G, Burke GL, et al. Ethnic differences in hypertension incidence among middle-aged and older adults: the multi-ethnic study of atherosclerosis. Hypertension 2011;57:1101–7.
17. Dyer AR, Liu K, Walsh M, et al. Ten-year incidence of elevated blood pressure and its predictors: the CARDIA Study, Coronary Artery Risk Development in (Young) Adults. J Hum Hypertens 1999;13:13–21.
18. Etkin N, Mahoney J, Forsthoefel M, et al. Racial differences in hypertension-associated red cell sodium permeability. Nature 1982;297:588–9.
19. Liu X, Song P. Is the association of diabetes with uncontrolled blood pressure stronger in Mexican Americans and Blacks than in Whites among diagnosed hypertensive patients? Am J Hypertens 2013. [Epub ahead of print].
20. Ogden CL, Carroll MD, Kit BK, et al. Prevalence of obesity and trends in body mass index among US children and adolescents, 1999-2010. JAMA 2012;307:483–90.
21. TODAY Study Group. Rapid rise in hypertension and nephropathy in youth with type 2 diabetes: the TODAY clinical trial. Diabetes Care 2013;36:1735–41.
22. Massiera F, Bloch-Faure M, Ceiler D, et al. Adipose angiotensinogen is involved in adipose tissue growth and blood pressure regulation. FASEB J 2001;15:2727–9.
23. Boustany CM, Bharadwaj K, Daugherty A, et al. Activation of the systemic and adipose renin-angiotensin system in rats with diet-induced obesity and hypertension. Am J Physiol Regul Integr Comp Physiol 2004;287:R943–9.
24. Mehta PK, Griendling KK. Angiotensin II cell signaling: physiological and pathological effects in the cardiovascular system. Am J Physiol Cell Physiol 2007;292:C82–97.

25. Williams JS, Williams GH. 50th anniversary of aldosterone. J Clin Endocrinol Metab 2003;88:2364–72.
26. Whaley-Connell A, Johnson MS, Sowers JR. Aldosterone: role in the cardiometabolic syndrome and resistant hypertension. Prog Cardiovasc Dis 2010;52: 401–9.
27. Caprio M, Feve B, Claes A, et al. Pivotal role of the mineralocorticoid receptor in corticosteroid-induced adipogenesis. FASEB J 2007;21:2185–94.
28. Jeon JH, Kim KY, Kim JH, et al. A novel adipokine CTRP1 stimulates aldosterone production. FASEB J 2008;22:1502–11.
29. Cooper SA, Whaley-Connell A, Habibi J, et al. Renin-angiotensin-aldosterone system and oxidative stress in cardiovascular insulin resistance. Am J Physiol Heart Circ Physiol 2007;293:H2009–23.
30. Taniyama Y, Griendling KK. Reactive oxygen species in the vasculature: molecular and cellular mechanisms. Hypertension 2003;42:1075–81.
31. Madamanchi NR, Vendrov A, Runge MS. Oxidative stress and vascular disease. Arterioscler Thromb Vasc Biol 2005;25:29–38.
32. Dröge W. Free radicals in the physiological control of cell function. Physiol Rev 2002;82:47–95.
33. Johar S, Cave AC, Narayanapanicker A, et al. Aldosterone mediates angiotensin II-induced interstitial cardiac fibrosis via a Nox2-containing NADPH oxidase. FASEB J 2006;20:1546–8.
34. Barhoumi T, Kasal DA, Li MW, et al. T regulatory lymphocytes prevent angiotensin II-induced hypertension and vascular injury. Hypertension 2011;57: 469–76.
35. Brown NJ. Aldosterone and vascular inflammation. Hypertension 2008;51: 161–7.
36. Ferrannini E, Buzzigoli G, Bonadonna R, et al. Insulin resistance in essential hypertension. N Engl J Med 1987;317:350–7.
37. Bonora E, Capaldo B, Perin PC, et al. Hyperinsulinemia and insulin resistance are independently associated with plasma lipids, uric acid and blood pressure in non-diabetic subjects. The GISIR database. Nutr Metab Cardiovasc Dis 2008; 18:624–31.
38. Muniyappa R, Quon MJ. Insulin action and insulin resistance in vascular endothelium. Curr Opin Clin Nutr Metab Care 2007;10:523–30.
39. Vincent MA, Montagnani M, Quon MJ. Molecular and physiologic actions of insulin related to production of nitric oxide in vascular endothelium. Curr Diab Rep 2003;3:279–88.
40. Taniguchi CM, Emanuelli B, Kahn CR. Critical nodes in signalling pathways: insights into insulin action. Nat Rev Mol Cell Biol 2006;7:85–96.
41. Potenza MA, Marasciulo FL, Chieppa DM, et al. Insulin resistance in spontaneously hypertensive rats is associated with endothelial dysfunction characterized by imbalance between NO and ET-1 production. Am J Physiol Heart Circ Physiol 2005;289:H813–22.
42. Formoso G, Chen H, Kim JA, et al. Dehydroepiandrosterone mimics acute actions of insulin to stimulate production of both nitric oxide and endothelin 1 via distinct phosphatidylinositol 3-kinase- and mitogen-activated protein kinase-dependent pathways in vascular endothelium. Mol Endocrinol 2006;20: 1153–63.
43. Mukai Y, Wang CY, Rikitake Y, et al. Phosphatidylinositol 3-kinase/protein kinase Akt negatively regulates plasminogen activator inhibitor type-1 expression in vascular endothelial cells. Am J Physiol Heart Circ Physiol 2006;292:H1937–42.

44. Kim J, Montagnani M, Kwaug KK, et al. Reciprocal relationship between insulin resistance and endothelial dysfunction. Circulation 2006;113:1888–904.
45. Heagerty AM, Heerkens EH, Izzard AS. Small artery structure and function in hypertension. J Cell Mol Med 2010;14:1037–43.
46. Anderson EA, Hoffman RP, Balon TW, et al. Hyperinsulinemia produces both sympathetic neural activation and vasodilation in normal humans. J Clin Invest 1991;87:2246–52.
47. Landsberg L. Insulin-mediated sympathetic stimulation: role in the pathogenesis of obesity-related hypertension (or, how insulin affects blood pressure, and why). J Hypertens 2001;19:523–8.
48. Haynes WG, Morgan DA, Walsh SA, et al. Receptor-mediated regional sympathetic nerve activation by leptin. J Clin Invest 1997;100:270–8.
49. Song J, Hu X, Riazi S, et al. Regulation of blood pressure, the epithelial sodium channel (ENaC), and other key renal sodium transporters by chronic insulin infusion in rats. Am J Physiol Renal Physiol 2006;290:F1055–64.
50. Tiwari S, Sharma N, Gill PS, et al. Impaired sodium excretion and increased blood pressure in mice with targeted deletion of renal epithelial insulin receptor. Proc Natl Acad Sci U S A 2008;105:6469–774.
51. Muscelli E, Natali A, Bianchi S, et al. Effect of insulin on renal sodium and uric acid handling in essential hypertension. Am J Hypertens 1996;9:746–52.
52. Garcia-Touza M, Sowers JR. Evidence-based hypertension treatment in patients with diabetes. J Clin Hypertens (Greenwich) 2012;14:97–102.
53. Cushman WC, Evans GW, Byington RP, et al, ACCORD Study Group. Effects of intensive blood-pressure control in type 2 diabetes mellitus. N Engl J Med 2010; 362:1575–85.
54. American Diabetes Association. Standards of medical care in diabetes–2011. Diabetes Care 2011;34:S11–61.
55. UK Prospective Diabetes Study Group. Tight blood pressure control and risk of macrovascular and microvascular complications in type 2 diabetes: UKPDS 38. BMJ 1998;317:703–13.
56. Hansson L, Zanchetti A, Carruthers SG, et al. Effects of intensive blood pressure lowering and low-dose aspirin in patients with hypertension: principal results of the Hypertension Optimal Treatment (HOT) randomised trial. HOT Study Group. Lancet 1998;351:1755–62.
57. Tuomilehto J, Rastenyte D, Birkenhäger WH, et al. Effects of calcium-channel blockade in older patients with diabetes and systolic hypertension. Systolic Hypertension in Europe Trial Investigators. N Engl J Med 1999;340:677–84.
58. Curb JD, Pressel SL, Cutler JA, et al. Effect of diuretic-based antihypertensive treatment on cardiovascular disease risk in older diabetic patients with isolated systolic hypertension. JAMA 1996;276:1886–92.
59. Schrier RW, Estacio RO, Jeffers B. Appropriate blood pressure control in NIDDM (ABCD) trial. Diabetologia 1996;39:1646–54.
60. Cooper-DeHoff RM, Gong Y, Handberg EM, et al. Tight blood pressure control and cardiovascular outcomes among hypertensive patients with diabetes and coronary artery disease. JAMA 2010;304:61–8.
61. American Diabetes Association. Standards of medical care in diabetes-2013. Diabetes Care 2013;36:S11–66.
62. Redon J, Mancia G, Sleight P, et al, ONTARGET Investigators. Safety and efficacy of low blood pressures among patients with diabetes: subgroup analyses from the ONTARGET (Ongoing Telmisartan Alone and in combination with Ramipril Global Endpoint Trial). J Am Coll Cardiol 2012;59:74–83.

63. Bangalore S, Kumar S, Lobach I, et al. Blood pressure targets in subjects with type 2 diabetes mellitus/impaired fasting glucose: observations from traditional and bayesian random-effects meta-analyses of randomized trials. Circulation 2011;123:2799–810.

64. Kim YS, Davis SC, Truijen J, et al. Intensive blood pressure control affects cerebral blood flow in type 2 diabetes mellitus patients. Hypertension 2011;57: 738–45.

65. Cummings DM, Letter AJ, Howard G, et al. Generic medications and blood pressure control in diabetic hypertensive subjects: results from the REasons for Geographic And Racial Differences in Stroke (REGARDS) study. Diabetes Care 2013;36:591–7.

66. Tuomilehto J, Lindström J, Eriksson JG, et al, Finnish Diabetes Prevention Study Group. Prevention of type 2 diabetes mellitus by changes in lifestyle among subjects with impaired glucose tolerance. N Engl J Med 2001;344: 1343–50.

67. Sacks FM, Svetky LP, Vollmer WM, et al. Effects on blood pressure of reduced dietary sodium and the Dietary Approaches to Stop Hypertension (DASH) diet. DASH-Sodium Collaborative Research Group. N Engl J Med 2001;344:3–10.

68. Azadbakht L, Fard NR, Karimi M, et al. Effects of the dietary approaches to stop hypertension (DASH) eating plan on cardiovascular risks among type 2 diabetic patients. Diabetes Care 2011;34:55–7.

69. Azadbakht L, Surkan PJ, Esmaillzadeh A, et al. The dietary approaches to stop hypertension eating plan affects C-reactive protein, coagulation abnormalities, and hepatic function tests among type 2 diabetic patients. J Nutr 2011;141: 1083–8.

70. Noda K, Zhang B, Iwata A, et al, STYLIST Study Investigators. Lifestyle changes through the use of delivered meals and dietary counseling in a single-blind study. The STYLIST study. Circ J 2012;76:1335–44.

71. Cook NR, Cutler JA, Obarzanek E, et al. Long term effects of dietary sodium reduction on cardiovascular disease outcomes: observational follow-up of the trials of hypertension prevention (TOHP). BMJ 2007;334:885–8.

72. Cook NR, Kumanyika SK, Cutler JA. Effect of change in sodium excretion on change in blood pressure corrected for measurement error. The Trials of Hypertension Prevention, Phase I. Am J Epidemiol 1998;148:431–44.

73. Taylor RS, Ashton KE, Moxham T, et al. Reduced dietary salt for the prevention of cardiovascular disease: a meta-analysis of randomized controlled trials (Cochrane Review). Am J Hypertens 2011;24:843–53.

74. Rugale C, Oudot C, Desmetz C, et al. Sodium restriction prevents cardiovascular remodeling associated with insulin-resistance in the rat. Ann Cardiol Angeiol (Paris) 2013;62:139–43.

75. Whelton SP, Chin A, Xin X, et al. Effect of aerobic exercise on blood pressure: a metaanalysis of randomized, controlled trials. Ann Intern Med 2002;136: 493–503.

76. Hansson L, Lindholm LH, Niskanen L, et al. Effect of angiotensin-converting-enzyme inhibition compared with conventional therapy on cardiovascular morbidity and mortality in hypertension: the Captopril Prevention Project (CAPPP) randomized trial. Lancet 1999;353:611–6.

77. ALLHAT Collaborative Research Group. Major outcomes in high-risk hypertensive patients randomized to angiotensin-converting enzyme inhibitor or calcium channel blocker vs diuretic: the Antihypertensive and Lipid-Lowering Treatment to Prevent Heart Attack Trial (ALLHAT). JAMA 2002;288:2981–97.

78. The Heart Outcomes Prevention Evaluation Study Investigators. Effects of an angiotensin-converting-enzyme inhibitor, ramipril, on cardiovascular events in high risk patients. N Engl J Med 2000;342:145–53.

79. Heart Outcomes Prevention Evaluation (HOPE) Study Investigators. Effects of ramipril on cardiovascular and microvascular outcomes in people with diabetes mellitus: results of the HOPE study and MICRO-HOPE substudy. Lancet 2000; 355:253–9.

80. Lindholm LH, Ibsen H, Dahlöf B, et al, LIFE Study Group. Cardiovascular morbidity and mortality in patients with diabetes in the Losartan Intervention For Endpoint reduction in hypertension study (LIFE): a randomised trial against atenolol. Lancet 2002;359:1004–10.

81. Ogihara T, Nakao K, Fukui T, et al, Candesartan Antihypertensive Survival Evaluation in Japan Trial Group. Effects of candesartan compared with amlodipine in hypertensive patients with high cardiovascular risks: Candesartan Antihypertensive Survival Evaluation in Japan Trial. Hypertension 2008;51:393–8.

82. Fretheim A. VALUE: analysis of results. Lancet 2004;364:934–5.

83. Yusuf S, Teo KK, Pogue J, et al, ONTARGET Investigators. Telmisartan, ramipril, or both in patients at high risk for vascular events. N Engl J Med 2008;358: 1547–59.

84. Ruggenenti P, Perna A, Ganeva M, et al. Impact of blood pressure control and angiotensin-converting enzyme inhibitor therapy on new-onset microalbuminuria in type 2 diabetes: a post hoc analysis of the BENEDICT trial. J Am Soc Nephrol 2006;17:3472–81.

85. Haller H, Ito S, Izzo J, et al. Olmesartan for delay or prevention of microalbuminuria in type 2 diabetes. N Engl J Med 2011;364:907–17.

86. Bilous R, Chaturvedi N, Sjolie AK, et al. Effect of candesartan on microalbuminuria and albumin excretion rate in diabetes: three randomized trials. Ann Intern Med 2009;5:11–20.

87. Lastra G, Whaley-Connell A, Manrique C, et al. Low-dose spironolactone reduces reactive oxygen species generation and improves insulin-stimulated glucose transport in skeletal muscle in the TG(mRen2)27 rat. Am J Physiol Endocrinol Metab 2008;295:E110–6.

88. Lastra-Lastra G, Sowers JR, Restrepo-Erazo K, et al. Role of aldosterone and angiotensin II in insulin resistance: an update. Clin Endocrinol 2009;71:1–6.

89. Estacio RO, Jeffers BW, Hiatt WR, et al. The effect of nisoldipine as compared with enalapril on cardiovascular outcomes in patients with non-insulin-dependent diabetes and hypertension. N Engl J Med 1998;338:645–52.

90. Tatti P, Pahor M, Byington RP, et al. Outcome results of the Fosinopril Versus Amlodipine Cardiovascular Events Randomized Trial (FACET) in patients with hypertension and NIDDM. Diabetes Care 1998;21:597–603.

91. Leenen FH, Nwachuku CE, Black HR, et al, Antihypertensive and Lipid-Lowering Treatment to Prevent Heart Attack Trial Collaborative Research Group. Clinical events in high-risk hypertensive patients randomly assigned to calcium channel blocker versus angiotensin-converting enzyme inhibitor in the Antihypertensive and Lipid-lowering Treatment to Prevent Heart Attack trial. Hypertension 2006;48:374–84.

92. Julius S, Kjeldsen SE, Weber M, et al, VALUE Trial Group. Outcomes in hypertensive patients at high cardiovascular risk treated with regimens based on valsartan or amlodipine: the VALUE randomised trial. Lancet 2004;363:2022–31.

93. Berl T, Hunsicker LG, Lewis JB, et al, Irbesartan Diabetic Nephropathy Trial, Collaborative Study Group. Cardiovascular outcomes in the Irbesartan Diabetic

Nephropathy Trial of patients with type 2 diabetes and overt nephropathy. Ann Intern Med 2003;138:542–9.

94. Ostergren J, Poulter NR, Sever PS, et al, ASCOT Investigators. The Anglo-Scandinavian Cardiac Outcomes Trial: blood pressure-lowering limb: effects in patients with type II diabetes. J Hypertens 2008;26:2103–11.

95. Beckett NS, Peters R, Fletcher AE, et al, HYVET Study Group. Treatment of hypertension in patients 80 years of age or older. N Engl J Med 2008;358:1887–98.

96. Manrique C, Johnson M, Sowers JR. Thiazide diuretics alone or with beta-blockers impair glucose metabolism in hypertensive patients with abdominal obesity. Hypertension 2010;55:15–7.

97. Cooper-DeHoff RM, Wen S, Beitelshees AL, et al. Impact of abdominal obesity on incidence of adverse metabolic effects associated with antihypertensive medications. Hypertension 2010;55:61–8.

98. Raheja P, Price A, Wang Z, et al. Spironolactone prevents chlorthalidone-induced sympathetic activation and insulin resistance in hypertensive patients. Hypertension 2012;60:319–25.

99. Zhou X, Ma L, Habibi J, et al. Nebivolol improves diastolic dysfunction and myocardial remodeling through reductions in oxidative stress in the Zucker obese rat. Hypertension 2010;55:880–8.

100. Campbell JE, Drucker DJ. Pharmacology, physiology, and mechanisms of incretin hormone action. Cell Metab 2013;17:819–37.

101. Thorens B, Porret A, Buhler L, et al. Cloning and functional expression of the human islet GLP-1 receptor: demonstration that exendin-4 is an agonist and exendin-(9–39) an antagonist of the receptor. Diabetes 1993;42:1678–82.

102. Gros R, You X, Baggio LL, et al. Cardiac function in mice lacking the glucagon-like peptide-1 receptor. Endocrinology 2003;144:2242–52.

103. Grieve DJ, Cassidy RS, Green BD. Emerging cardiovascular actions of the incretin hormone glucagon-like peptide-1: potential therapeutic benefits beyond glycaemic control? Br J Pharmacol 2009;157:1340–51.

104. Ussher JR, Drucker DJ. Cardiovascular biology of the incretin system. Endocr Rev 2012;33:187–215.

105. Horton ES, Silberman C, Davis KL, et al. Weight loss, glycemic control, and changes in cardiovascular biomarkers in patients with type 2 diabetes receiving incretin therapies or insulin in a large cohort database. Diabetes Care 2010;33:1759–65.

106. Mistry GC, Maes AL, Lasseter KC. Effect of sitagliptin, a dipeptidyl peptidase-4 inhibitor, on blood pressure in nondiabetic patients with mild to moderate hypertension. J Clin Pharmacol 2008;48:592–8.

107. Aroor AR, Sowers JR, Bender SB, et al. Dipeptidylpeptidase inhibition is associated with improvement in blood pressure and diastolic function in insulin-resistant male Zucker obese rats. Endocrinology 2013;154:2501–13.

108. Liu L, Liu J, Wong WT, et al. Dipeptidyl peptidase 4 inhibitor sitagliptin protects endothelial function in hypertension through a glucagon-like peptide 1-dependent mechanism. Hypertension 2012;60:833–41.

109. Ossum A, van Deurs U, Engstrøm T, et al. The cardioprotective and inotropic components of the postconditioning effects of GLP-1 and GLP-1(9-36)a in an isolated rat heart. Pharmacol Res 2009;60:411–7.

110. Girardi AC, Fukuda LE, Rossoni LV, et al. Dipeptidyl peptidase IV inhibition downregulates Na+ - H+ exchanger NHE3 in rat renal proximal tubule. Am J Physiol Renal Physiol 2008;294:F414–22.

111. Pacheco BP, Crajoinas RO, Couto GK, et al. Dipeptidyl peptidase IV inhibition attenuates blood pressure rising in young spontaneously hypertensive rats. J Hypertens 2011;29:520–8.

112. Sharma AM, Bakris G, Neutel JM, et al. Single-pill combination of telmisartan/amlodipine versus amlodipine monotherapy in diabetic hypertensive patients: an 8-week randomized, parallel-group, double-blind trial. Clin Ther 2012;34:537–51.

113. Weber MA, Bakris GL, Jamerson K, et al, ACCOMPLISH Investigators. Cardiovascular events during differing hypertension therapies in patients with diabetes. J Am Coll Cardiol 2010;56:77–85.

114. Dahlof B, Swever PS, Poulter NR, et al, ASCOT Investigators. Prevention of cardiovascular events with an antihypertensive regimen of amlodipine adding perindopril as required versus atenolol adding bendroflumethiazide as required, in the Anglo-Scandinavian Cardiac Outcomes Trial-Blood Pressure Lowering Arm (ASCOT-BPLA); a multicenter randomised controlled trial. Lancet 2005;366:895–906.

115. Gupta AK, Arshad S, Poulter NR. Compliance, safety, and effectiveness of fixed-dose combinations of antihypertensive agents: a meta-analysis. Hypertension 2010;55:399–407.

116. Chrysant SG, Littlejohn T 3rd, Izzo JL Jr, et al. Triple-combination therapy with olmesartan, amlodipine, and hydrochlorothiazide in black and non-black study participants with hypertension: the TRINITY randomized, double-blind, 12-week, parallel-group study. Am J Cardiovasc Drugs 2012;12:233–43.

117. Wakefield BJ, Holman JE, Ray A, et al. Effectiveness of home telehealth in comorbid diabetes and hypertension: a randomized, controlled trial. Telemed J E Health 2011;17:254–61.

118. Johns EJ, Abdulla MH. Renal nerves in blood pressure regulation. Curr Opin Nephrol Hypertens 2013;22:504–10.

119. Symplicity HTN-2 Investigators, Esler MD, Krum H, et al. Renal sympathetic denervation in patients with treatment-resistant hypertension (The Symplicity HTN-2 Trial): a randomised controlled trial. Lancet 2010;376:1903–9.

120. Mahfoud F, Schlaich M, Kindermann I, et al. Effect of renal sympathetic denervation on glucose metabolism in patients with resistant hypertension: a pilot study. Circulation 2011;123:1940–6.

121. Mahfoud F, Ukena C, Schmieder RE, et al. Ambulatory blood pressure changes after renal sympathetic denervation in patients with resistant hypertension. Circulation 2013;128:132–40.

122. Fagard RH, Celis H, Thijs L, et al. Daytime and nighttime blood pressure as predictors of death and cause-specific cardiovascular events in hypertension. Hypertension 2008;51:55.

123. Pickering TG, Shimbo D, Haas D. Ambulatory blood-pressure monitoring. N Engl J Med 2006;354:2368–74.

Polycystic Ovary Syndrome

Anindita Nandi, MD[a], Zijian Chen, MD[a], Ronak Patel, MD[a],
Leonid Poretsky, MD[b],*

KEYWORDS

- Polycystic ovary syndrome • Risk factors • Long-term effects • Insulin resistance

KEY POINTS

- Risk factors for polycystic ovary syndrome (PCOS) include genetics, metabolic profiles, and the in utero environment.
- Long-term consequences of PCOS include metabolic complications such as diabetes, obesity, and cardiovascular disease.
- Dysregulation of insulin action is closely linked to the pathogenesis of PCOS.

HISTORY OF POLYCYSTIC OVARY SYNDROME

It is unclear when polycystic ovary syndrome (PCOS) was first described, but there are some clues in the Egyptian papyri to suggest the presence of PCOS-like syndrome. Hippocrates (460–377 BC) noted "but those women whose menstruation is less than 3 days or is meager, are robust, with a healthy complexion and a masculine appearance; yet they are not concerned about bearing children nor do they become pregnant."[1] Soranus of Ephesus (ca. 98–138 AD) noted that "sometimes it is also natural not to menstruate at all. It is natural too in persons whose bodies are of a masculine type. We observe that the majority of those not menstruating are rather robust, like mannish and sterile women."[2] Moises Maimonides (1135–1204 AD) reported "there are women whose skin is dry and hard, and whose nature resembles the nature of a man. However, if any woman's nature tends to be transformed to the nature of a man, this does not arise from medications, but is caused by heavy menstrual activity."[3] Achard and Thiers[4] observed a similar relationship between hyperandrogenism and diabetes in their study of the "bearded woman." These historical statements compile a variety of signs that are suggestive of PCOS.

In 1721, Italian scientist Antonio Vallisneri made a connection between masculine features and abnormal morphology of ovaries: "young married peasant women,

[a] Division of Endocrinology and Metabolism, Beth Israel Medical Center, Albert Einstein College of Medicine, New York, NY 10003, USA; [b] Division of Endocrinology and Metabolism, Department of Medicine, Gerald J. Friedman Diabetes Institute, Beth Israel Medical Center, Albert Einstein College of Medicine, 317 East 17th Street, 7th Floor, New York, NY 10003, USA
* Corresponding author.
E-mail address: lporetsk@chpnet.org

Endocrinol Metab Clin N Am 43 (2014) 123–147
http://dx.doi.org/10.1016/j.ecl.2013.10.003
0889-8529/14/$ – see front matter © 2014 Elsevier Inc. All rights reserved.

moderately obese and infertile, with 2 larger than normal ovaries, bumpy and shiny, whitish, just like pigeon eggs."[5] In 1935, Stein and Leventhal[6] ultimately formally described a syndrome of amenorrhea and polycystic ovaries (**Fig. 1**); they further depicted this syndrome, which bore their name, as one that involves masculine features, such as acne and hirsutism.

DEFINITION OF PCOS

Today this syndrome is termed PCOS. It is one of the most prevalent disorders, affecting about 5% of women of reproductive age.[7] At present, 3 definitions of PCOS are most commonly cited (**Box 1**). These definitions were proposed by National Institute of Child Health and Human Development (NICHD) in 1990, the European Society for Human Reproduction and Embryology and American Society for Reproductive Medicine (ESHRE/ASRM or Rotterdam) in 2003, and Androgen Excess Society (AES) in 2006. Each of these definitions underlines the importance of excluding other causes of androgen excess and anovulatory fertility before diagnosing PCOS.

The NICHD criteria were an important first step toward establishing a universally accepted definition of PCOS. However, this definition was based on majority opinion and not on clinical trial evidence. PCOS is defined as the presence of both androgen excess and oligo-anovulation. In subsequent years it was realized that the clinical presentation of PCOS was much more variable than the NICHD criteria suggested, and polycystic ovarian morphology was often present in women with biochemical and clinical findings of PCOS. In 2003, the revised Rotterdam consensus definition included polycystic ovaries as a third diagnostic marker for PCOS. Based on this definition, a woman with the diagnosis of PCOS should meet 2 of the 3 following criteria: (1) presence of oligo-anovulation or chronic anovulation, (2) clinical and/or biochemical signs suggesting hyperandrogenism, and (3) polycystic ovaries on ultrasonographic examination. The Rotterdam definition of PCOS broadened the phenotypic expression of the syndrome and redefined PCOS as primarily a syndrome of ovarian dysfunction.[8] The Rotterdam definition quickly became controversial, as PCOS could now be defined even in the absence of androgen excess or menstrual irregularity. In 2006, the Androgen Excess Society formed a task force to review existing data on PCOS. It was concluded that evidence to support features of PCOS in women with polycystic

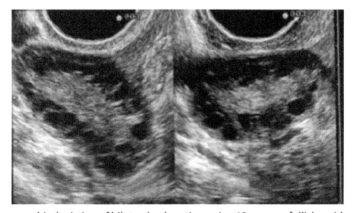

Fig. 1. Sonographic depiction of bilateral polycystic ovaries: 10 or more follicles with peripheral distribution. (*From* Balen AH, Laven JS, Tan SL, et al. Ultrasound assessment of the polycystic ovary: international consensus definitions. Hum Reprod Update 2003;9:505–14; with permission.)

> **Box 1**
> **Definitions of PCOS**
>
> *National Institutes of Health*
>
> 1990 National Institute of Child Health and Human Development (NICHD) Guidelines
>
> Patient demonstrates both:
>
> 1. Clinical and/or biochemical signs of hyperandrogenism
>
> 2. Oligo-anovulation or chronic anovulation
>
> Exclusion of other causes of androgen excess and anovulatory infertility is necessary.
>
> *Rotterdam*
>
> 2003 European Society for Human Reproduction and Embryology and American Society for Reproductive Medicine (ESHRE/ASRM or Rotterdam) Guidelines
>
> Patient demonstrates 2 of 3 criteria:
>
> 1. Oligo-anovulation or chronic anovulation
>
> 2. Clinical and/or biochemical signs of hyperandrogenism
>
> 3. Polycystic ovaries
>
> Exclusion of other causes of androgen excess and anovulatory infertility is necessary.
>
> *Androgen Excess Society (AES) Guidelines*
>
> In 2006 the AES suggested tightening of diagnostic criteria.
>
> Patient demonstrates both:
>
> 1. Hirsutism and/or hyperandrogenemia
>
> 2. Oligo-anovulation and/or polycystic ovaries
>
> Exclusion of other causes of androgen excess and anovulatory infertility is necessary.

ovaries and ovulatory dysfunction in the absence of clinical or biochemical signs of hyperandrogenism was conflicting.[9,10] The AES proposed definition that takes into account the wide heterogeneity of PCOS and the variable prevalence of polycystic ovarian morphology. It requires the presence of both hirsutism or hyperandrogenism and either oligo-ovulation or polycystic ovaries.

CLINICAL FEATURES OF PCOS

PCOS is a heterogeneous and chronic condition. This syndrome can be divided into 3 broad segments: reproductive manifestations, metabolic features, and psychological sequelae. The spectrum of clinical features varies across the life cycle. In adolescence PCOS exhibits reproductive and psychological manifestations, which over time transition to frank infertility and metabolic complications. However, in obese adolescent metabolic implications of PCOS such as impaired glucose tolerance (IGT), diabetes mellitus (DM) and metabolic syndrome can be present.

REPRODUCTIVE FEATURES OF PCOS

Ovarian dysfunction commonly manifests as oligomenorrhea or amenorrhea, this being a result of chronic anovulation.[11] However, dysfunctional uterine bleeding can be present in women with prolonged anovulation, mimicking regular menstrual cycles. Up to 70% to 80% of women with PCOS have ovarian dysfunction suggested by oligomenorrhea or amenorrhea. Among those with oligomenorrhea, 80% to 90% will be diagnosed with PCOS.[11] Only 40% of women with amenorrhea will be diagnosed as having PCOS.[12] Menstrual irregularities can be masked by use of oral contraceptive pills (OCPs). Cessation of OCPs results in recurrence of underlying irregular cycles. Unopposed estrogen and endometrial hyperplasia in these patients can also present as menorrhagia. Even with regular menstrual cycles PCOS can be diagnosed, based on newer diagnostic criteria (see **Box 1**).[13]

PCOS is the most common cause of anovulatory infertility. Approximately 90% to 95% of women attending infertility clinics have PCOS. Although 60% of women with PCOS are fertile (able to conceive within 12 months), the time to conception is often increased.[11] Obesity is seen in up to 90% of women with PCOS, and infertility and is an independent risk factor for infertility. It also reduces the efficacy of infertility treatments and increases pregnancy-related complications including miscarriage.[11] Weight optimization before pregnancy should ideally be recommended. It is important that family planning discussions are pursued in a timely manner, as age-related infertility exacerbates PCOS-related infertility.

Clinical hyperandrogenism generally manifests as hirsutism, acne, and male pattern alopecia.[13] About 60% of PCOS patients have hirsutism, but the prevalence varies significantly with race and obesity.[13] Hirsutism can be assessed with a standardized scoring system, such as the Ferriman-Gallwey assessment (**Fig. 2**). Approximately one-third of cases are affected by acne.[14] Although alopecia is commonly seen, male pattern hair loss requires a strong familial predisposition and is less frequent in PCOS. Presence of virilization, especially in the presence of clitoromegaly or ambiguous genitalia, warrants exclusion of other causes such as adrenal or ovarian androgen-secreting tumors. Biochemical patterns of hyperandrogenism seen in PCOS include increased total and free testosterone and dehydroepiandrosterone, often accompanied by a decreased level of sex hormone–binding globulin (SHBG).[14]

METABOLIC FEATURES OF PCOS

Dyslipidemia is common in PCOS, the usual pattern of which shows elevated triglycerides with a low level of high-density lipoprotein (HDL).[15] The causes of dyslipidemia are multifactorial and seem to be independent of body mass index.[15,16] Insulin resistance that eventually affects the expression of lipoprotein and hepatic lipase along with stimulation of lipolysis is important in the pathophysiology of dyslipidemia in PCOS.[15]

Insulin resistance, relatively reduced secretion of insulin, reduced hepatic insulin extraction, impaired suppression of hepatic gluconeogenesis, and abnormalities in insulin receptor signaling are the most important causes of abnormal glucose metabolism in PCOS.[17–21] Insulin resistance is present in about 50% to 80% of PCOS women.[22] Compared with obese women, lean women have less severe insulin resistance.[23] Women with PCOS are at a higher risk of developing IGT and type 2 DM (DM2) than their age-matched and weight-matched normal counterparts.[24] The prevalence of IGT and DM2 in PCOS women is 31.3% and 7.5%, respectively.[24] The rate of conversion from IGT to DM2 has not been uniformly reported, but based on 2 Australian studies could range from 2.9% per year to 8.7% per year.[25,26] Women with PCOS are also at higher risk of developing gestational diabetes (GDM), independent of weight status. However, obesity does seem to exacerbate the development of GDM in PCOS.[24,27] PCOS is considered by the International Diabetes Federation to be a nonmodifiable risk factor associated with DM2.[28]

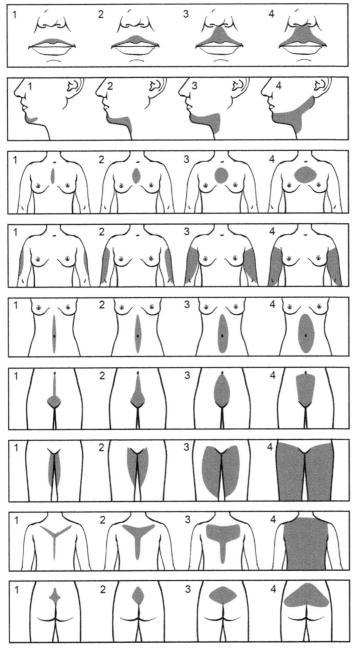

Fig. 2. Ferriman-Gallwey scale. Severity of hirsutism is graded progressively from 1 to 4 at different body locations. (*From* Hatch R, Rosenfield RL, Kim MH, et al. Hirsutism: implications, etiology, and management. Am J Obstet Gynecol 1981;140:815–30; with permission.)

PSYCHOLOGICAL FEATURES OF PCOS

The concerns that arise from phenotypic changes in PCOS (acne, hirsutism, obesity) along with infertility and long-term health can compromise quality of life and adversely affect psychological health. Women with PCOS are more prone to poor self-esteem, negative body image, anxiety, and depression.[29,30] It is extremely important to evaluate and address these issues as a part of PCOS management.

RISK FACTORS FOR PCOS

Although there have been limited studies regarding ethnic differences in the presentation and prevalence of PCOS, some data suggest variable phenotypes in different ethnic lineages. PCOS appears to be more prevalent in African Americans than Caucasians, with prevalence of 8% versus 4.8%.[31] Asian women present with similar testosterone levels but less hirsutism than counterparts in other populations.[32] Insulin resistance seems more prevalent in certain ethnic groups, such as those of Latino, Caribbean, and South Asian origin.[33] The diversity in presentation among different ethnicities suggests genetic differences in the etiology of PCOS.

Further evidence that genetic factors play a large role in the development of PCOS is found in the familial aggregation of disease incidence. Although there is significant heterogeneity in study design, current data suggest an autosomal dominant mode of inheritance of genetic determinants.[33] In addition to reproductive abnormalities and hirsutism, there is an increased risk of insulin resistance and metabolic disturbances in first-degree relatives, implicating a genetic link between PCOS and metabolic changes.[34] Twin studies evaluating differences between monozygotic twins and dizygotic twins, however, indicate that there is a more complex genetic presentation. Discordance between twins in PCOS symptoms suggests a polygenic inheritance pattern or influence of environmental factors.[35]

Premature pubarche in adolescents is often linked to later development of PCOS.[36] Menarche in these girls is accompanied by several features of PCOS including insulin resistance, dyslipidemia, and elevated androgens.[37] These adolescents develop ovarian hyperandrogenism at a much higher rate than the general population (45% vs 3%–6%).[38] Evaluation of girls with premature pubarche using stimulation with gonadotropin-releasing hormone analogue shows a greater increase in ovarian and adrenal androgens than is seen in girls without hyperandrogenism.[39] Similar trends are seen with corticotropin stimulation.[40] This finding suggests an abnormal activity of ovarian and adrenal 17α-hydroxylase and 17,20-lyase functions.[41] These data support a pubertal onset of ovarian and adrenal hyperandrogenism in at least some patients.

In addition to the influences throughout life, the in utero environment is implicated in the increased risk of development of PCOS. This process is an example of the Barker hypothesis of fetal programming: insults occurring at certain gestational stages can permanently alter tissue structure and function.[42] It is hypothesized that intrauterine growth restriction may affect in utero programming of PCOS. Restriction of uterine growth has been associated with the development of PCOS in the Spanish population.[43,44] These women often also may have a history of precocious puberty. Similar development of PCOS-like traits has been shown in animal models such as sheep and rodents.[45,46] Large studies in the Finnish and Dutch population, however, fail to support such an association.[47,48]

It is also hypothesized that fetal undernutrition selects for the thrifty genotype: genes that are important in energy conservation.[49] One can see that activation of such genes would be beneficial in times of famine, but can lead to obesity and diabetes in times of plenty. Barker[42] suggests that the fetal response to undernutrition leads to organized development that supports brain development above other organ systems. The link between PCOS and insulin regulation is again seen with intrauterine growth restriction. In addition to the increased risk of development of PCOS, intrauterine growth restriction also predisposes an individual to subsequent development of hypertension, insulin resistance, DM2, and cardiovascular disease.

Prenatal exposure to androgens may also play a role in the later development of PCOS. In animal models of PCOS, symptomatology is often due to prenatal exposure of females to androgens. Of note, these females do not exhibit low birth weights. Age of menarche is also delayed, in contrast to the precocious puberty seen in the low-birth-weight model. Prenatally androgenized female rhesus monkeys ovulate at 50% to 60% of the frequency of normal females; 33% to 40% are anovulatory.[50] Despite the decreased ovulation rates, these animals also demonstrate double the normal incidence of polyfollicular ovaries.[50,51] Such effects are seen with androgen exposure during all periods of gestation.

Although hirsutism is difficult to assess in the rhesus monkey, it has been shown that circulating testosterone levels are elevated in females treated prenatally with androgens in the early phase.[52,53] However, the testosterone response to recombinant human chorionic gonadotropin (rhCG) is similarly elevated in both early and late prenatally androgen-treated females.[50,54] Even in this model of prenatal exposure to androgens, insulin resistance seems to play a pathophysiologic role, as treatment of these monkeys with insulin sensitizers also improves the anovulatory state.[55]

Prenatally treated female rhesus monkeys, like women with PCOS, show impaired oocyte development in response to controlled ovarian hyperstimulation. There is decreased intrafollicular steroidogenesis and impaired blastocyst formation. This phenotype is more dramatic in early-treated females.[56,57] Abnormal follicle differentiation and oocyte maturation in early-treated but not late-treated females is associated with hypersecretion of luteinizing hormone (LH) and failure to suppress insulin levels during treatment with recombinant human follicle-stimulating hormone for oocyte retrieval.[56]

Other long-term metabolic outcomes seen in PCOS women are also noted in prenatally androgenized female monkeys. As with the reproductive outcomes, prenatally treated monkeys show more severely impaired metabolic phenotypes than late-treated females, including insulin resistance, insulin secretion, and accumulation of visceral fat.[50,58,59] Treatment with insulin sensitizers, either metformin or thiazolidinediones, improves insulin regulation in androgenized females.[55] Male relatives of women with PCOS demonstrate features consistent with metabolic syndrome.[60,61] Adult male monkeys who have been exposed to androgens during gestation also demonstrate insulin resistance and decreased pancreatic function.[62]

LONG-TERM CONSEQUENCES OF PCOS
Insulin Resistance and Risk of Diabetes

PCOS is not only a disorder of hyperandrogenemia and anovulation; it is also associated with several long-term health consequences. Women with PCOS have a higher frequency of hyperinsulinemia and insulin resistance than age-matched and weight-matched controls.[63,64] However, insulin resistance is not seen in all patients with PCOS. Anovulatory women have a greater degree of insulin resistance than those with menstrual regularity.[19,65] Insulin resistance has also been correlated with androgen levels in women with PCOS.[20] Because insulin resistance is a precursor of diabetes and cardiovascular disease, it is not surprising that women with PCOS are also at risk for these entities. The risk of developing diabetes in women with PCOS is increased 3- to 7-fold.[24,63] The prevalence of IGT is also increased in comparison with women without PCOS (31%–35%).[66] Glucose intolerance is seen at an earlier age in the third to fourth decade of life.[24,66] It has been observed that women with PCOS have increased mortality from complications of diabetes.[67]

Obesity

Women with PCOS have a higher prevalence of obesity, as high as 40% in the United States. There is some variation with regard to geographic location and ethnicity. For example, the prevalence is 35% to 38% in the European population and 10% to 38% in the Mediterranean population. There is a predisposition to accumulation of central or visceral fat. Obese women with PCOS have a more severely affected reproductive phenotype, and tend to have higher rates of menstrual irregularity, infertility, and hirsutism. The free testosterone levels are higher and SHBG is lower. These women also have poor outcomes with ovulation induction and higher rates of miscarriage. Weight loss can reverse the degree of reproductive irregularities and minimize the metabolic sequelae of obesity, including dyslipidemia and insulin resistance.[68,69]

Hyperlipidemia

Mixed hyperlipidemia is common in women with PCOS. Elevations are seen in levels of low-density lipoprotein (LDL), very LDL, and triglycerides, and a decrease in HDL level is commonly present. Moreover, the LDL particles are predominantly small dense LDL, which has increased atherogenic potential. A greater number of abnormalities are seen, even after controlling for degree of obesity.[70,71] The difference in lipid levels is more pronounced at an earlier age. Lipid abnormalities are not consistently correlated with hyperinsulinemia or central adiposity.[71,72] Androgen levels are correlated with elevated triglycerides, but not with other lipid abnormalities.[73] Of note, women with hirsutism and regular cycles often do not demonstrate hyperlipidemia. However, women with both hirsutism and irregular menses have lower HDL and higher triglyceride levels.[74]

Cardiovascular Disease

In addition to hyperlipidemia, there is an increased prevalence of other cardiovascular risk factors, such as hypertension, endothelial dysfunction, and inflammation. Obese women with PCOS were found to have higher systolic blood pressures when compared with weight-matched control women. Women with oligomenorrhea and hirsutism have raised systolic and diastolic blood pressures.[73,74] Markers of abnormal endothelium and inflammation can be seen through increased levels of C-reactive protein and endothelin-1 in women with PCOS, independent of obesity.[75–78] However, there is variability in study results.

Women with PCOS are at increased risk for premature atherosclerosis and cardiovascular events. Carotid intima media thickness (IMT) indicates an increased risk for atherosclerosis. Difference in mean carotid IMT is seen only in women older than 45 years.[79] Premenopausal women with PCOS also have higher rates of coronary artery calcium, a marker for coronary atherosclerosis.[80] However, it is difficult to differentiate the effects of obesity and metabolic syndrome from those of PCOS in this patient population. The presence of these risk factors in women with PCOS would predict a higher rate of cardiovascular events. In fact, mathematical modeling assessing risk-factor variables in comparison with a reference population suggests a relative risk of 7.4 for myocardial infarction in women with PCOS.[81] However, an increased risk for cardiovascular disease has not been clearly demonstrated.[68,82]

Endometrial Cancer

PCOS is a state of recurrent anovulation, resulting in unopposed estrogen exposure to the endometrium. In a retrospective study of 345 women with PCOS, a significantly increased risk of endometrial cancer was seen (odds ratio 5.3). Obesity could not be ruled out as a confounding factor.[82] One study has shown that the risk of endometrial cancer is increased only in the obese subset of anovulatory women.[83] Studies looking at the risk for endometrial cancer are difficult to interpret, as results are often contradictory and lacking in relative risk assessment.[84] It is suggested that menses or withdrawal bleeding should be induced every 3 months in women with anovulation to decrease their risk of developing endometrial hyperplasia or cancer.[68]

Pregnancy Complications

Along with difficulty in achieving and maintaining successful gestation, patients with PCOS are susceptible to several pregnancy complications. There are increased risks for gestational diabetes, pregnancy-induced hypertension, and preeclampsia. However, there is significant heterogeneity in the rates of complications between studies. The diverse phenotypes and severity of PCOS are likely contributors to this heterogeneity. Although in some studies PCOS is linked to increased preterm delivery and cesarean sections, other meta-analyses have failed to show a significant difference. There is also some controversy over whether PCOS leads to an increased risk of low birth weight in infants.[85]

Animal studies suggest that some of these pregnancy complications may be related to or caused by hyperinsulinemia or insulin resistance. Animal models with altered insulin signaling in *Caenorhabditis elegans*, *Drosophila*, and mice show decreased fertility or sterility phenotypes.[86–88] In one study, hyperinsulinemia in female mice, independent of obesity and hyperglycemia, correlated with increased pregnancy terminations and low birth weight in progeny.[89] Outcomes of treating women with insulin sensitizers also suggest that pregnancy complications in women with PCOS may be due in part to insulin resistance. Treatment of women with metformin throughout pregnancy results in lower rates of early pregnancy loss, preterm delivery, preeclampsia, and restriction of fetal growth. There has been no evidence of teratogenic effects or developmental delays in offspring from pregnancies treated with metformin.[90–92]

PCOS IN ADOLESCENCE

PCOS is increasingly seen in the adolescent population, although the diagnosis of the disorder in this group of patients can be challenging. First, menstrual irregularity is common in girls in the first years after menarche. Up to 59% of cycles may be anovulatory 3 years post menarche. Moreover, acne and mild hirsutism are fairly common in peripuberty because of increased adrenal and ovarian androgen production. Imaging ovaries can also present confusion, as polycystic ovaries (defined by the presence of 12 follicles 2–9 mm in diameter) can frequently be seen in adolescents both with and without PCOS. Therefore the application of the Rotterdam criteria may lead to overdiagnosis of PCOS in this population. It is recommended that all 3 of the Rotterdam criteria be used to diagnose PCOS. If only 2 are present, the patient should be followed for possible development of PCOS. Treatment of PCOS in adolescents is similar to that in adults. Lifestyle intervention should be the first line of therapy.[93]

Adolescents with PCOS are also at risk for the development of metabolic sequelae such as diabetes and hyperlipidemia. There is a higher prevalence of the metabolic syndrome in adolescents with PCOS than without (26%–35% vs 15%).[94–97] In comparison with control groups, adolescents with PCOS have higher fasting and stimulated insulin responses to intravenous glucose tolerance test,[94,95] and have a higher prevalence of IGT and DM2.[93,98] Circulating lipid levels have been reported to be either within the normal range or have varied elevations of specific lipids.[93] Blood pressure tends to remain normal, but there can be absence of the typical decline in nocturnal blood pressure.

INSULIN RESISTANCE AND PCOS

The literature describes the occurrence of insulin resistance concurrently with the phenotype of PCOS, most notably of hyperandrogenism.[99] Type A and type B syndromes of insulin resistance feature extreme insulin resistance in conjunction with hyperandrogenism and reproductive disorder. There is insulin resistance secondary to reduction in several insulin receptors, or the presence of insulin receptor autoantibodies. In addition, hyperinsulinemia and its association with hyperandrogenism is also present in nearly 5% of obese women.[100,101] The cause of their hyperinsulinemia is secondary to the downregulation of the insulin receptor, which normalizes with caloric restriction.[102,103] Therefore it is reasonable to propose that if the mechanism behind the association of insulin resistance and hyperandrogenism is discovered, it is likely that within this interaction one can glean the pathway to the pathogenesis of PCOS. An extensive review of insulin action in the ovary can be found in a previous review of diabetes and the female reproductive system.[104] Here the in vitro and in vivo literature on insulin resistance, ovarian function, and hyperandrogenism is briefly reviewed.

In Vitro Models

Insulin receptors are found throughout ovarian tissue in the granulosa, thecal, and stromal compartments. In vitro studies have shown that the binding of insulin causes phosphorylation of these receptors or the tyrosine residues of the β subunits.[105,106] In addition, exposure to insulin has been shown to increase the production of androgens, estrogens, and progesterone by the granulosa and thecal cells. Finally, steroidogenesis can be blocked in both granulosa and thecal cells in women with PCOS through the administration of anti-insulin receptor antibodies.[107,108] This finding shows that insulin is integral in the physiology of the ovary, especially in relation to steroidogenesis (**Table 1**).

Insulin-like growth factor–binding proteins (IGFBP) are a family of proteins that regulate the bioavailability of insulin-like growth factors (IGFs). Insulin downregulates the production of IGFBP-1 via reduced production in both liver and ovarian cells. The reduction in the concentration of IGFBP-1 leads to an increase in free IGF-1 levels.[109] IGF-1 in turn stimulates DNA synthesis and estrogen secretion via both granulosa and luteal cells. IGF-1 also inhibits IGFBP-1 production while augmenting estrogen and progesterone production.[110,111] IGF-2 stimulates the aromatization of androgens, as well as increasing the basal secretion of progesterone and estrogen. Both IGF-1 and IGF-2 act on human thecal cells in vitro to enhance androgen production. Hyperinsulinemia can produce amplification of IGF-1 effects by regulating IGF receptors in the ovary and modulating IGFBP-1 production (**Fig. 3**).[109,112–114]

A study of skin fibroblast insulin receptors from women with PCOS showed no change in insulin binding or receptor affinity in comparison with controls. However, basal autophosphorylation of the insulin receptor was increased with minimal further stimulation from insulin, which was different from controls. Isolates from skeletal muscle of women with PCOS showed a similar defect.[115,116] This observation is significant in that it shows a generalized change in the physiology of insulin receptors in PCOS. In

Table 1
Insulin action on ovarian growth and function

Effect	Organ
Directly stimulates steroidogenesis	Ovary
Acts synergistically with LH and FSH to stimulate steroidogenesis	Ovary
Stimulates 17α-hydroxylase	Ovary
Stimulates or inhibits aromatase	Ovary, adipose tissue
Upregulates LH receptors	Ovary
Promotes ovarian growth and cyst formation synergistically with LH/hCG	Ovary
Downregulates insulin receptors	Ovary
Upregulates type 1 IGF receptors or hybrid insulin/type 1 IGF receptors	Ovary
Inhibits IGFBP-1 production	Ovary, liver
Potentiates the effect of GnRH on LH and FSH	Pituitary
Inhibits SHBG production	Liver
Upregulates PPARγ	Ovary
Activates StAR protein	Ovary

Abbreviations: FSH, follicle-stimulating hormone; GnRH, gonadotropin-releasing hormone; hCG, human chorionic gonadotropin; IGF, insulin-like growth factor; IGFBP, IGF-binding protein; LH, luteinizing hormone; PPAR, peroxisome proliferator–activated receptor; SHBG, sex hormone–binding globulin; StAR, steroidogenic acute regulatory.

Adapted from Poretsky L, Cataldo NA, Rosenwaks Z, et al. The insulin-related ovarian regulatory system in health and disease. Endocr Rev 1999;20(4):535–82; with permission.

addition, this early change in the insulin signaling pathway is important. The insulin receptor phosphorylation activates downstream targets such as insulin receptor substrate 1 (IRS1) or phosphatidylinositide-3-kinase (PI3K), which are linked to insulin resistance in some women with PCOS.[117]

Although the exact biochemical pathway is still unclear, there is certainly a link between the phenotype found in PCOS, hyperinsulinemia, and glucose metabolism. The interaction between the insulin receptor and steroidogenesis or hyperandrogenism is present. The exact relationship, however, remains obscure. One of the competing

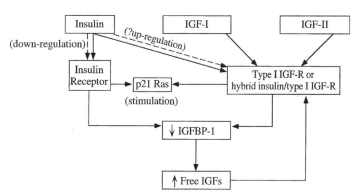

Fig. 3. Amplification of effects of insulin-like growth factor 1 (IGF-I) after regulation of IGF receptors in the ovary and modulation of the production of IGF-binding protein 1 (IGFBP-I). R, receptor.

theories is that hyperandrogenism leads to insulin resistance. This notion is supported by the observation that androgen antagonists, estrogens, and progesterone can cause the remission of insulin resistance in PCOS patients. Another theory proposes that hyperinsulinemia, caused by insulin resistance, leads to ovarian hyperstimulation resulting in hyperandrogenism. However, although there is a relationship between hyperinsulinemia and hyperandrogenism, once again the mechanism behind this phenomenon is currently unknown.[118,119]

In Vivo Models

Various models have been used to elicit the change in insulin activity in the setting of PCOS. Yan and colleagues[119] showed that the exposure of prenatal rates to androgens caused metabolic derangements in the female offspring. On exposure to 5α-dihydrotestosterone during gestation, prenatally androgenized offspring (PNA) develop increased numbers of atretic and cystic follicles with morphologic changes similar to those seen in rodents and humans with PCOS. In addition, PNA rats also exhibited elevated levels of fasting glucose, fasting insulin, and leptin. Finally, there was an increase in weight gain in PNA rats when compared with controls. Laboratory testing shows that these animals are more insulin resistant than littermate controls, with higher 30-minute and 60-minute glucose values during glucose tolerance test.[116] These data are congruent with separate studies by Lewy and colleagues[120] and Sir-Petermann and colleagues,[121] which have shown that pubertal daughters of women with PCOS have higher insulin levels and prevalence of glucose intolerance compared with controls.

During biochemical analysis of cell signaling intermediates, it was also found that insulin-stimulated Akt phosphorylation was significantly reduced in PNA rat skeletal muscle. In addition, IRS1 and IRS2 were both reduced.[121] These findings are similar to those in PCOS patients who have also been shown to have impaired insulin-mediated phosphorylation of Akt.[122] These results suggest a possible molecular basis for insulin resistance in PCOS phenotypes.

Insulin secretion in women with PCOS has been shown to be relatively decreased given the presence of insulin resistance. Euglycemic clamping performed in patients with PCOS reveals a decrease in insulin-mediated glucose disposal. The magnitude of the decrease is similar to that of patients who have non–insulin dependent DM. In addition, when PCOS patients are matched with weight and body-type controls, they still demonstrate a reduction in glucose clearance mediated by insulin. Although this does not reveal the etiology of insulin resistance, it confirms that insulin resistance as an integral entity of PCOS.[19]

Genetics

The genetic predisposition of both PCOS and insulin resistance has been suggested in the literature. Rare syndromes of extreme insulin resistance and hyperandrogenism have been described. It can be postulated that mutations can occur in the insulin receptor as well as in its signaling pathway. These mutations can alter how an individual processes insulin signal and can cause the other defects such as hyperandrogenism and ovarian dysfunction. The phenotype observed in extreme insulin resistance syndromes is an exaggeration of that seen in PCOS. Furthermore, families with multiple members affected by PCOS have been described, suggesting a possible genetic cause.[123,124]

Many approaches have been taken in the search of genetic linkage and susceptibility to the development of PCOS. First, there is a focus on the genes leading to rare insulin-resistance syndromes. Because there is a similarity between the phenotype of these syndromes and PCOS, there may exist specific characteristic gene mutations on the insulin receptor itself that can link insulin resistance with PCOS. The second avenue of investigation consists of case-control studies investigating genes in the insulin metabolic signaling pathway and their association with PCOS. A third approach focuses on the familial genetics of PCOS. Given the possible genetic link in PCOS, a reasonable approach to the discovery of genetics of PCOS would be the usage of genome-wide association studies (GWAS) to delineate susceptible genes for complex traits, thought to be caused by defects in multiple genes or loci.[125]

Identification of genetic mutations within the insulin receptor has shown mixed results. Whereas some studies, focused on women with both insulin resistance and PCOS, did not discover any mutations in the insulin receptor, others have found certain mutations that may be associated with the syndrome. Mutations of the insulin receptor or related molecules (INSR, VNTR, IRS1/2, PPARγ, and PPP1R3) have all been found to be associated with PCOS.[126,127] However, the exact mechanism of the linkage has not been entirely elucidated.

Case-control genetic studies have also found candidate genes linking PCOS, the insulin receptor, and the regulation of metabolism. One of the most intriguing is the transforming growth factor β (TGFβ) family of signaling molecules, including follistatin and myostatin. The TGFβ signaling pathway is found to be important in the control of folliculogenesis and the development of pancreatic islets.[128,129] In addition, it has been shown to be involved in the regulation of adipogenesis. The summation of the metabolic derangements that are observed with the defects in this pathway can produce both the reproductive and metabolic phenotypes of PCOS.

Studies using GWAS are able to map regions which have variations that may ultimately determine the phenotype expressed. The use of GWAS to discover these variations is another approach to the search for genetic origins of complex disease states. GWAS has thus far identified several candidates that may be contributory to the genesis of PCOS. Of these, the LHCGR gene, which encodes the receptor for LH and hCG, is promising as a gene that can likely alter reproductive physiology. In addition, derangements in the THADA gene are associated with increased LH and testosterone in subjects with PCOS, and DENND1A gene variations are associated with insulin resistance.[130,131]

Although it has not discovered a definitive cause for PCOS, GWAS is nonetheless an important tool in the search of the genetic factors for PCOS. Not only can its use identify the loci associated with disease as described previously, it can also be used in the analysis of different ethnic populations. Comparison of GWAS cohorts from different ethnic backgrounds can further discern whether each of the ethnic backgrounds shares the same PCOS susceptibility, thus allowing for the discovery of how early in human history the genetics of PCOS first occurred. Although powerful, there are certain pitfalls to this technique. To gain significance, GWAS necessitates a large number of individuals. In addition, genes that are identified may not always confer significant risk for the trait being studied, perhaps because the identified genes form a common pathway for the pathogenesis of many disease states.[132,133]

Syndromes of Severe Insulin Resistance

The genetic syndromes of insulin resistance are a group of rare disorders that share the commonalities of hyperinsulinemia and abnormal glucose homeostasis with ovarian dysfunction, hyperandrogenism, and acanthosis. It is interesting that these genetic syndromes are a phenotype consisting of exaggerated symptoms seen in PCOS. The evaluation of the genetic basis for these syndromes may give us a glimpse of the genetic and molecular mechanisms behind PCOS.[124] Insulin resistance syndromes can be subcategorized by the type of defect that leads to the severe insulin resistance. These defects include mutations in the insulin receptor, signaling pathway defects downstream from the insulin receptor, and mutations in adipose tissue which then cause insulin resistance.

The defects of the insulin receptors were reported by Kadowaki and colleagues[132] and Yoshimasa and colleagues.[133] The spectrum of disease seen with these mutations ranges from early onset to severe. The genes are associated with hypoglycemia, postprandial hyperglycemia, and extreme hyperinsulinemia. There can also be accompanying mental retardation, changes in tissue development, and aberrant sexual development. Less severe insulin receptor mutations are more common, with manifestation of disease appearing during the peripubertal period. The symptoms of oligomenorrhea, hyperandrogenism, and acanthosis can be very similar to those seen in PCOS.[134,135]

Insulin receptor autoantibodies are a rare cause of insulin resistance, with a mechanism similar to that of insulin receptor defect. The autoantibodies target the insulin receptor and block insulin action, leading to suppressed biological response to the insulin signal. In turn, this causes a compensatory elevation of serum insulin levels. The mechanisms of action of the autoantibodies are varied, and include direct binding-site inactivation, accelerated receptor degradation, or inhibition of conformational change within the receptor after binding. The clinical picture is one of insulin resistance and hyperglycemia, with prominent acanthosis nigricans and a history of autoimmunity.[134] Reproductive dysfunction similar to PCOS is seen in this disorder. Only a small number of patients exhibit this syndrome, so no uniform therapy exists. Improvement has been observed on high-dose steroids, plasma exchange, and metformin in select case studies and series.[124]

Defects in the insulin signaling pathway causing severe insulin resistance are a rare category of mutations. The AKT2 mutation, which encodes a serine/threonine kinase within the signal transduction pathway downstream from the insulin receptor, is one such mutation. Phenotypically the affected individuals have acanthosis nigricans, ovarian hyperandrogenism, and DM. In addition there is lipodystrophy, signifying the importance of insulin in adipogenesis. Another such mutation in the downstream insulin signaling pathway is the AS160 nonsense mutation, which encodes for a guanosine triphosphatase–activating protein that forms the link between insulin signaling and glucose uptake by the GLUT4 transporter. Individuals with this mutation have the phenotype of acanthosis nigricans and hyperinsulinemia.[135,136]

Disorders relating to lipodystrophy and severe insulin resistance are most common. Many defects have been discovered in this subgroup. These mutations have been classified as congenital generalized lipodystrophy and familial partial lipodystrophy. Individuals afflicted with this group of disorders exhibit dyslipidemia or nonalcoholic fatty liver disease accompanied by severe insulin resistance and reproductive dysregulation. The pathologic features of this group of disorders stem from adipose tissue deficiency, which is either generalized or partial. This derangement in adipose tissue leads to the eventual development of hyperinsulinemia and insulin resistance.[137]

TREATMENT OF PCOS

Because polycystic ovary syndrome manifests as a multifaceted disease entity encompassing hyperandrogenism, anovulation or oligomenorrhea, infertility, and insulin resistance or glucose dysregulation, the treatment goals are to ameliorate 1 or more facets of this disease. Even though this is primarily a disease of reproductive abnormalities, the defects of insulin action in the pathophysiology of the disease are important. It is not surprising, then, that treatment options to improve hyperinsulinemia or insulin resistance play a role in the treatment recommendations for PCOS.

The initial approach to PCOS includes lifestyle modification. Obesity is associated with worsening severity of symptoms in this disease. Calorie restriction with weight loss of 5% or greater can lead to changes in insulin, IGF-1, SHBG, and menstrual irregularities.[138] Changes in insulin level are accompanied by a decrease in androgenic parameters such as androstenedione, testosterone levels, and LH levels.[139,140] It has been reported that even a 2% to 5% change in weight can effectively restore ovulation.[41] When diet and exercise are not effective, surgical modalities such as gastric banding, gastroplasty, and Roux-en-Y procedure can be considered to reduce weight. It is once again postulated that the resultant decrease in insulin levels leads to improvement in ovulation rates and hyperandrogenism.[141]

If weight loss alone is not effective, insulin sensitizers such as metformin and thiazolidinediones are an effective alternative. Metformin is a biguanide that functions by suppressing hepatic gluconeogenesis and increasing fat and muscle sensitivity to insulin. A series of 14 studies with metformin has shown that 50% of women have improvement in ovulation rates with treatment.[142,143] This improvement may be weight independent, as lean women also show improvement in hyperandrogenism and menstrual irregularity with lowering of insulin levels.[144] Although most studies to date have been short-term evaluations, long-term studies have also verified these findings.[145]

Thiazolidinediones are peroxisome proliferator–activated receptor γ (PPARγ) agonists. Use of these insulin-sensitizing agents has shown improvement in ovulation, insulin resistance, hyperandrogenism, and hirsutism in both overweight and lean women.[41,146] Efficacy has been shown with all agents in this class of medications, including troglitazone, pioglitazone, and rosiglitazone.[146–148] Thiazolidinediones affect ovarian function by decreasing circulating insulin levels as well as through direct insulin-independent effects on the ovary itself (**Table 2**).[149] Both insulin signaling and PPARγ activation leads to stimulation of the expression of steroidogenic acute

---

Table 2
Direct and insulin-mediated effects of thiazolidinediones on ovarian function

1. Direct Can be observed in vitro, may be present in vivo	2. Indirect Observed in vivo; are due to systemic insulin-sensitizing action and reduction of hyperinsulinemia
A. Insulin-independent	
↑ Progesterone production	↓ Testosterone production
↓ Testosterone production	↓ Estradiol production
↓ E2 production	↑ IGFBP-1 production
↑ IGFBP-1 production in the absence of insulin	↑ SHBG ↓ Free testosterone
B. Insulin-sensitizing (enhanced insulin effect)	
↓ IGFBP-1 production	
↑ Estradiol production (in vivo, in a setting of high-dose insulin infusion)	

Adapted from Seto-Young D, Paliou M, Schlosser J, et al. Direct thiazolidinedione action in the human ovary: insulin-independent and insulin-sensitizing effects on steroidogenesis and insulin-like growth factor binding protein-1 production. J Clin Endocrinol Metab 2005;90:6099–105; with permission.

regulatory protein. In turn, this stimulates progesterone synthesis in ovarian cells.[41] However, because of the effects of thiazolidinediones on aromatase, estrogen production is reduced.

OCPs are an alternative treatment option that works independently of insulin resistance. OCPs provide direct negative feedback to LH secretion, leading to reduced androgen production by the ovary. OCPs also lead to increased SHBG levels; this then binds to androgens, effectively decreasing the levels of circulating free androgen.[41] When choosing OCPs, it is recommended to provide patients with one that has low androgenic potential.

Although weight loss, insulin sensitizers, and OCPs can all lead to reduced androgen levels, antiandrogenic compounds can be more effective in this regard. These agents, including spironolactone, cyproterone acetate, flutamide, and finasteride, should be given along with pregnancy counseling. Pregnancy should be avoided during the use of these agents, as they may have adverse effects on the male fetus.[41] Cosmetic methods, such as waxing, depilatories, electrolysis, and laser treatment, can also be used to treat hirsutism.

When single modalities are not effective in the treatment of PCOS, combination therapies can be used. Comparison of metformin and ethinylestradiol/cyproterone acetate with OCP alone showed greater decreases in androgen levels and an increase in SHBG level in the combination arm.[150] The combined group also showed a greater decrease in body mass index and insulin levels. A study by Lemay and colleagues[151] was designed to assess the efficacy of combining rosiglitazone and ethinylestradiol/cyproterone acetate. Patients were given either agent for 6 months then the combined therapy for the following 6 months. Patients receiving the combination achieved greater reductions in androgen levels and had an increase in SHBG levels. Increased insulin sensitivity was not consistently noted in this group. A recent study evaluated the combination of metformin and low-dose spironolactone in comparison with either drug alone. The combination group showed greater improvement in menstrual cycles, testosterone levels, and hyperinsulinemia.[152]

This article covers treatment options in the management of menstrual irregularity, hyperandrogenism, hyperinsulinemia, and insulin resistance. The extensive literature on ovulation induction and infertility treatment in PCOS is not reviewed here, but has been covered in recent publications that discuss infertility treatment and address optimal therapy throughout gestation in women with PCOS.[102,153]

SUMMARY

The syndrome of PCOS is strongly associated with states of insulin resistance and hyperinsulinemia. In vitro and in vivo data appear to support this link between insulin action and ovarian function. Risk factors and long-term consequences of this disease entity strongly resemble those of metabolic syndrome. Treatment of insulin resistance/hyperinsulinemia can lead to amelioration of not only the metabolic dysregulation but also the hyperandrogenism and reproductive dysfunction. However, whether insulin resistance is the causative factor in the development of PCOS remains to be ascertained. Moreover, the mechanism by which insulin resistance may lead to reproductive dysfunction requires further elucidation.

REFERENCES

1. Hanson AE. Hippocrates: diseases of women 1. Signs (Chic) 1975;1:567–84.
2. Temkin O. Soranus' gynecology. Baltimore (MD): The Johns Hopkins University Press; 1991.

3. Rosner F, Munter S. The medical aphorism of Moses Maimonides, vol. 2. New York: Yeshiva University Press; 1971.

4. Achard EC, Thiers J. Le virilisme et son association a l'insuffisnace glycolytique (diabete des femme a barbe). Bull Acad Natl Med 1921;86:51.

5. Kovacs C, Smith J. A guide to the polycystic ovary: its effects on health and fertility. Castle Hill Barns (United Kingdom): TFM Publishing; 2002.

6. Stein IF, Leventhal ML. Amenorrhea associated with bilateral polycystic ovaries. Am J Obstet Gynecol 1935;29:181–91.

7. Carmina E, Lobo R. Polycystic ovary syndrome (PCOS): arguably the most common endocrinopathy is associated with significant morbidity in women. J Clin Endocrinol Metab 1999;84:1897–9.

8. Azziz R. Diagnostic criteria for polycystic ovary syndrome: a reappraisal. Fertil Steril 2005;83(5):1343–6.

9. Michelmore K, Ong K, Mason S, et al. Clinical features in women with polycystic ovaries: relationships to insulin sensitivity, insulin gene VNTR and birth weight. Clin Endocrinol (Oxf) 2001;55(4):439–46.

10. Norman RJ, Hague WM, Masters SC, et al. Subjects with polycystic ovaries without hyperandrogenaemia exhibit similar disturbances in insulin and lipid profiles as those with polycystic ovary syndrome. Hum Reprod 1995;10(9): 2258–61 [PubMed: 8530647].

11. Brassard M, AinMelk Y, Baillargeon JP, et al. Basic infertility including polycystic ovary syndrome. Med Clin North Am 2008;92:1163–92, Xi.

12. Azziz R, Carmina E, Dewailly D, et al. Task force on the phenotype of the polycystic ovary syndrome of the Androgen Excess and PCOS Society: the Androgen Excess and PCOS Society criteria for the polycystic ovary syndrome: the complete task force report. Fertil Steril 2009;91:456–88.

13. Azziz R, Carmina E, Dewailly D, et al. Androgen Excess Society: position statement: criteria for defining polycystic ovary syndrome as a predominantly hyperandrogenic syndrome: an Androgen Excess Society guideline. J Clin Endocrinol Metab 2006;91:4237–45.

14. Norman RJ, Dewailly D, Legro RS, et al. Polycystic ovary syndrome. Lancet 2007;370:685–97.

15. Wild RA, Painter PC, Coulson PB, et al. Lipoprotein lipid concentrations and cardiovascular risk in women with polycystic ovary syndrome. J Clin Endocrinol Metab 1985;61:946–51.

16. Wild RA, Bartholomew MJ. The influence of body weight on lipoprotein lipids in patients with polycystic ovary syndrome. Am J Obstet Gynecol 1988;159: 423–7.

17. Dunaif A, Finegood DT. Beta-cell dysfunction independent of obesity and glucose intolerance in the polycystic ovary syndrome. J Clin Endocrinol Metab 1996;81:942–7.

18. O'Meara N, Blackman JD, Ehrmann DA. Defects in beta-cell function in functional ovarian hyperandrogenism. J Clin Endocrinol Metab 1993;76: 1241–7.

19. Dunaif A, Segal KR, Futterweit W, et al. Profound peripheral insulin resistance, independent of obesity, in polycystic ovary syndrome. Diabetes 1989;38: 1165–74.

20. Dunaif A. Insulin resistance and the polycystic ovary syndrome: mechanism and implications for pathogenesis. Endocr Rev 1997;18:774–800.

21. Diamanti-Kandarakis E, Papavassiliou AG. Molecular mechanisms of insulin resistance in polycystic ovary syndrome. Trends Mol Med 2006;12:324–32.

22. Legro RS, Castracane VD, Kauffman RP. Detecting insulin resistance in polycystic ovary syndrome: purposes and pitfalls. Obstet Gynecol Surv 2004;59: 141–54.

23. Vrbikova J, Cibula D, Dvorakova K, et al. Insulin sensitivity in women with polycystic ovary syndrome. J Clin Endocrinol Metab 2004;89:2942–5.

24. Legro RS, Kunselman AR, Dodson WC, et al. Prevalence and predictors of risk for type 2 diabetes mellitus and impaired glucose tolerance in polycystic ovary syndrome: a prospective, controlled study in 254 affected women. J Clin Endocrinol Metab 1999;84:165–9.

25. Barr EL, Magliano DJ, Zimmet PZ, et al. AusDiab 2005: the Australian diabetes, obesity and lifestyle study. Melbourne (Australia): International Diabetes Institute; 2006.

26. Legro RS, Gnatuk CL, Kunselman AR, et al. Changes in glucose tolerance over time in women with polycystic ovary syndrome: a controlled study. J Clin Endocrinol Metab 2005;90:3236–42.

27. Boudreaux MY, Talbott EO, Kip KE, et al. Risk of T2DM and impaired fasting glucose among PCOS subjects: results of an 8-year follow-up. Curr Diab Rep 2006;6:77–83.

28. Alberti KG, Zimmet P, Shaw J. International Diabetes Federation: a consensus on Type 2 Diabetes prevention. Diabet Med 2007;24:451–63.

29. Coffey S, Mason H. The effect of polycystic ovary syndrome on health-related quality of life. Gynecol Endocrinol 2003;17:379–86.

30. Deeks A, Gibson-Helm M, Teede H. Anxiety and depression in polycystic ovary syndrome (PCOS): a comprehensive investigation. Fertil Steril 2010;93:2421–3.

31. Azziz R, Woods KS, Reyna R, et al. The prevalence and features of the polycystic ovary syndrome in an unselected population. J Clin Endocrinol Metab 2004; 89(6):2745–9.

32. Carmina E, Koyama T, Chang L, et al. Does ethnicity influence prevalence of adrenal hyperandrogenism and insulin resistance in polycystic ovary syndrome. Am J Obstet Gynecol 1992;167(6):1807–12.

33. Legro RS. Phenotype and genotype in polycystic ovary syndrome. In: Kovacs G, Norman R, editors. Polycystic ovary syndrome. Cambridge (United Kingdom): Cambridge University Press; 2007. p. 25–41.

34. Legro RS, Driscoll D, Strauss JF Jr, et al. Evidence for a genetic basis for hyperandrogenemia in polycystic ovary syndrome. Proc Natl Acad Sci U S A 1998;95: 14956–60.

35. Jahantar S, Eden JA, Warren P, et al. A twin study of polycystic ovary syndrome. Fertil Steril 1995;63:478–86.

36. Ibanez L, DiMartino-Nardi J, Potau N, et al. Premature adrenarche: normal variant or forerunner of adult disease? Endocr Rev 2000;21:671–96.

37. Ibanez L, Potau N, Chacon P, et al. Hyperinsulinemia, dyslipidemia, and cardiovascular risk in girls with a history of premature pubarche. Diabetologia 1998;41: 1057–63.

38. Ibanez L, Potau N, Zampolli M, et al. Hyperinsulinemia and decreased insulin-like growth factor binding protein-I are common features in prepubertal and pubertal girls with a history of premature pubarche. J Clin Endocrinol Metab 1999; 82:2283–8.

39. Ibanez L, Potau N, Zampolli M, et al. Girls diagnosed with premature pubarche show an exaggerated ovarian androgen synthesis from the early stages of puberty: evidence from gonadotropin-releasing hormone agonist testing. Fertil Steril 1997;67:849–55.

40. Ibanez L, Potau N, Zampolli M, et al. Source localization of androgen excess in adolescent girls. J Clin Endocrinol Metab 1994;79:1778–84.
41. Zweig SB, Tolentino MC, Strizhevsky M, et al. Polycystic ovary syndrome. In: Poretsky L, editor. Principles of diabetes mellitus. New York: Springer; 2010. p. 515–30.
42. Barker DJ. The developmental origins of chronic adult disease. Acta Paediatr Suppl 2004;93:26–33.
43. Ibanez L, Potau N, Francois J, et al. Pubarche, hyperinsulinism, and ovarian hyperandrogenism in girls: relation to reduced fetal growth. J Clin Endocrinol Metab 1998;83:3558–62.
44. Ibanez L, Potau N, Zampolli M, et al. Hyperinsulinemia in post pubertal girls with a history of premature pubarche and functional ovarian hyperandrogenism. J Clin Endocrinol Metab 1996;81:1237–43.
45. Manikkam M, Crespi EJ, Doop DD, et al. Fetal programming: prenatal testosterone excess leads to fetal growth retardation and postnatal catch up growth in sheep. Endocrinology 2004;145:790–8.
46. Slob AK, denHamer R, Woutersen PJ, et al. Prenatal testosterone propionate and postnatal ovarian activity in the rat. Acta Endocrinol 1983;103:420–7.
47. Laitinen J, Taponen S, Martikainen H, et al. Body size from birth to adulthood as a predictor of self-reported polycystic ovary syndrome symptoms. Int J Obes Relat Metab Disord 2003;27:710–5.
48. Sadrzadeh S, Klip WA, Broekmans FJ, et al. Birth weight and age at menarche in patients with polycystic ovary syndrome or diminished ovarian reserve, in a retrospective cohort. Hum Reprod 2003;18:2225–30.
49. Prentice AM. Early influences on human energy regulation(CHECK):thrifty genotype and thrifty phenotypes. Physiol Behav 2005;86:640–5.
50. Abbott DH, Barnett DK, Bruns CM, et al. Androgen excess fetal programming of female reproduction: a developmental etiology for polycystic syndrome? Hum Reprod Update 2005;11:257–74.
51. Abbott DH, Eisner JR, Colman RJ, et al. Prenatal androgen excess programs for PCOS in female rhesus monkey. In: Chang RJ, Dunaif A, Hiendel J, editors. Polycystic ovary syndrome. New York: Marcel Dekker; 2002. p. 119–33.
52. Abbott GH, Dumesic DA, Eisner JR, et al. Insights into the development of PCOS from studies of prenatally androgenized female rhesus monkey. Trends Endocrinol Metab 1998;9:62–4.
53. Dumesic DA, Abbott DH, Eisner JR, et al. Prenatal exposure of female rhesus monkeys to testosterone propionate increases serum luteinizing hormone levels in adulthood. Fertil Steril 1997;67:155–63.
54. Eisner JR, Barnett MA, Dumesic DA, et al. Ovarian hyperandrogenism in adult female rhesus monkeys exposed to prenatal androgen excess. Fertil Steril 2002;77:167–72.
55. Abbott DH, Foong SC, Barnett DK, et al. Nonhuman primates contribute unique understanding to anovulatory infertility in women. ILAR J 2004;45:116–31.
56. Dumesic DA, Schramm RD, Peterson E, et al. Impaired developmental competence of oocytes in adult prenatally androgenized female rhesus monkeys undergoing gonadotropin stimulation for in vitro fertilization. J Clin Endocrinol Metab 2002;87:1111–9.
57. Dumesic DA, Schramm RD, Peterson E, et al. Reduced intrafollicular androstenedione and estradiol levels in early treated prenatally androgenized female rhesus monkeys receiving FSH therapy for in vitro fertilization. Biol Reprod 2003; 69:1213–9.

58. Eisner JR, Dumesic DA, Kemnitz JW, et al. Timing of prenatal androgen excess determines differential impairment in insulin secretion and action in adult female rhesus monkeys. J Clin Endocrinol Metab 2000;85:1206–10.

59. Eisner JR, Dumesic DA, Kemnitz JW, et al. Increased adiposity in female rhesus monkeys exposed to androgen excess during early gestation. Obes Res 2003; 11:279–86.

60. Yildiz BO, Yarali H, Oguz H, et al. Glucose intolerance, insulin resistance, and hyperandrogenemia in first degree relatives of women with polycystic ovary syndrome. J Clin Endocrinol Metab 2003;88:2031–6.

61. Kaushal R, Parchure N, Bano G, et al. Insulin resistance and endothelial dysfunction in the brothers of Indian subcontinent Asian women with polycystic ovaries. Clin Endocrinol 2004;60:322–8.

62. Bruns CM, Baum ST, Colman RJ, et al. Insulin resistance and impaired insulin secretion in prenatally androgenized male rhesus monkeys. J Clin Endocrinol Metab 2004;89:6218–23.

63. Dunaif A, Graf M, Mandeli J, et al. Characterization of groups of hyperandrogenic women with acanthosis nigricans, impaired glucose tolerance, and/or hyperinsulinemia. J Clin Endocrinol Metab 1987;65:499–507.

64. Liao E, Poretsky L. Polycystic ovary syndrome and its complications. In: Mantzoros CS, editor. Contemporary diabetes: obesity and diabetes. New Jersey: Humana Press Inc; 2006. p. 255–76.

65. Robinson S, Kiddy D, Gelding SV, et al. The relationship of insulin sensitivity to menstrual pattern in women with hyperandrogenism and polycystic ovaries. Clin Endocrinol 1993;39:351–5.

66. Ehmann DA, Barnes RB, Rosenfield RL, et al. Prevalence of impaired glucose tolerance and diabetes in women with polycystic ovary syndrome. Diabetes Care 1999;22:141–6.

67. Pierpoint T, McKeigue DM, Isaacs AJ, et al. Mortality of women with polycystic ovary syndrome at long-term follow up. J Clin Epidemiol 1998;51:581–6.

68. Kousta E, Franks S. Long term health consequences of polycystic ovary syndrome. In: Kovacs G, Norman R, editors. Polycystic ovary syndrome. Cambridge (United Kingdom): Cambridge University Press; 2007. p. 81–101.

69. Salehi M, Bravo-Vera A, Sheikh A, et al. Pathogenesis of polycystic ovary syndrome: what is the role of obesity? Metabolism 2004;53:358–76.

70. Vrbikova J, Cifkova R, Jirkovska A, et al. Cardiovascular risk factors in young Czech females with polycystic ovary syndrome. Hum Reprod 2003;18:980–4.

71. Mather KJ, Kwan F, Corenblum B, et al. Hyperinsulinemia in polycystic ovary syndrome correlates with increased cardiovascular risk independent of obesity. Fertil Steril 2000;73:150–6.

72. Pirwany IR, Fleming R, Greer IA, et al. Lipids and lipoprotein subfractions in women with PCOS: relationship to metabolic and endocrine parameters. Clin Endocrinol 2001;54:447–53.

73. Legro RS, Kunselman AR, Dunaif A. Prevalence and predictors of dyslipidemia in women with polycystic ovary syndrome. Am J Med 2001;111:607–13.

74. Taponen S, Martikainen H, Jarvelin MR, et al. Metabolic cardiovascular disease risk factors in women with self reported symptoms of oligomenorrhea and/or hirsutism: Northern Finland Birth Cohort 1996 Study. J Clin Endocrinol Metab 2004; 89:2114–8.

75. Diamanti-Kandarakis E, Spina G, Kouli C, et al. Increased endothelin-1 levels in women with polycystic ovary syndrome and the beneficial effect of metformin therapy. J Clin Endocrinol Metab 2001;86:4666–73.

76. Orio F Jr, Palomba S, Cascella T, et al. Early impairment of endothelial structure and function in young normal-weight women with polycystic ovary syndrome. J Clin Endocrinol Metab 2004;89:4588–93.

77. Kelly C, Lyall H, Petrie JR, et al. Low grade chronic inflammation in women with polycystic ovarian syndrome. J Clin Endocrinol Metab 2001;86:2453–5.

78. Tarkun I, Arslan BC, Canturk Z, et al. Endothelial dysfunction in young women with polycystic ovary syndrome: relationship with insulin resistance and low-grade chronic inflammation. J Clin Endocrinol Metab 2004;89:5592–6.

79. Talbott EO, Guzick DS, Sutton-Tyrell K, et al. Evidence for association between polycystic ovary syndrome and premature carotid atherosclerosis in middle-aged women. Arterioscler Thromb Vasc Biol 2000;20:2414–21.

80. Christian RC, Dumesic DA, Behrenbeck T, et al. Prevalence and predictors of coronary artery calcification in women with polycystic ovary syndrome. J Clin Endocrinol Metab 2003;88:2562–8.

81. Dahlgren E, Janson PO, Johansson S, et al. Polycystic ovary syndrome and risk for myocardial infarction, evaluated from a risk factor model based on a prospective population study of women. Acta Obstet Gynecol Scand 1992;71:599–604.

82. Wild S, Pierpont T, McKeigue P, et al. Cardiovascular disease in women with polycystic ovary syndrome at long-term follow up: a retrospective cohort study. Clin Endocrinol (Oxf) 2000;52:595–600.

83. Coulam CB, Annegers JF, Kranz JS. Chronic anovulation syndrome and associated neoplasia. Obstet Gynecol 1983;61:403–47.

84. Hardiman P, Pillay OC, Atiomo W. Polycystic ovary syndrome and endometrial carcinoma. Lancet 2003;361:1810–2.

85. Jun ZQ, Pang LH, Li MJ, et al. Obstetric complications in women with polycystic ovary syndrome: a systematic review and meta-analysis. Reprod Biol Endocrinol 2013;11:56.

86. Hsin H, Kenyon C. Signals from the reproductive system regulate the lifespan of C. elegans. Nature 1999;399:362.

87. Bohni R, Riesgo-Escovar J, Oldham S, et al. Autonomous control of cell and organ size by CHICO, a Drosophila homologue of vertebrate IRS1-4. Cell 1999;97(7):865.

88. Withers DJ. Insulin receptor substrate proteins and neuroendocrine function. Biochem Soc Trans 2001;29:525.

89. Nandi A, Wang X, Accili D, et al. The effect of insulin signaling on female reproductive function independent of adiposity and hyperglycemia. Endocrinology 2010;151(4):1863–71.

90. Lautatzis ME, Goulis DG, Vrontakis M. Efficacy and safety of metformin during pregnancy in women with gestational diabetes mellitus or polycystic ovary syndrome: a systematic review. Metabolism 2013;62(11):1522–34.

91. Zheng J, Shan PF, Gu W. The efficacy of metformin in pregnant women with polycystic ovary syndrome: a meta-analysis of clinical trials. J Endocrinol Invest 2013. [Epub ahead of print].

92. Glueck CJ, Goldenberg N, Pranikoff J, et al. Effects of metformin-diet intervention before and throughout pregnancy on obstetric and neonatal outcomes in patients with polycystic ovary syndrome. Curr Med Res Opin 2013;29(1):55–62.

93. Roldan B, Escobar-Morreale HF. The pediatric origins of polycystic ovary syndrome. In: Kovacs G, Norman R, editors. Polycystic ovary syndrome. Cambridge (United Kingdom): Cambridge University Press; 2007. p. 233–61.

94. Rackow BW. Polycystic ovary syndrome in adolescents. Curr Opin Obstet Gynecol 2012;24:281–7.

95. Nicandri KF, Hoeger K. Treatment and diagnosis of PCOS in adolescents. Curr Opin Endocrinol Diabetes Obes 2012;19:497–504.

96. Apter D, Butzon T, Laughlin GA, et al. Metabolic features of polycystic ovary syndrome are found in adolescent girls with hyperandrogenism. J Clin Endocrinol Metab 1995;80:2966–73.

97. Mauras N, Welch S, Rini A, et al. Ovarian hyperandrogenism is associated with insulin resistance to both peripheral carbohydrate and whole body protein metabolism in post pubertal young females: a metabolic study. J Clin Endocrinol Metab 1998;83:1900–5.

98. Arsalanian SA, Lewy VD, Danadian K. Glucose intolerance in obese adolescents with polycystic ovary syndrome: roles of insulin resistance and B cell dysfunction and risk of cardiovascular disease. J Clin Endocrinol Metab 2001; 86:66–71.

99. Frank S. Polycystic ovary syndrome. N Engl J Med 1995;333:853–61.

100. Kahn CR, Flier JS, Bar RS, et al. Antibodies that impair insulin receptor binding in an unusual diabetic syndrome with severe insulin resistance. Science 1975;190:63–5.

101. Kahn CR, Flier JS, Bar RS, et al. The syndromes of insulin resistance and acanthosis nigricans. Insulin-receptor disorders in man. N Engl J Med 1976;294: 739–45.

102. Poretsky L, Bhargava G, Kalin MF, et al. Regulation of insulin receptors in the human ovary: in vitro studies. J Clin Endocrinol Metab 1988;67:774–8.

103. Poretsky L, Bhargava G, Saketos M, et al. Regulation of human ovarian insulin receptors in vivo. Metabolism 1990;39:161–6.

104. Nandi A, Poretsky L. Diabetes and the female reproductive system. Endocrinol Metab Clin North Am, in press.

105. Poretsky L, Smith D, Seibel M, et al. Specific insulin binding sites in human ovary. J Clin Endocrinol Metab 1984;59:809–11.

106. Poretsky L, Grigorescu F, Seibel M, et al. Distribution and characterization of insulin and insulin-like growth factor I receptors in normal human ovary. J Clin Endocrinol Metab 1985;61:728–34.

107. Barbieri RL, Makris A, Ryan KJ. Effects of insulin on steroidogenesis in cultured porcine ovarian theca. Fertil Steril 1983;40:237–41.

108. Willis D, Franks S. Insulin action in human granulosa cells from normal and polycystic ovaries is mediated by the insulin receptor and not the type-I insulin-like growth factor receptor. J Clin Endocrinol Metab 1995;80:3788–90.

109. Poretsky L, Cataldo NA, Rosenwaks Z, et al. The insulin-related ovarian regulatory system in health and disease. Endocr Rev 1999;20(4):535.

110. Voutilainen R, Franks S, Mason HD, et al. Expression of insulin-like growth factor (IGF), IGF binding protein, and IGF receptor messenger ribonucleic acids in normal and polycystic ovaries. J Clin Endocrinol Metab 1996;81(3):1003.

111. Rosenfeld RG, Rosenbloom AL, Guevara-Aguirre J. Growth hormone (GH) insensitivity due to primary GH receptor deficiency. Endocr Rev 1994;15(3):369.

112. Poretsky L, Chun B, Liu HC, et al. Insulin-like growth factor II (IGF-II) inhibits insulin-like growth factor binding protein I (IGFBP-1) production in luteinized human granulosa cells with a potency similar to insulin-like growth factor I (IGF-I). J Clin Endocrinol Metab 1996;81(9):3412.

113. Damario MA, Bogovixh K, Hung-Ching L, et al. Synergistic effects of insulin-like growth factor-I and human chorionic gonadotropin in the rat ovary. Metabolism 2000;49:314–20.

114. Poretsky L. Commentary: polycystic ovary syndrome—increased or preserved ovarian sensitivity to insulin? J Clin Endocrinol Metab 2006;91:2859–60.
115. Dunaif A, Xia J, Book CB, et al. Excessive insulin receptor serine phosphorylation in cultured fibroblasts and in skeletal muscle. J Clin Invest 1995;96:801–10.
116. Cheatham B, Kahn CR. Insulin action and the insulin signaling network. Endocr Rev 1995;16:117–42.
117. Nestler JE, Jakubowicz DJ, de Vargas AF, et al. Insulin stimulates testosterone biosynthesis by human thecal cells from women with polycystic ovary syndrome by activating its own receptor and using inositolglycan mediators as the signal transduction system. J Clin Endocrinol Metab 1998;83(6):2001.
118. Shoupe D, Lobo RA. The influence of androgens on insulin resistance. Fertil Steril 1984;41(3):385.
119. Yan X, Dai X, Wang J, et al. Prenatal androgen excess programs metabolic derangements in pubertal female rats. J Endocrinol 2013;217:119–29.
120. Lewy VD, Danadian K, Witchel SF, et al. Early metabolic abnormalities in adolescent girls with polycystic ovarian syndrome. J Pediatr 2001;138:38–44.
121. Sir-Petermann T, Codner E, Perez V, et al. Metabolic and reproductive features before and during puberty in daughters of women with polycystic ovary syndrome. J Clin Endocrinol Metab 2009;94:1923–30.
122. Hojlund K, Glintborg D, Andersen NR, et al. Impaired insulin-stimulated phosphorylation of Akt and AS160 in skeletal muscle of women with polycystic ovary syndrome is reversed by pioglitazone treatment. Diabetes 2008;57:357–66.
123. Semple R, Savage D, Cochran E, et al. Genetic syndromes of severe insulin resistance. Endocr Rev 2011;32:498–514.
124. Diamanti-Kandarakis E, Dunaif A. Insulin resistance and the polycystic ovary syndrome revisited: an update on mechanisms and implications. Endocr Rev 2012;33:981–1030.
125. Shi Y, Massagué J. Mechanisms of TGF-β signaling from cell membrane to the nucleus. Cell 2003;113:685–700.
126. Chang H, Brown CW, Matzuk MM. Genetic analysis of the mammalian transforming growth factor-β superfamily. Endocr Rev 2002;23:787–823.
127. Miralles F, Czernichow P, Scharfmann R. Follistatin regulates the relative proportions of endocrine versus exocrine tissue during pancreatic development. Development 1998;125:1017–24.
128. Gonzalez-Cadavid NF, Bhasin S. Role of myostatin in metabolism. Curr Opin Clin Nutr Metab Care 2004;7:451–7.
129. Chen ZJ, Zhao H, He L, et al. Genome-wide association study identifies susceptibility loci for polycystic ovary syndrome on chromosome 2p16.3, 2p21 and 9q33.3. Nat Genet 2011;43:55–9.
130. Goodarzi MO, Jones MR, Li X, et al. Replication of association of DENND1A and THADA variants with polycystic ovary syndrome in European cohorts. J Med Genet 2012;49:90–5.
131. Jones MR, Chua AK, Mengesha EA, et al. Metabolic and cardiovascular genes in polycystic ovary syndrome: a candidate-wide association study (CWAS). Steroids 2012;77:317–22.
132. Kadowaki T, Bevins CL, Cama A, et al. Two mutant alleles of the insulin receptor gene in a patient with extreme insulin resistance. Science 1988;240:787–90.
133. Yoshimasa Y, Seino S, Whittaker J, et al. Insulin resistant diabetes due to a point mutation that prevents insulin proreceptor processing. Science 1988;240:784–7.
134. Magsino C, Spencer J. Insulin receptor antibodies and insulin resistance. South Med J 1999;92:717–9.

135. George S, Rochford JJ, Wolfrum C, et al. A family with severe insulin resistance and diabetes due to a mutation in AKT2. Science 2004;304:1325–8.
136. Dash S, Sano H, Rochford JJ, et al. A truncation mutation in TBC1D4 in a family with acanthosis nigricans and postprandial hyperinsulinemia. Proc Natl Acad Sci U S A 2009;106:9350–5.
137. Garg A. Lipodystrophies: genetic and acquired body fat disorders. J Clin Endocrinol Metab 2011;96:3313–25.
138. Caballero E. Diabetes in culturally diverse populations: from biology to culture. In: Poretsky L, editor. Principles of diabetes mellitus. New York: Springer; 2010. p. 129–46.
139. Bates GW, Whitworth NS. Effect of body weight reduction on plasma androgens in obese fertile women. Fertil Steril 1982;38:406–9.
140. Pasquali R, Antenucci D, Casimirri F, et al. Clinical and hormonal characteristics of obese and amenorrheic women before and after weight loss. J Clin Endocrinol Metab 1989;68:173–9.
141. Clark DO. Physical activity efficacy and effectiveness among older adults and minorities. Diabetes Care 1997;20:1176–82.
142. Katsiki N, Hatzitolios A. Insulin-sensitizing agents in the treatment of polycystic ovary syndrome: an update. Curr Opin Obstet Gynecol 2010;22:466.
143. Bloomgarden ZT, Futterwiet W, Poretsky L. The use of insulin-sensitizing agents in patients with polycystic ovary syndrome. Endocr Pract 2001;7:279–86.
144. Nestler JE, Jakubowicz DJ. Decreases in ovarian cytochrome p450c17 alpha activity and serum free testosterone after reduction of insulin secretion in polycystic ovary syndrome. N Engl J Med 1996;335:617–23.
145. Moghetti P, Castello R, Negri C, et al. Metformin effects on clinical features, endocrine and metabolic profiles, and insulin sensitivity in polycystic ovary syndrome: a randomized, double-blind, placebo-controlled 6-month trial, followed by open, long-term clinical evaluation. J Clin Endocrinol Metab 2000;85(1): 139–46.
146. Azziz R, Ehrmann D, Legro RS, et al. Troglitazone improves ovulation and hirsutism in polycystic ovary syndrome: a multi-center, double blind placebo-controlled trial. J Clin Endocrinol Metab 2001;86:1626–32.
147. Brettenthaler N, De Geyter C, Huber P, et al. Effect of insulin sensitizer pioglitazone on insulin resistance, hyperandrogenism, and ovulatory dysfunction in women with polycystic ovary syndrome. J Clin Endocrinol Metab 2004;89: 3835–40.
148. Garmes H, Tambascia M, Zantut-Wittmann P. Endocrine-metabolic effects of the treatment with pioglitazone in obese patients with polycystic ovary syndrome. Gynecol Endocrinol 2005;21:317–23.
149. Seto-Young D, Paliou M, Schlosser J, et al. Thiazolidinedione action in the human ovary: insulin-independent and insulin sensitizing effects of steroidogenesis and insulin-like growth factor binding protein-1 production. J Clin Endocrinol Metab 2005;90:6099–105.
150. Elter K, Imir G, Durmusoglu F. Clinical, endocrine and metabolic effects of metformin added to ethinyl estradiol-cyproterone acetate in non-obese women with polycystic ovary syndrome: a randomized and control study. Hum Reprod 2002; 17(7):1729.
151. Lemay A, Dodin S, Turcot L, et al. Rosiglitazone and ethinyl-estradiol/cyproterone acetate as single and combined treatment of overweight women with polycystic ovary syndrome and insulin resistance. Hum Reprod 2006; 21(1):121.

152. Ganie MA, Khurana ML, Nisar S, et al. Improved efficacy of low-dose spirono-lactone and metformin combination than either drug alone in the management of women with polycystic ovary syndrome: a six month, open-label randomized study. J Clin Endocrinol Metab 2013;98:3599-607.
153. Araki T, Elias R, Rosenwaks Z, et al. Achieving a successful pregnancy in women with polycystic ovary syndrome. Endocrinol Metab Clin North Am 2011;40:865-94.

Peripheral Arterial Disease

Janice V. Mascarenhas, MBBS[a,b], Mostafa A. Albayati, BSc, MBBS[c],
Clifford P. Shearman, BSc, MBBS, MS, FRCS[c],
Edward B. Jude, MD, MRCP[a,b],*

KEYWORDS

- Endothelial dysfunction • Ankle brachial pressure index • Intermittent claudication
- Critical limb ischemia

KEY POINTS

- Peripheral arterial disease (PAD) is a common comorbid condition frequently encountered in patients with diabetes.
- The unfavorable metabolic milieu in diabetes favors the development of PAD.
- Ankle brachial pressure index is a good screening tool for detection of PAD.
- Lifestyle modification and antiplatelet therapy continue to be the standard therapy for the management of PAD.

INTRODUCTION

Peripheral arterial disease (PAD) is a chronic atherosclerotic process that causes narrowing of the peripheral arterial vasculature, predominantly of the lower limbs. It has an estimated worldwide prevalence of up to 10%, increasing to nearly 30% in patients more than 50 years of age.[1] Critical limb ischemia (CLI), the most severe manifestation of the disease, can result in limb loss, or even death, if not treated promptly.

The clinical importance of diabetes in PAD is several-fold. Patients with diabetes have a 4-fold increased risk of developing PAD,[2] which presents at an earlier stage and progresses more rapidly than in people without diabetes. In addition, the outcome after surgical revascularization is often worse in diabetic patients with PAD because of a delay in diagnosis and this group is 10 to 16 times more likely to undergo major (above the ankle) amputation.[3] The outlook for patients after amputation is generally poor and approximately 30% ambulate with a prosthetic limb and 50% die within 2 years. The subsequent financial, social, and psychological implications on patients

[a] Department of Endocrinology, Tameside Hospital NHS Foundation Trust, Fountain Street, Ashton-Under-Lyne, Lancashire OL6 9RW, UK; [b] University of Manchester, Oxford Road, Manchester M13 9PL, UK; [c] Department of Vascular Surgery, University Hospital Southampton NHS Foundation Trust, Southampton General Hospital, Tremona Road, Southampton, Hampshire SO16 6YD, UK
* Corresponding author. Department of Endocrinology, Tameside Hospital NHS Foundation Trust, Fountain Street, Ashton-Under-Lyne, Lancashire OL6 9RW.
E-mail address: edward.jude@tgh.nhs.uk

Endocrinol Metab Clin N Am 43 (2014) 149–166
http://dx.doi.org/10.1016/j.ecl.2013.09.003
0889-8529/14/$ – see front matter © 2014 Elsevier Inc. All rights reserved.

and health care providers can be profound and highlight the need to develop strategies for the early diagnosis and treatment of patients with PAD, in particular those with diabetes.

This article reviews the pathophysiology of PAD focusing on the effect of diabetes and provides an up-to-date overview of the diagnosis and management of this common condition.

RISK FACTORS AND PATHOGENESIS

Atherosclerosis is characterized by intimal lesions called atheroma, or atheromatous or fibrofatty plaques, which protrude into and obstruct vascular lumen and weaken the underlying media.[4] In atherosclerotic PAD of the lower limbs, arterial stenoses result in a gradual reduction of blood supply to the limbs, which eventually manifests clinically as pain and tissue loss. Many patients with PAD are asymptomatic and the earliest manifestation of the condition is pain on walking, known as intermittent claudication (IC). In addition, if untreated, patients may develop pain at rest and tissue loss or gangrene.

The global distribution of atherosclerosis causes other serious complications, and many patients with PAD also have clinically relevant cerebral or coronary artery disease, which is reflected in the 6-fold increase in mortality from cardiovascular disease compared with patients without PAD.[5]

Risk Factors for PAD

The atherosclerotic risk factors responsible for PAD and other cardiovascular diseases are common to all these conditions. These predisposing risk factors have been identified by means of several well-defined prospective studies such as the Framingham Heart Study and the Multiple Risk Factor Intervention Trial.[6]

Age, sex, and ethnicity

The incidence and prevalence of PAD increase with age. The Framingham Offspring Study showed that the odds ratio of PAD was 2.6 for each 10 years of age.[7] Although some studies have found the prevalence to be similar between both sexes, the male/female ratio is commonly reported as 2:1. This finding may partly be explained by the protective effects of estrogen in premenopausal women. Black ethnicity is also an independent risk factor for PAD, with an odds ratio of 2.8.[8]

Cigarette smoking

Smoking is the most important modifiable risk factor for developing PAD, and this relationship has been recognized for several decades after findings that IC (leg pain on walking) was 3 times more common among smokers than nonsmokers.[1] Public health strategies to reduce cigarette smoking have therefore long been advocated for patients with IC. The Edinburgh Artery Study showed a 4-fold risk increase in IC in smokers than in nonsmokers.[9] In addition, a meta-analysis of 29 studies found that the failure rate of surgical bypass grafts is 3 times greater in patients who continue to smoke.[10] These complications of smoking may be attributed to the endothelial dysfunction and proinflammatory and thrombotic states that develop following the increased oxidative stress.[11]

Diabetes

Along with smoking, diabetes is a major risk factor for PAD, mainly affecting the infrapopliteal arteries in these patients. For every 1% increase in hemoglobin A_{1c} (HbA_{1c}) there is a corresponding 26% increased risk of PAD[12] and, in addition to severity of hyperglycemia, the United Kingdom Prospective Diabetes Study (UKPDS) found that duration of hyperglycemia is also associated with an increased risk for PAD independently of other factors.[13] These findings emphasize that early diagnosis of diabetes and strict glycemic control are of paramount importance to minimizing the onset and/or progression of PAD.

PAD in patients with diabetes is aggressive and more rapidly progressive than in nondiabetic counterparts, which is reflected in the significantly higher incidence of major amputation in this group. One of the commonest and most costly causes of hospital admission for a person with diabetes is foot ulceration and infection. In the United Kingdom, the National Institute for Health and Clinical Excellence (NICE) has produced specific guidance on managing patients with diabetes and foot ulceration, recommending urgent referral to a multidisciplinary diabetic foot team without delay and preferably within 24 hours.[14]

Hypertension
The UKPDS also found that increased systolic blood pressure (SBP) was an independent risk factor for PAD. Each 10 mm Hg increase in SBP was associated with a 25% increased risk for developing PAD.[13] The Framingham Heart Study identified that a blood pressure greater than 160/95 mm Hg increased the risk of IC approximately 3-fold to 4-fold.[15] In other studies, the prevalence of PAD among hypertensive and nonhypertensive subjects was 6.9% versus 2.2%, respectively.[8] However, the relative risk for developing PAD is less for hypertension than diabetes or smoking.

Hyperlipidemia
Hyperlipidemia also represents an independent risk factor for developing PAD and data from the Framingham Heart Study showed that a fasting cholesterol concentration of greater than 7 mmol/L (270 mg/dL) conferred a 2-fold increase in the risk of IC. Previous studies have found that for every 10 mg increase in total cholesterol there is a 5% to 10% increment in the subsequent risk of PAD.[2]

Other factors
Chronic renal insufficiency, increased hematocrit resulting in a hyperviscosity state, and hyperhomocysteinemia also seem to be linked to an increased risk of PAD, although it is unclear whether these links are causal. Some recent studies have also shown that C-reactive protein (CRP) is increased in patients with PAD,[16] but the evidence for this link remains limited at present.

ATHEROSCLEROSIS IN PAD

The overwhelming importance of atherosclerosis has stimulated efforts to study its cause, resulting in several hypotheses for atherogenesis. The contemporary view of the pathogenesis of atherosclerosis incorporates elements from 3 components: (1) biological environment (ie, risk factors previously discussed), (2) hemodynamic factors (eg, low wall shear stresses at bifurcation regions), and (3) genetic or inherited factors.

The key processes in atherosclerosis are intimal thickening and lipid accumulation in large and medium-sized arteries initiated by low-grade injury to the endothelium caused by the known risk factors of atherosclerosis. The resultant endothelial dysfunction causes increased permeability to, and accumulation of, plasma lipoproteins (mainly low-density lipoprotein [LDL]) in the intimal wall, which are oxidized by free radicals generated in macrophages, endothelial cells, and smooth muscle cells (SMCs).[4] The subsequent oxidized LDL causes endothelial surface expression of vascular cell adhesion molecules (VCAMs), specifically VCAM-1 and P-selectin, which bind to monocytes in the general circulation.[17] It also stimulates the release of chemo-kines such as monocyte chemoattractant protein-1 (MCP-1), which is involved in recruiting monocytes into the tunica intima. After entering the intima, monocytes differentiate into lipid-laden macrophages, which internalize the oxidized LDL to form foam cells.[18] Proinflammatory cytokines, such as tumor necrosis factor (TNF)-alpha and interleukin (IL)-1β, released from macrophages, increase expression of LDL receptors at the endothelial surface.[19] A vicious cycle thus ensues, whereby more lipid-laden foam cells accumulate in the arterial wall leading to more inflammation (**Fig. 1**).

Oxidized LDL also causes the release of growth factors, including platelet-derived growth factor (PDGF), fibroblast growth factor (FGF), and transforming growth factor (TGF) alpha, which cause the migration of SMCs from the tunica media into the intima, where they proliferate and deposit extracellular matrix (ECM) components over the core of the fatty streak to form a thick fibrous cap and prevent progression to a

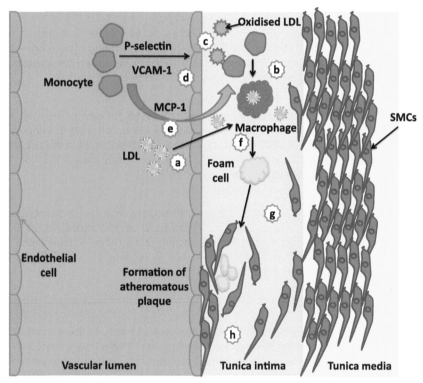

Fig. 1. Pathogenesis of atherosclerosis. (a) Accumulation of LDL within the intima as a result of endothelial dysfunction. (b) Oxidation of LDL by free radicals produced by endothelial cells, macrophages, and SMCs. (c) Oxidized LDL causes increased expression of cell adhesion molecules over the endothelial surface (VCAMs, P-selectin). (d) VCAMs facilitate adherence of circulating monocytes to endothelium. (e) Migration of monocytes into the intima by MCP-1. (f) Differentiation of monocytes into macrophages that imbibe the oxidized LDL to form foam cells. (g) Migration of SMCs from media to intima under the influence of growth factors (platelet-derived growth factor, fibroblast growth factor, and transforming growth factor alpha). (h) Proliferation of SMCs and extracellular matrix deposition around the foam cells leads to the formation of an atheromatous plaque within the vessel wall.

complicated lesion.[4] This growth in size of the atheromatous plaque causes stenosis and a gradual occlusion of the affected artery, resulting in tissue ischemia.

As a physiologic adaptation, the collateral lower limb arteries increase both in diameter and number (angiogenesis). Although these adaptations can help restore resting blood flow, the collateral circuitry is not an effective substitute to accommodate the higher flows necessary during activity[20] and eventually many patients develop a shift from asymptomatic to symptomatic PAD. This shift initially manifests as IC and progresses to CLI (rest pain and/or tissue loss) depending on the severity and duration of arterial occlusion.

The eventual depletion of matrix components by matrix metalloproteinases (MMPs), released from SMCs, leads to cap thinning and predisposes to plaque rupture.[21] Sudden rupture of a vulnerable plaque may occur spontaneously without obvious triggers. By contrast, it may occur following disruption caused by increased mechanical or hemodynamic forces, for instance during increased physical activity. Rupture of the plaque exposes the ECM, particularly collagen, to platelets and proteins in the coagulation pathway. Platelets undergo adhesion, aggregation, and activation and release potent vasospastic substances (thromboxane-A2, serotonin, and platelet factors 3 and 4) as well as coagulation factors (factor V) and plasminogen activator inhibitor (PAI)-1,[4] which initiate the coagulation cascade leading to deposition of a fibrin thrombus and worsening of the luminal occlusion. Fragments of the thrombus may also embolize into the distal circulation. Rapid exacerbation of symptoms and a sudden onset of IC are important warning signs because they may indicate new arterial occlusion caused by rupture of an atherosclerotic plaque or emboli from more proximal arterial sites in the lower limb or aorta.

Pathogenesis of the Complications of Diabetes in PAD

In patients with diabetes, atherosclerosis has several specific biologic and clinical differences from the disease in nondiabetic patients. Vascular disease in diabetes affects both the microcirculation (arterioles and capillaries) and macrocirculation (large and medium-sized arteries). In PAD, diabetes predominantly affects the medium-sized arteries and is caused by the abnormal metabolic state that prevails in the condition. The most important aberrations are chronic hyperglycemia, dyslipidemia, and a prothrombotic state, which cause accelerated atherosclerosis in these patients.

Hyperglycemia

Hyperglycemia is the most important metabolic cause of endothelial dysfunction in people with diabetes, which is associated with increased monocyte-vascular endothelial interaction; an early step in the development of atherosclerosis. This process is partly caused by the effect on nitric oxide (NO) production, which is involved in preventing adherence of circulating monocytes to vascular endothelium and also hinders the activation of nuclear factor kappa B (NF-κB), a proinflammatory and proatherosclerotic gene regulator in endothelial cells, vascular SMCs, and macrophages.[22]

Hyperglycemia also causes changes in proteins, producing advanced glycation end products (AGEs). These AGEs are formed by nonenzymatic reactions between intracellular glucose-derived dicarbonyl precursors and the amino group of both intracellular and extracellular proteins.[23] AGEs have several biologic and chemical properties that are detrimental to atherosclerosis. Their formation on extracellular matrix components, such as collagen, causes cross-linking between polypeptides and decreases arterial wall elasticity, which may predispose the vessel to shear stress and endothelial injury.

In addition, the binding of an AGE to its receptor (located on several cell types including endothelial cells, mesangial cells, and macrophages), stimulates the activation of NF-κB, generating a variety of cytokines, growth factors, and other proinflammatory molecules that contribute to intimal thickening and plaque growth.[24] Other effects of AGE-receptor signaling include increased endothelial permeability, increased procoagulant activity (induction of thrombomodulin and tissue factor), and enhanced proliferation and synthesis of extracellular matrix by fibroblasts and SMCs.[4]

Activation of intracellular protein kinase C (PKC) by calcium ions and diacylglycerol (DAG) is an important signal transduction pathway in many cellular systems. Intracellular hyperglycemia can also stimulate the synthesis of DAG and PKC activation, which can result in increased production of endothelin-1, a potent vasoconstrictor, and decreased activity of the vasodilator endothelial nitric oxide synthase (eNOS). Other untoward reactions of augmented PKC activity include increased deposition of extracellular matrix and basement membrane material through induced expression of TGF-β, fibronectin, and collagen. Production of the procoagulant plasminogen activator inhibitor (PAI)-1 molecule leads to reduced fibrinolysis and increases the risk of vascular occlusive episodes.[25]

Impaired lipid metabolism

Impaired glucose homeostasis also has a marked effect on lipid metabolism, resulting in an atherogenic dyslipidemia, which is strongly associated with the development of atherosclerosis and can occur without significantly increased total serum cholesterol.[26] The abnormal lipid profile in diabetes is characteristic of a low high-density lipoprotein and increased small dense LDL. Hyperglycemia causes auto-oxidation of LDL. Small dense LDL binds avidly to proteoglycans within the intima. Increased vascular permeability to small dense LDL facilitates its uptake by macrophages to form foam cells.[27]

Hypercoagulability and platelet dysfunction

Diabetes is also associated with a prothrombotic state with increases in fibrinogen, factor VII activity, plasminogen activator inhibitor-1, and platelet aggregation. Calcium hemostasis regulating platelet shape, secretion, aggregation, and thromboxane production is disturbed in diabetes. Platelet expression of receptor proteins for von Willebrand factor (vWF) and fibrin products is increased.[28] Platelet activation (during endothelial injury or plaque rupture) results in translocation of adhesion molecules (P-selectin) to the surface membrane, which is accompanied by conformational changes in glycoprotein IIb-IIIa (GPIIb-IIIa) complex on the plasma membrane.[29] Hyperaggregability is augmented by the interaction of vWF with GPIIb-IIIa complexes. This increase in intrinsic platelet activity contributes to a state of enhanced thrombotic potential in diabetic atherosclerotic lesions.

Because of the pathologic processes discussed earlier, examination of atherosclerotic plaque in people with diabetes shows markedly different composition to nondiabetic plaque. Increased thrombus formation, inflammation, and neovascularization in diabetic lesions make them more unstable and prone to rupture. Calcification is particularly common, which has significant implications for treatment, making the artery more fragile and prone to cracking and disruption.[26]

PREDICTORS OF DISEASE PROGRESSION

Accumulating data indicate that insights gained from the link between inflammation and atherosclerosis can potentially yield clinically important predictive and prognostic information of future PAD. Several biochemical markers have been investigated, including acute-phase reactant proteins, plasma glycoproteins, fibrin degradation products, amino acids, and lipoproteins.

C-reactive Protein

CRP is an acute-phase reactant protein frequently present in inflammatory states including PAD and diabetes. It has been investigated extensively in patients with PAD, and seems to present in increased serum levels compared with patients who do not have PAD. Some studies have related CRP to the severity of PAD, showing a relation to future hemodynamic function and cardiovascular events in patients with PAD,[16] although its role as an independent marker of the extent of atherosclerosis in patients with PAD is still unclear.

Fibrinogen

Fibrinogen, another acute-phase reactant that is synthesized by the liver, is an independent predictor of cardiovascular mortality.[26] Elevated fibrinogen levels in patients with PAD have also been found to increase risk for poor outcome.[30]

D-dimer

D-dimer, a plasmin-derived degradation product of cross-linked fibrin, is another potential biochemical marker for predicting the risk of PAD. Increased D-dimer levels have been correlated with reduced ankle brachial pressure index values (ABPI; an index of severity of PAD) and some studies suggest that D-dimer could have a role as a short-term predictor for all-cause mortality among patients with PAD.[31]

Hyperhomocysteinemia

Homocysteine is an amino acid derivative of methionine. Increased homocysteine levels are detected in cystathionine β-synthase deficiency, vitamin B and folic acid deficiency, hypothyroidism, aging, and menopause. Homocysteine provokes atherosclerosis through increased oxidative stress and endothelial dysfunction.[28] Numerous studies have replicated the association between hyperhomocysteinemia and PAD. Hyperhomocysteinemia is also a predictor of both cardiovascular and all-cause mortality in patients with PAD.[32] However, in the Heart Outcomes Prevention Evaluation Study, vitamin B supplementation intended to normalize homocysteine levels was not associated with cardiovascular risk reduction.[33]

Lipoprotein (a)

Lipoprotein (a), also known as Lp(a), is a lipoprotein similar to LDL (both possess surface apolipoprotein B-100). However, Lp(a) contains a unique glycoprotein apo(a) that resembles plasminogen and hence competes with it at the plasminogen receptor. Lp(a) exerts its atherogenic effects by stimulating PAI-1 activity, suppressing plasminogen activity and promoting vascular SMC proliferation.[34]

Lp(a) may represent an independent marker for development of PAD. The investigators of the Invecchiare in Chianti (InCHIANTI) Study in Italy concluded that Lp(a) is an independent PAD correlate in their cross-sectional evaluation.[35] However, prospective studies in larger populations and longer follow-up are needed to firmly establish this association.

CLINICAL PRESENTATION

Most patients with PAD are initially asymptomatic (up to 75%) and are diagnosed following ABPI measurements of less than 0.9. However, even asymptomatic patients have an increased cardiovascular risk and often the PAD is unmasked by the development of a nonhealing foot wound in people with diabetes. Other patients may present with symptoms of IC or CLI.

Intermittent Claudication

IC is characterized by tight, cramplike muscular pain on walking that generally develops over months or years with a gradual reduction in pain-free walking distance. The distribution of the pain is usually determined by the site of disease, and, because PAD most commonly affects the infrainguinal arteries (and infrageniculate arteries in diabetic patients), pain is usually felt in the calf (distal to the site of stenosis or occlusion). This pain is also typically worse on uphill walking and is characteristically relieved by rest. More proximal disease involving the common femoral and iliac arteries may cause pain in the thigh or buttock, respectively. The presence of bilateral symptoms may indicate aortic disease. The severity of IC is classified according to the Fontaine or the more recent Rutherford (**Table 1**) systems.

Most patients with IC do not deteriorate and, in many, their walking spontaneously improves. Only round 2% to 3% per year deteriorate and need revascularization to prevent limb loss, which is important to recognize when planning interventional treatment.

Critical Limb Ischemia

CLI is a term that was developed to identify patients whose circulation is reduced to a level that, without revascularization, would cause them to lose a leg. This concept has proved difficult to define accurately because patients with PAD may be offered amputation of a limb for a range of reasons including infection and poorly controlled pain as well as poor circulation. The Transatlantic Inter-Society Consensus for the Management of Peripheral Arterial Disease (TASC II) suggests that a patient with persistent pain for more than 2 weeks, ulcers or gangrene, with proven arterial disease should be considered to have CLI.[1] Although the diagnosis can be confirmed by an ABPI of less than 0.5, this is not always the case for diabetic patients who may exhibit values of greater than 1.0 because of calcified vessels. The term severe limb ischemia is sometimes used to denote that the patient is considered to need revascularization to avoid amputation.

Patients with CLI face an overwhelming cardiovascular risk and 50% die within 1 year of diagnosis. Patients with CLI have a high prevalence of diabetes. In the Bypass versus Angioplasty in Severe Ischaemia of the Leg (BASIL) trial, 42% of patients at that time (more than 12 years ago) with CLI had diabetes.[36] The need to urgently intervene in this group of patients is important because a significant proportion deteriorate with amputation or death.

Table 1 Rutherford classification		
Grade	**Category**	**Manifestation**
0	0	Asymptomatic
I	1	Mild claudication
I	2	Moderate claudication
I	3	Severe claudication
II	4	Ischemic rest pain
III	5	Minor tissue loss
IV	6	Ulceration or gangrene

Adapted from Norgren L, Hiatt WR, Dormandy JA, et al, TASC II Working Group. Inter-society consensus for the management of peripheral arterial disease (TASC II). Eur J Vasc Endovasc Surg 2007;33(Suppl 1):S1–75; with permission.

DIAGNOSIS OF PAD
Clinical Examination

Once a diagnosis of PAD is suspected from the history, a full cardiovascular examination is performed to detect other manifestations of cardiovascular disease. Upper limb peripheral pulses should be palpated and the blood pressure checked. Cardiac auscultation should also be performed to establish the cardiac rhythm. An abdominal examination is important to identify an abdominal aortic aneurysm, which may be felt as a pulsatile and expansile mass above the level of the umbilicus.

Examination of the peripheral circulation should begin with adequate exposure of both lower limbs from the pelvis to the feet to allow detailed inspection for clinical signs such as cracked skin, hair loss, nail damage, ulceration, and gangrene (**Table 2**). In a patient with diabetes, it is also important to look for signs of abnormal foot shape and callus formation.[37] Limb temperature and capillary refill time should also be assessed.

The key component to a peripheral vascular examination is peripheral pulse palpation. In the lower limb, from proximal to distal, this includes the femoral, popliteal, posterior tibial, and anterior tibial/dorsalis pedis pulses. In 10% to 15% of the population there is a congenital absence of the dorsalis pedis, therefore its absence on examination needs to be taken into context with the history and other examination findings. In clinical practice, eliciting lower limb pulses is often difficult, so ankle pressure should also be measured.

It is also important to examine for more subtle signs of ischemia, which can be done by performing the Buerger test. First, with the patient supine, the legs are elevated to an angle of 45° and held for 1 to 2 minutes. The onset of pallor indicates ischemia, which occurs when the peripheral arterial pressure is inadequate to overcome the effects of gravity. The second part of the test involves returning the leg from the raised position and hanging it over the side of the bed. In a patient with PAD, the leg revert to its normal pink color more slowly. In addition, the affected limb may develop a deep red color because of arteriolar dilatation. In patients with diabetic autonomic neuropathy a similar appearance can occur with normal circulation.

ABPI Measurement

The ABPI measurement is an important component to the diagnosis and monitoring of PAD, and is expressed as the ratio of the ankle pressure to the brachial pressure. An ABPI of less than or equal to 0.9 is usually considered abnormal. As previously stated,

Table 2 The University of Texas wound classification system			
Stages **Grade 0**	**Grade I**	**Grade II**	**Grade III**
Stage A Preulcerative or postulcerative lesion completely epithelialized	Superficial wound, not involving tendon, capsule, or bone	Wound penetrating to tendon or capsule	Wound penetrating to bone or joint
Stage B Infection +	Infection +	Infection +	Infection +
Stage C Ischemia +	Ischemia +	Ischemia +	Ischemia +
Stage D Infection and ischemia +	Infection and ischemia +	Infection and ischemia +	Infection and ischemia +

Adapted from Lavery LA, Armstrong DG, Harkless LB. Classification of diabetic foot wounds. J Foot Ankle Surg 1996;35:528–31; with permission.

in diabetic patients the peripheral arteries may be stiff or calcified, often giving an artificially high ankle pressure. In this group, measurement of toe pressures provides an accurate alternative option. Toe pressure is calculated as the ratio of toe pressure to brachial artery pressure, and an abnormal value is defined as less than 0.7.

Measuring ABPI requires an 8-MHz Doppler ultrasound probe, sphygmomanometer, and cuff. The patient is positioned supine with the legs at the same level as the heart. The cuff is secured around the arm and gel is applied over the brachial pulse followed by the Doppler probe over the pulse at an angle of approximately 60°. The cuff is inflated until the arterial signal disappears and, on deflation, the pressure at which the signal returns is taken as the pressure. This procedure is repeated on the other arm to acquire the higher reading of the two. The same steps are repeated for the dorsalis pedis and posterior tibial arteries in the lower limb, again using the higher value to calculate the ABPI. The peroneal artery should also be insonated because in people with diabetes it is often the only major calf vessel supplying the foot, via its anterior and posterior communicating branches.

In symptomatic patients with an ABPI of less than 0.9 there is a 95% sensitivity for diagnosing PAD.[37] This high sensitivity, together with its noninvasive approach, has made it an effective screening tool for PAD. According to the American Diabetes Association (ADA), ABPI measurements should be performed routinely in people with diabetes aged more than 50 years. If normal, the ABPI should then be repeated every 5 years. A screening ABPI is recommended in diabetic patients aged less than 50 years in the presence of other cardiovascular risk factors (**Table 3**).[38]

Treadmill Exercise Testing

One limitation of ABPI testing is that some patients with IC may have no pressure decreases across a stenotic area at rest and therefore a normal ABPI. However, with exercise the increased inflow velocity makes such lesions more hemodynamically significant. Exercise testing involves observation of the patient walking and determining the distance to the onset of pain. A decrease in ABPI of 15% to 20% after exercise is diagnostic of PAD.[1] Few patients need this level of investigation, and this test is now largely used to evaluate new treatments and in patients with diagnostic doubt after initial examination.

Transcutaneous Oxygen Pressure Measurement

The measurement of transcutaneous oxygen pressure (TcPo$_2$), a noninvasive method to quantify skin oxygenation, may be useful in the advanced stages of lower limb ischemia for assessing the likelihood of healing of ischemic ulcers. A TcPo$_2$ of less than 30 mm Hg is associated with poor wound healing. In the past, some groups

Table 3 ABPI criteria for the diagnosis of peripheral vascular disease	
ABPI	**Inference**
0.91–1.3	Normal
0.7–0.9	Mild obstruction
0.4–0.69	Moderate obstruction
<0.4	Severe obstruction
>1.3	Poorly compressible

Data from American Diabetes Association. Peripheral arterial disease in people with diabetes. Diabetes Care 2003;26:3336.

have observed that a TcPo$_2$ of less than 20 mm Hg confers a several-fold increase in early wound healing failure among diabetic patients with foot ulcers.[39] However, in clinical practice TcPo$_2$ has not been widely adopted because it tends to be variable.

Duplex Ultrasound Scanning

The primary purpose of imaging is to identify an arterial lesion that is suitable for revascularization. In a few patients in whom the diagnosis is of doubt after initial examination it can be used to confirm the presence of PAD. Duplex ultrasound scanning (DUS) is a noninvasive imaging technique that determines the direction and velocity of blood flow through a vessel. This ability to identify areas of turbulence and determine the velocity shift across a diseased segment provides an objective evaluation of the hemodynamic severity and extent of PAD. The runoff vessels can also be scanned. This information can be used to guide the type of intervention that is applicable to a patient (eg, angioplasty or bypass surgery) and, in many patients with clear scans, no further imaging is required. Because it is noninvasive, readily available, and has a high sensitivity (88%–90%) and specificity (96%–99%), it has been promoted by NICE as the first-line imaging investigation in the United Kingdom for all patients for whom revascularization is being considered.[40,41]

Angiography

Depending on the pattern of disease and nature of the planned intervention, more detailed information may be required. Angiography is considered the gold standard imaging test for PAD. Although digital subtraction angiography (DSA) was initially a popular method, it is now rarely used because of its invasiveness, high cost, and risk of contrast-induced nephrotoxicity.

DSA has now been largely superseded by multislice computed tomography angiography (CTA) and magnetic resonance angiography (MRA). In many units, CTA is the preferred mode of imaging, owing to its relative noninvasiveness, rapid image acquisition times, and the familiarity of computed tomography technology. Its major limitations include the use of intravenous contrast medium and its high radiation exposure, which can be problematic for patients requiring repeated scans. MRA does not involve the use of iodinated contrast or exposure to radiation and is now the preferred second-line investigation for PAD (**Fig. 2**). However, the use of gadolinium contrast is associated with the complication systemic nephrogenic interstitial fibrosis, which although rare can be fatal and is more common in patients with impaired renal function. Caution is exercised, especially in patients receiving metformin therapy, to avoid lethal lactic acidosis. In such circumstances the drug is discontinued for 48 hours before the procedure. Serum creatinine should be assessed 24 to 48 hours following the procedure and, if normal, then metformin therapy can be resumed.

MANAGEMENT

The purpose of management of patients with PAD is 3-fold: (1) to improve symptoms and pain-free walking distance, (2) to prevent amputation, and (3) to prevent further cardiovascular morbidity. Treatment can be divided into 3 categories: lifestyle/risk factor modifications, drug therapy, and surgical intervention.

Lifestyle and Risk Modifications

Cigarette smoking

Smoking is recognized as the single most important risk factor for the development of atherosclerotic PAD. Not only does it increase the risk of developing PAD but the

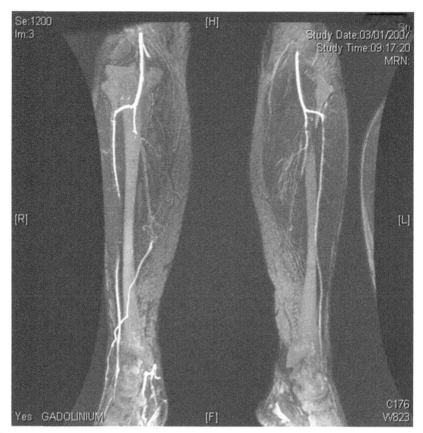

Fig. 2. Magnetic resonance angiogram in a patient with diabetes showing diffuse disease of the calf blood vessels.

evidence also suggests it reduces the success of surgical intervention and increases the risk of amputation. Smoking cessation advice, combined with nicotine replacement therapy, therefore represents the cornerstone of PAD management and should be offered to all smokers.

Hyperglycemia

Optimizing glycemic control in diabetic patients is also important. Although studies of diabetic patients have yielded no evidence that aggressive glycemic control reduces the risk of PAD,[41] given the important role of hyperglycemia in atherogenesis every attempt should be made to optimize diabetic control in patients with PAD. The current ADA guidelines recommend an HbA_{1c} of less than 7% as a target for all diabetic patients in general.[42]

Hypercholesterolemia

There is strong direct evidence supporting the use of statins to reduce LDL cholesterol levels in patients with PAD. The Heart Protection Study showed that patients with PAD who took simvastatin 40 mg for hypercholesterolemia had a 17% and 16% reduction in cardiovascular mortality and need for noncoronary revascularization, respectively.[43] Based on this, all patients with PAD should be offered statin therapy unless contraindicated or not tolerated. The mounting evidence that statins contribute to atherosclerotic plaque stability further supports their use in PAD.

Hypertension
In the UKPDS, strict blood pressure control conferred a 50% risk reduction for PAD.[44] Hypertension guidelines recommend a goal of less than 140/90 mm Hg in all patients with atherosclerosis and less than 130/80 mm Hg if the patient is diabetic.[45] The Heart Outcomes Study revealed that the angiotensin-converting enzyme inhibitor, ramipril, reduced cardiovascular events by 22% in patients with PAD. Therefore, in hypertensive patients with PAD, ramipril should be considered as first-line therapy. Its use in nonhypertensive diabetic patients who may have renal impairment should be limited because of its effect on renal function.

Exercise
Exercise is now widely thought to be of benefit to patients with PAD, not only helping to improve pain-free walking distance but also possibly contribute to reducing cardiovascular-related death. A Cochrane Review of 22 studies concluded that exercise programs of 2 or more exercise sessions per week improves walking distance by 50% to 200% in claudicants.[46] Several mechanisms have been proposed for this benefit including metabolic adaptation of the muscle, transformation of muscle fiber type, and increased capillary blood flow. Given the strong evidence, NICE therefore recommended that all patients with IC be offered supervised exercise classes. However, only 27% of vascular surgeons in the United Kingdom currently have access to such programs.[47]

Drug Therapy

Antiplatelet agents
The rationale behind the use of antiplatelet agents is based on their suppression of platelet hyperactivity in the atherosclerotic process that leads to thrombus formation at the site of plaques.

The Antithrombotic Trialists' Collaboration meta-analysis identified that antiplatelet agents, particularly aspirin (a salicylate drug), reduced cardiovascular events by 23% in patients with PAD.[48] Clopidogrel, a theopyridine derivative, had a 24% relative risk reduction in cardiovascular events (stroke, myocardial infarction, or vascular death) compared with aspirin in the PAD subgroup of the Clopidogrel versus Aspirin in Patients at Risk of Ischaemic Events trial.[49] It is now becoming the preferred agent for patients with PAD. Dual antiplatelet therapy is associated with an excessive risk of bleeding complications that outweigh the cardiovascular benefits in patients with PAD and so cannot be recommended at present.

Vasoactive agents
Two agents, pentoxifylline and cilostazol, are available for the treatment of IC in the United Kingdom. Pentoxifylline reduces blood viscosity and fibrinogen levels and has an antiplatelet action. The results of this agent in IC studies are varied; although early trials were positive, several meta-analyses showed only modest improvement in walking distance and questioned the drug's overall clinical benefit (including its safety profile).[50] Cilostazol acts by inducing vasodilation and indirectly inhibits platelet aggregation. A meta-analysis of 6 randomized, controlled trials showed a net benefit of cilostazol compared with placebo in treadmill performance and an improvement in quality-of-life measures.[51]

However, the improvement in walking offered by these drugs is modest, there are few long-term follow-up data, and their cost-effectiveness remains questionable. As a result, NICE have recently evaluated these drugs along with 2 other vasoactive agents, naftidrofuryl oxalate and inositol nicotinate, concluding that if vasoactive drugs are indicated then naftidrofuryl should be used given its cost-effectiveness compared with the other agents.[52] It is important to evaluate treatment after 3 months and, if the patient has not benefitted, then to stop the drug.

Surgical Intervention

Surgical intervention to revascularize and reperfuse the limb can be achieved by open surgical (bypass or endarterectomy) or endovascular techniques, such as angioplasty with or without a stent. This type of intervention should be considered when conservative measures have failed to resolve lifestyle-limiting IC or if there is evidence of CLI (eg, ulceration and tissue loss).

For patients with IC, because the disease is often limited to a single arterial segment, angioplasty with or without stenting is often the first-line treatment.[53] Surgical bypass for claudicants is generally reserved for those with debilitating symptoms and a disease pattern that is not amenable to angioplasty. Patients with CLI typically have more widespread disease involving multiple segments and in these patients surgical bypass is usually more appropriate, although advances in endovascular technology and improved stent design over the last decade have fueled greater enthusiasm for endovascular intervention in CLI. However, the only randomized controlled trial to have compared bypass surgery with angioplasty in patients with CLI, the BASIL trial (452 patients with CLI randomized to a surgery-first or angioplasty-first strategy with follow-up of 5 years or more in many patients) found no difference in amputation-free survival and overall survival between the techniques at 1 year.[36] For patients who survived to 2 years, a survival advantage was seen in the bypass-first group with a trend to improved amputation-free survival. The investigators concluded that bypass surgery offered the best long-term outcomes and is the preferred intervention strategy for patients expected to survive 2 years or more.

Although the BASIL trial is the only level 1 evidence available, it is important to highlight that the trial was performed more than 8 years ago and therefore may not accurately reflect the results that are achievable with current catheter devices and grafts. In current clinical practice, the choice of intervention is largely influenced by the patient's premorbid condition and estimated durability of treatment. The TASC II document has outlined its own treatment recommendations according to lesion site and morphology.[1]

At present, the best option for diabetic patients with PAD is unclear. Excellent results from distal angioplasty have been shown from single centers with 5-year patency rates of 88%.[54] However, again, the BASIL trial showed a similarity in limb salvage rates for both interventions in the diabetic group, who comprised more than 40% of study participants. What is apparent in diabetic patients is the higher reintervention rate caused by restenosis.

NEW THERAPIES AND FUTURE OPPORTUNITIES
Spinal Cord Stimulation

Spinal cord stimulation is a technique that involves modulating the neurophysiology of the spinal tract pathways to change the perception of pain. It has been used in the management of chronic pain for many disease states for several years, including angina pectoris and PAD. For PAD, the method involves implanting an electrical lead(s) into the epidural space of the spinal cord at the level of L3 to L4 to change or modulate the neurologic signals to the brain, producing a sensation of warmth and paresthesia in the limb. It is used primarily for intractable pain in patients with nonreconstructible PAD. Apart from managing pain, this method has not been shown to reduce amputation or mortality in previous randomized controlled studies.[55]

Intermittent Pneumatic Compression

Intermittent pneumatic compression of the calf and foot has been shown to increase popliteal artery blood flow and distal limb pressure indices. The mechanism for this is unclear, but it is thought that compression of the foot reduces venous leg pressure, thereby increasing the arteriovenous pressure gradient. One study showed sustained benefits in walking ability up to 12 months.[56] As a low-risk domestic treatment with a high compliance,[57] it may become a useful therapy in the future.

Angiogenesis

Over the last decade the development of new blood vessels in ischemic tissue, termed therapeutic angiogenesis, has gained strong interest as an alternative noninterventional therapy for PAD. Several proangiogenic growth factors have been identified and it is hypothesized that increasing the levels of these may stimulate new blood vessel formation.[58] Much research has been directed toward gene therapy, which involves inserting a gene coding for a growth factor into a DNA plasmid either via direct injection into the muscle of the ischemic limb or a viral vector, or cell therapy whereby cells attracted to areas of ischemia are injected intramuscularly.[59] At present, these studies are largely in the early preclinical phase and it is therefore too early to judge their clinical significance.

SUMMARY

PAD is an atherosclerotic-driven condition that is common but remains underdiagnosed and undertreated, partly because of a lack of awareness of its significance among both clinicians and the public. In diabetic patients, PAD begins early, progresses more rapidly, and is frequently asymptomatic (owing to coexisting neuropathy), making it difficult to diagnose in this group. Strict management of the metabolic instigators and use of screening techniques for PAD in diabetes can facilitate its early diagnosis and reduce its progression.

In addition to best medical therapy, exercise seems to be an equally effective treatment option in improving walking distance and should therefore be offered to patients as early as possible. Moreover, early revascularization has been shown to reduce the risk of amputation and must be offered early in suitable patients. Although there is no strong evidence to support surgical bypass rather than endovascular revascularization at present, these techniques are complementary and the choice of intervention should be applied appropriately by a multidisciplinary vascular team on a selective, patient-specific basis.

REFERENCES

1. Norgren L, Hiatt WR, Dormandy JA, et al, TASC II Working Group. Inter-society consensus for the management of peripheral arterial disease (TASC II). Eur J Vasc Endovasc Surg 2007;33(Suppl 1):S1–75.
2. Newman AB, Siscovick DS, Manolio TA, et al. Ankle-arm index as a marker of atherosclerosis in the Cardiovascular Health Study. Cardiovascular Heart Study (CHS) Collaborative Research Group. Circulation 1993;88:837–45.
3. Al-Delaimy WK, Merchant AT, Rimm EB, et al. Effect of type 2 diabetes and its duration on the risk of peripheral arterial disease among men. Am J Med 2004;116:236–40.

4. Kumar V, Abbas A, Fausto N. Pathological basis of disease. 7th edition. Philadelphia: Elsevier Saunders; 2005.
5. Criqui MH, Langer RD, Fronek A, et al. Mortality over a period of 10 years in patients with peripheral arterial disease. N Engl J Med 1992;326:381–6.
6. Kannel WB, Wilson PW. An update on coronary risk factors. Med Clin North Am 1995;75:951–71.
7. Murabito JM, Evans JC, Nieto K, et al. Prevalence and clinical correlates of peripheral arterial disease in the Framingham Offspring Study. Am Heart J 2002;143:961–5.
8. Selvin E, Erlinger TP. Prevalence of and risk factors for peripheral arterial disease in the United States: results from the National Health and Nutrition Examination Survey, 1999-2000. Circulation 2004;110:738–43.
9. Fowkes FG, Housley E, Cawood EH, et al. Edinburgh Artery Study: prevalence of asymptomatic and symptomatic peripheral arterial disease in the general population. Int J Epidemiol 1991;20:384–92.
10. Willigendael EM, Teijink JA, Bartelink ML, et al. Smoking and the patency of lower extremity bypass grafts: a meta-analysis. J Vasc Surg 2005;42:67–74.
11. Ambrose JA, Barua RS. The pathophysiology of cigarette smoking and cardiovascular disease: an update. J Am Coll Cardiol 2004;43(10):1731–7.
12. Selvin E, Marinopoulos S, Berkenblit G, et al. Meta-analysis: glycosylated hemoglobin and cardiovascular disease in diabetes mellitus. Ann Intern Med 2004; 141(6):421–31.
13. Adler AI, Stevens RJ, Neil A, et al. UKPDS 59: hyperglycemia and other potentially modifiable risk factors for peripheral vascular disease in type 2 diabetes. Diabetes Care 2002;25:894–9.
14. National Institute for Health and Clinical Excellence. Diabetic foot problems: inpatient management. CG119. 2011. Available at: www.nice.org.uk/CG119. Accessed August 28, 2013.
15. Murabito JM, D'Agostino RB, Silbershatz H, et al. Intermittent claudication. A risk profile from The Framingham Heart Study. Circulation 1997;96:44–9.
16. Vainas T, Stassen FR, de Graaf R, et al. C-reactive protein in peripheral arterial disease: relation to severity of the disease and future cardiovascular events. J Vasc Surg 2005;42:243–51.
17. Marui N, Offermann MK, Swerlick R, et al. VCAM-1 gene transcription and expression are regulated through an antioxidant-sensitive mechanism in human vascular endothelial cells. J Clin Invest 1993;92:1866–74.
18. Libby P. Inflammation in atherosclerosis. Nature 2002;420:868–74.
19. Farzaneh-Far A, Rudd J, Weissberg PL. Inflammatory mechanisms: ischaemic heart disease. Br Med Bull 2001;59:55–68.
20. Murrant CL. Structural and functional limitations of the collateral circulation in peripheral artery disease. J Physiol 2008;586:5845.
21. Shah PK. Mechanisms of plaque vulnerability and rupture. J Am Coll Cardiol 2003;41:15–22.
22. Veves A, Akbari CM, Primavera J, et al. Endothelial dysfunction and the expression of endothelial nitric oxide synthetase in diabetic neuropathy, vascular disease, and foot ulceration. Diabetes 1998;47:457–63.
23. Eckel RH, Wassef M, Chait A, et al. Prevention conference VI: diabetes and cardiovascular disease: writing group II: pathogenesis of atherosclerosis in diabetes. Circulation 2002;105:e138–43.
24. Brownlee M. Biochemistry and molecular cell biology of diabetic complications. Nature 2001;414:813–20.

25. Giacco F, Brownlee M. Textbook of diabetes. 4th edition. Hoboken (NJ): Wiley-Blackwell; 2010.
26. Albayati MA, Shearman CP. Peripheral arterial disease and bypass surgery in the diabetic lower limb. Med Clin North Am 2013;97:821–34.
27. Steinberg HO, Baron AD. Vascular function, insulin resistance and fatty acids. Diabetologia 2002;45:623–34.
28. Jude EB, Eleftheriadou I, Tentolouris N. Peripheral arterial disease in diabetes—a review. Diabet Med 2010;27:4–14.
29. Schneider DJ. Factors contributing to increased platelet reactivity in people with diabetes. Diabetes Care 2009;32:525–7.
30. Doweik L, Maca T, Schillinger M, et al. Fibrinogen predicts mortality in high risk patients with peripheral artery disease. Eur J Vasc Endovasc Surg 2003;26:381–6.
31. Vidula H, Tian L, Liu K, et al. Biomarkers of inflammation and thrombosis as predictors of near-term mortality in patients with peripheral arterial disease: a cohort study. Ann Intern Med 2008;148:85–93.
32. Taylor LM Jr, Moneta GL, Sexton GJ, et al. Prospective blinded study of the relationship between plasma homocysteine and progression of symptomatic peripheral arterial disease. J Vasc Surg 1999;29:8–19.
33. Lonn E, Yusuf S, Arnold MJ, et al. Homocysteine lowering with folic acid and B vitamins in vascular disease. N Engl J Med 2006;354:1567–77.
34. Khawaja FL, Kullo IJ. Novel markers of peripheral arterial disease. Vasc Med 2009;14:381–92.
35. Volpato S, Vigna GB, McDermott MM, et al. Lipoprotein(a), inflammation, and peripheral arterial disease in a community-based sample of older men and women (the InCHIANTI study). Am J Cardiol 2010;105:1825–30.
36. Adam DJ, Beard JD, Cleveland T, BASIL Trial Participants. Bypass versus angioplasty in severe ischaemia of the leg (BASIL): multicentre, randomised controlled trial. Lancet 2005;366:1925–34.
37. Bhattacharya V, Stansby G. Postgraduate vascular surgery: the candidate's guide to the FRCS. Cambridge (United Kingdom): Cambridge University Press; 2010.
38. American Diabetes Association. Peripheral arterial disease in people with diabetes. Diabetes Care 2003;26:3333–41.
39. Pecoraro RE, Ahroni JH, Boyko EJ, et al. Chronology and determinants of tissue repair in diabetic lower-extremity ulcers. Diabetes 1991;40:1305–13.
40. Collins R, Burch J, Cranny G, et al. Duplex ultrasonography, magnetic resonance angiography, and computed tomography angiography for diagnosis and assessment of symptomatic, lower limb peripheral arterial disease: systematic review. BMJ 2007;334:1257.
41. Holman RR, Paul SK, Bethel MA, et al. 10-year follow-up of intensive glucose control in type 2 diabetes. N Engl J Med 2008;359:1577–89.
42. American Diabetes Association. Standards of medical care in diabetes. Diabetes Care 2006;29:S4–42.
43. Heart Protection Study Group Collaborators Group. MRC/BHF heart protection study of cholesterol lowering with simvastatin in 20,536 high-risk individuals: randomised placebo controlled trial. Lancet 2002;360:7–22.
44. Holman RR, Paul SK, Bethel MA, et al. Long-term follow-up after tight control of blood pressure in type 2 diabetes. N Engl J Med 2008;359:1565–76.
45. European Society of Hypertension/European Society of Cardiology. ESH/ESC guidelines for the management of arterial hypertension. J Hypertens 2003;2:1011–53.

46. Watson L, Ellis B, Leng GC. Exercise for intermittent claudication. Cochrane Database Syst Rev 2008;(4):CD000990.

47. Beard JD, Gaines PA. Vascular and endovascular surgery: a companion to specialist surgical practice. 4th edition. Edinburgh (United Kingdom): Elsevier Saunders; 2009.

48. Antithrombotic Trialists' Collaboration. Collaborative meta-analysis of randomised trials of antiplatelet therapy for the prevention of death, myocardial infarction, and stroke in high risk patients. BMJ 2002;324:71–86.

49. CAPRIE Steering Committee. A randomised, blinded, trial of clopidogrel versus aspirin in patients at risk of ischaemic events (CAPRIE). Lancet 1996;348: 1329–39.

50. Moher D, Pham B, Ausejo M, et al. Pharmacological management of intermittent claudication: a meta- analysis of randomised trials. Drugs 2000;59:1057–70.

51. Regensteiner J, Ware JI, McCarthy W, et al. Effect of cilostazol on treadmill walking, community-based walking ability, and health-related quality of life in patients with intermittent claudication due to peripheral arterial disease: meta-analysis of six randomized controlled trials. J Am Geriatr Soc 2002;50:1939–46.

52. National Institute for Health and Clinical Excellence. Technology Appraisal Guidance 223. Cilostazol, naftidrofuryl oxalate, pentoxifylline and inositol nicotinate for the treatment of intermittent claudication in people with peripheral arterial disease. Available at: www.nice.org.uk/guidance/TA223. Accessed August 29, 2013.

53. National Institute for Health and Clinical Excellence. Lower limb peripheral arterial disease: diagnosis and management. Available at: www.nice.org.uk/nicemedia/live/13856/60428/60428.pdf. Accessed August 25, 2013.

54. Faglia E, Dalla Paola L, Clerici G, et al. Peripheral angioplasty as the first choice revascularisation procedure in diabetic patients with critical limb ischaemia: prospective study of 993 consecutive patients hospitalised and followed between 1999-2003. Eur J Vasc Endovasc Surg 2005;29:620–7.

55. Klomp HM, Spincemaille GH, Steyerberg EW, et al. Spinal cord stimulation in critical limb ischaemia: a randomised trial. Lancet 1999;353:1040–4.

56. Ramaswami G, D'Ayala M, Hollier LH, et al. Rapid foot and calf compression increases walking distance in patients with intermittent claudication: results of a randomized study. J Vasc Surg 2005;41:794–801.

57. Delis KT, Nicolaides AN. Effect of intermittent pneumatic compression of foot and calf on walking distance, hemodynamics and quality of life in patients with arterial claudication: a prospective randomized controlled study with 1-year follow-up. Ann Surg 2005;241:431–41.

58. Dubsky M, Jirkovska A, Bem R, et al. Both autologous bone marrow mononuclear cell and peripheral blood progenitor cell therapies similarly improve ischaemia in patients with diabetic foot in comparison with control treatment. Diabetes Metab Res Rev 2013;29:369–76.

59. Grochot-Przeczek A, Dulak J, Jozkowicz A. Therapeutic angiogenesis for revascularization in peripheral artery disease. Gene 2013;525:220–8.

Diabetes and Cancer

Zara Zelenko, BA, PhD(c), Emily Jane Gallagher, MD*

KEYWORDS

- Diabetes mellitus • Obesity • Metabolic syndrome • Cancer • Hyperinsulinemia
- Hyperglycemia • Inflammation

KEY POINTS

- Type 2 diabetes, obesity, and the metabolic syndrome are associated with an increased risk of cancer development.
- Proposed mechanisms to link type 2 diabetes and cancer include insulin resistance, hyperinsulinemia, insulin-like growth factor-1, hyperglycemia and dyslipidemia, inflammatory cytokines, and adipokines.
- Hyperinsulinemia, insulin receptor expression, and insulin receptor signaling are associated with increased tumor growth and metastasis.
- Hyperglycemia can contribute to the development and progression of cancers by promoting transformation of cancer cells, providing an energy source and allowing for cell survival and resistance to chemotherapy.
- Chronic inflammation leads to increased levels of circulating interleukin (IL)-1β, IL-6, and tumor necrosis factor-α that can promote invasion of tumor cells.

INTRODUCTION

Type 2 diabetes (T2D) and obesity are both associated with reduced life expectancy and have been correlated with an increased risk of cancer development. Obesity, the metabolic syndrome, and T2D are also associated with more advanced stage of certain cancers at presentation, resistance to therapy, and recurrence; factors that contribute to greater cancer mortality.[1–4] There are many biologic factors common to obesity and T2D that may contribute to cancer risk. In this review, we discuss the links between T2D and cancer and the various biologic mechanisms associated with T2D, the metabolic syndrome, and obesity that may be promote cancer development, growth, and metastases.

Disclosure: Authors have nothing to disclose.
Division of Endocrinology, Diabetes and Bone Diseases, Icahn School of Medicine at Mount Sinai, One Gustave L. Levy Place, Box 1055, New York, NY 10029, USA
* Corresponding author.
E-mail address: emily.gallagher@mssm.edu

Endocrinol Metab Clin N Am 43 (2014) 167–185
http://dx.doi.org/10.1016/j.ecl.2013.09.008
0889-8529/14/$ – see front matter © 2014 Elsevier Inc. All rights reserved.

EPIDEMIOLOGY OF DIABETES AND CANCER
Diabetes, Obesity, and the Metabolic Syndrome

The prevalence of T2D has been growing steadily over the past decade. In 2004, it was predicted that the number of people diagnosed with T2D would rise to 366 million by 2030; however, the numbers are rising more rapidly than predicted. Current estimates from the International Diabetes Federation (IDF), report that 366 million people worldwide had diabetes in 2011, and the projected number of people with diabetes by 2030 is 552 million. Many years before the development of hyperglycemia, the hallmark of diabetes, insulin resistance develops in metabolic tissues and consequently hyperinsulinemia occurs, due to beta cell compensation.[5,6] Eventually, beta cell failure occurs and patients develop hyperglycemia.[7] At this point, diabetes may be diagnosed, although the individual has most likely had insulin resistance and hyperinsulinemia for many preceding years.

Type 1 diabetes mellitus (T1D) results from the autoimmune destruction of the insulin-producing beta cells, which leads to severe insulin deficiency. T1D accounts for about 5% to 10% of diabetes. Various epidemiologic studies have been conducted to investigate the link between T1D and overall cancer incidence.[8] A study conducted in Denmark found that there was no overall increase in cancer cases among individuals with T1D,[8] whereas a Swedish study found a 17% increase in cancer risk in individuals with T1D.[9] This study reported an increased risk of leukemia and skin and stomach cancers.[9] A follow-up study by the same group observed an association between early-onset leukemia and T1D.[10] The highest incidence of acute myeloid leukemia and acute lymphoblastic leukemia in patients with T1D was observed in patients diagnosed with T1D between the ages of 10 and 20 years.[10] Whether the increase in cancer in these patients with T1D is due to a viral etiology or insulin therapy remains to be determined.[10]

The metabolic syndrome is a syndrome of insulin resistance that is associated with a greater risk of developing T2D. The metabolic syndrome is diagnosed by dyslipidemia and hypertension, in addition to abdominal obesity and abnormal glucose homeostasis.[11] The dyslipidemia and hypertension associated with the metabolic syndrome are thought to occur as a consequence of insulin resistance.[11] The Metabolic Syndrome and Cancer (Me-Can) Project in Austria, Sweden, and Norway has examined the association between the syndrome as a whole and its components with cancer risk. The investigators have reported that a higher composite metabolic syndrome score is associated with increased risk of liver cancer as well as bladder cancer in men and postmenopausal breast cancer in women.[12–14] They have also reported an increase in the risk of certain cancers associated with higher glucose levels, hypertriglyceridemia, and hypertension.[15–17]

Obesity, whether defined as a body mass index (BMI) of 30 kg/m² or higher or by increased waist circumference ($\geq$102 cm in men or $\geq$ 88 cm in women),[18] also is associated with an increased risk of certain cancers.[19] In 2008, the World Health Organization (WHO) reported that 10% of men and 14% of women worldwide were obese. In the WHO Region of the Americas, 26% of individuals were obese (www.who.int). Obesity is associated with many comorbid conditions, including the metabolic syndrome and T2D. The risk of developing T2D increases with higher BMI levels and with longer duration of obesity. Abdominal obesity is specifically associated with insulin resistance and the metabolic syndrome.[11] A meta-analysis of 221 datasets found that a 5 kg/m² increase in BMI was associated with an increased risk of developing esophageal, thyroid, colon, and renal carcinoma and multiple myeloma in men and women, in addition to hepatocellular and rectal cancer, and malignant melanoma in men, and endometrial, gallbladder, postmenopausal breast, and pancreatic cancer and leukemia in women.[19] The

Cancer Prevention Study II reported that obesity was associated with a significant increase in mortality from many similar cancers, including esophageal, colorectal, liver, gallbladder, pancreatic, breast, endometrial, cervical, ovarian, renal, brain, kidney and prostate cancer, non-Hodgkin's lymphoma, and multiple myeloma.[4] Obesity is usually defined by BMI in these epidemiologic studies; however, in certain ethnic groups, such as in individuals from Southeast Asia, insulin resistance may occur at a lower BMI, and waist circumference with race-specific cutoff values is considered to be a better measure of obesity.[11] There is a relative lack of prospective cohort studies examining the association between waist circumference and cancer risk; therefore, BMI is currently used to assess cancer risk associated with obesity.

Diabetes and Cancer Incidence

As for obesity and the metabolic syndrome, T2D has been associated with an increase in the incidence of many cancers and greater cancer mortality.[7,20–23] The association between diabetes and cancer risk is independent of BMI (**Table 1**). Many case-control and cohort studies have been performed in different populations examining the relative risk (RR) of different cancers in individuals with diabetes. Meta-analyses of these studies have reported an increased risk of liver, pancreatic, renal, endometrial, colorectal, bladder, and breast cancer, as well as an increase in the incidence of non-Hodgkin lymphoma.[7,21–24] For those with T2D compared with those without diabetes, the greatest increase in risk is for hepatocellular carcinoma (RR 2.5, 95% confidence interval [CI] 1.8–3.5), with the RR of cancer at other sites being between 1.18 (95% CI 1.05–1.32) for breast cancer and 2.22 (95% CI 1.8–2.74) for endometrial cancer in those with diabetes.[24] Some meta-analyses have addressed whether diabetes increases the risk of specific cancers after adjustment for other factors. Boyle and colleagues[25] examined 39 independent studies investigating women with and without T2D and found that postmenopausal women with T2D had an elevated risk of developing breast cancer compared with women without diabetes, but no increased risk in premenopausal breast cancer was observed in this study. Other cancers, such as hepatocellular cancer, have major risk factors, including infection with hepatitis B or hepatitis C virus.[26] Hepatitis C infection is found in 90% of patients with hepatocellular carcinoma in Japan, and although those with hepatitis C are 15 to 20 times more likely to develop hepatocellular carcinoma than those without, in a recent study of approximately 4000 individuals with treated hepatitis C, T2D was associated with a further 1.7-fold increased risk of developing hepatocellular carcinoma.[27] Notably, the risk

Table 1		
Cancer incidence in type 2 diabetes		
Cancer Type	**RR**	**(95% CI)**
Liver	2.5	(1.8–3.5)
Pancreas	1.9	(1.7–2.3)
Colorectal	1.3	(1.2–1.4)
Endometrium	2.2	(1.8–2.7)
Breast	1.2	(1.1–1.3)
Bladder	1.2	(1.1–1.4)
Prostate	0.9	(0.7–1.2)
All cancer	1.1	(1.0–1.2)

Abbreviations: CI, confidence interval; RR, relative risk.
  Data from Refs.[7,20–23]

of developing prostate cancer has been found to be lower in individuals with diabetes (RR 0.89, 95% CI 0.72–1.11).

Most studies examining the association between T2D and cancer have been performed in individuals of European descent. Fewer studies have been conducted in populations from different ethnic/racial groups and in different countries, where the incidence of certain cancers differ. For example, squamous cell cancer of the esophagus has a higher prevalence in East Asia, and African American men have a higher incidence of prostate cancer than men from European populations.[28,29] A study using Taiwan's Longitudinal Health Insurance Database found a positive association between T2D and the incidence of colorectal cancer.[30] However, in a case-control study in Taiwan, no association between esophageal carcinoma was found.[29] Another retrospective study examined a population of Chinese individuals with T2D and a mean BMI of 23.6 kg/m^2.[22] The study included men and women from a Chinese registry database. The investigators found that both men and women with T2D had increased risks of pancreatic cancers. Furthermore, men had an elevated risk of liver and kidney cancers, whereas women had an elevated risk of breast cancer and leukemia.[22] Although Asian and Western cultures traditionally differ in lifestyles and diets, many developing and industrializing countries are undergoing major changes in diet and lifestyle patterns and adopting a more Western lifestyle.[31] This entails reduced intake of vegetables and whole grains, and increasing the intake of fast foods and processed meats, as well as decreased physical activity.[31] This shift has contributed to the increasing rate of obesity and diabetes worldwide.[32] Therefore, further epidemiologic studies should be conducted in different populations worldwide to determine whether T2D increases the risk of site-specific cancers in individuals of different ethnic/racial background.

Diabetes and Cancer Mortality

Diabetes is associated with a greater mortality from many cancers (**Table 2**). Analysis of prospective data from more than 1 million US men and women followed for 26 years in the prospective Cancer Prevention Study II revealed that after adjustment for age, BMI, and other variables, diabetes was associated with a higher risk of mortality from hepatocellular, pancreatic, endometrial, colon, and breast cancer in women and breast, liver, oral cavity and pharynx, pancreas, and bladder cancer in men.[3] A large meta-analysis performed by the Emerging Risk Factors Collaboration examined the risk of death from cancer in individuals with and without diabetes in 97 prospective studies.[33] They reported that diabetes was associated with death from cancers of

Table 2 Cancer mortality in type 2 diabetes		
Cancer Type	**HR**	**(95% CI)**
Liver	2.2	(1.6–2.9)
Pancreas	1.2	(1.0–1.3)
Colorectal	1.4	(1.1–1.7)
Endometrium	1.4	(1.0–1.8)
Breast	1.4	(1.2–1.6)
Bladder	1.4	(1.0–2.0)
Prostate	1.6	(1.1–1.2)
All cancer	1.4	(1.0–1.8)

Abbreviations: CI, confidence interval; HR, hazard ratio.
   Data from Refs.[7,31,32,36,37]

the liver, pancreas, ovary, colon/rectum, lung, bladder, and breast.[33] Other studies have had similar findings. A retrospective study found that the 5-year overall survival rate of patients with endometrial cancer with T2D was significantly lower than for patients with endometrial cancer without T2D.[34] The patients with endometrial cancer with diabetes were older, had a more advanced stage at diagnosis, and had other complications compared with the patients with endometrial cancer without diabetes.[34] Even after the adjustments for these confounding factors, there was a significant effect of T2D affecting the mortality rate in the patients with endometrial cancer.[34] The study concluded that patients with endometrial cancer with T2D have worse survival rates than patients with endometrial cancer without T2D, 84% versus 68% mortality, respectively.[34] Another retrospective study found similar results between T2D and pancreatic cancer.[35] Patients with pancreatic adenocarcinoma and T2D had greater mortality rates than patients with pancreatic cancer without T2D.[35] Pancreatic cancer has long been associated with diabetes, and a new diagnosis of diabetes may be the first sign of undiagnosed pancreatic cancer. Therefore, many studies on individuals with pancreatic cancer exclude those who are diagnosed with pancreatic cancer within the 5 years of the diagnosis of diabetes. A study by Redaniel and colleagues[36] used the UK General Practice Research Database to investigate the link between T2D and treatment, with breast cancer risk and mortality. They found that women with T2D had a 49% increased mortality rate than women with breast cancer without T2D.[36] Diabetes has been associated with a more advanced stage at diagnosis and an increased risk of breast cancer recurrence after treatment.[1,37] Although men with diabetes have a lower incidence of prostate cancer, those with diabetes are more likely to have high-grade prostate cancer at presentation,[38] and studies have reported more advanced stage in men with diabetes.[2] Some studies also have reported a greater prostate cancer–specific mortality for individuals with diabetes and prostate cancer.[2,39] Others, however, have reported an increase in all-cause mortality in men with prostate cancer and diabetes, but not cancer-specific mortality,[40] and certain studies have shown a decrease in mortality in individuals with diabetes and prostate cancer.[3] A meta-analysis performed in 2010 of 4 studies reported a hazard ratio of 1.57 (95% CI 1.12–1.20) for prostate cancer mortality in men with preexisting diabetes.[41] Differences in study design, different populations, and time of diagnosis of diabetes relative to prostate cancer diagnosis and treatment and possibly diabetes treatments likely account the different results of these studies. Some of the increased cancer mortality associated with diabetes has been attributed to lower rates of cancer screening and more advanced stage at diagnosis.[7] Additionally, some studies have not distinguished cancer-specific mortality from all-cause mortality. These issues have been addressed in some recent studies that have reported greater cancer-specific mortality in individuals with diabetes and a number of different cancers.[2] However, further well-designed prospective epidemiologic studies need to be performed to clarify these issues and to determine the risks of cancer mortality associated with T2D. Many biologic mechanisms may account for the increased cancer incidence and mortality associated with obesity, the metabolic syndrome, and T2D.

BIOLOGIC MECHANISMS LINKING DIABETES AND CANCER

Various aspects of T2D have been suggested as potential mechanisms to promote cancer development (**Fig. 1**).[42–44] The increased risk of cancer with obesity, T2D, and the metabolic syndrome and their relationship to each other suggests common factors may explain the increased risk of cancer in these conditions. Potential

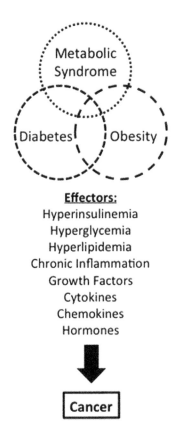

Effectors:
Hyperinsulinemia
Hyperglycemia
Hyperlipidemia
Chronic Inflammation
Growth Factors
Cytokines
Chemokines
Hormones

Cancer

Fig. 1. Aspects of T2D, obesity, and the metabolic syndrome affecting cancer development. The effectors through which T2D, obesity, and the metabolic syndrome may promote cancer development.

mechanisms to explain the relationship between T2D and cancers include insulin resistance, hyperinsulinemia, insulin-like growth factor-1 (IGF-1), hyperglycemia, and dyslipidemia (**Fig. 2**).[36,42,45] Inflammatory cytokines and adipokines also may contribute to metabolic dysfunction and promote cancer development.[34,43] Normal cells have to undergo morphologic changes before tumor growth, invasion, and metastasis occur. T2D can influence these changes either through IGF-1, hyperinsulinemia, hyperglycemia, or chronic inflammation.[44] It is thought that normal cells that have obtained oncogenic mutations are susceptible to the effects of T2D, the metabolic syndrome, and obesity, enabling cancer progression. The various mechanisms through which T2D, the metabolic syndrome, and obesity can promote tumorigenesis will be described in the following sections.

IGF-1, INSULIN, AND GLUCOSE
IGF-1

IGF-1 plays an important role in regulating cell proliferation, differentiation, and apoptosis. Many studies have reported that individuals with higher serum levels of IGF-1 are at an increased risk of developing cancers, such as prostate, colon, cervical, ovarian, and breast.[46] In addition, IGF-1 is expressed in stromal cells adjacent to normal breast epithelial cells.[47] The liver primarily produces IGF-1 and its production

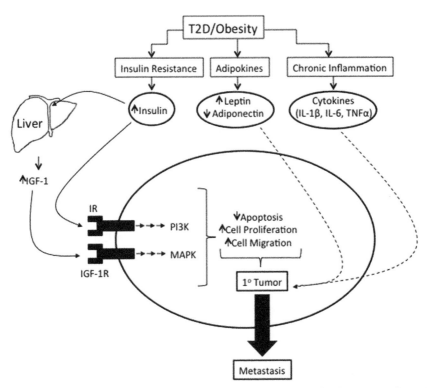

Fig. 2. Potential mechanisms of T2D and obesity leading to cancer development. Schematic representation of aspects of T2D and obesity that suggests insulin resistance and inflammation may promote primary tumor growth. Binding of insulin and IGF-1 to the IR/IGF-1R receptors leads to the activation of the PI3K and MAPK pathways. These signaling pathways promote cell proliferation and cell migration, and inhibit apoptosis, thus enhancing primary tumor progression. Chronic inflammation is associated with increased production of inflammatory cytokines that can directly act on the primary tumor. Furthermore, increased leptin and decreased adiponectin also can promote the development of the primary tumor.

is stimulated by growth hormone (GH) and insulin. IGF-1 binds to the extracellular subunit domain of the IGF-1 receptor (IGF-1R), which is a receptor tyrosine kinase (RTK).[48] The binding of IGF-1 to the receptor activates this RTK, which transduces a series of signaling cascades that activate mitogen-activated protein kinase (MAPK) and the phosphoinositide-3-kinase (PI3K)/Akt pathway.[48] MAPK activation leads to increased cell proliferation, whereas Akt activation leads to increased cell survival and migration.[49] This activation of the IGF-1R receptor has been linked to increased disease progression and poor prognosis in breast cancer.[50]

IGF-1 has been associated with breast cancer progression due to its mitogenic and antiapoptotic effects on mammary epithelial cells.[51] In vitro studies showed that it was possible to induce a transformed phenotype in human immortalized but untransformed mammary epithelial cells (MCF-10A cells), by overexpressing the IGF-1R in these cell lines. The cells adopted a more transformed phenotype, exhibiting growth factor–independent proliferation, lack of contact inhibition, anchorage-independent growth, and tumorigenesis in vivo.[52] The cells also demonstrated characteristics of epithelial-to-mesenchymal transition (EMT). They exhibited downregulation of epithelial markers, such as E-cadherin, β-catenin, and α-catenin, and upregulation of mesenchymal markers, such as vimentin, N-cadherin, and fibronectin. An increase of *snail* mRNA, which represses the transcription of *E-cadherin*, was also seen.[53] Furthermore, treating the malignant estrogen receptor–positive MCF-7 breast cancer cells, with IGF-1 and transforming growth factor β (TGF-β), it is possible to shift these cells from their epithelial nature to a more mesenchymal morphology.[51] Moreover, the gene expression of epithelial markers, *E-cadherin* and *Occludin*, became downregulated and upregulation of the expression of mesenchymal markers, *N-cadherin* and *vimentin* was observed.[51] These in vitro studies demonstrate that IGF-1 and IGF-1R signaling contribute to EMT. EMT is a biologic process in which polarized epithelial cells undergo various changes to take on a mesenchymal phenotype. This phenotype includes increased migratory capacity, invasiveness, resistance to apoptosis, and elevated production of extracellular matrix components.[54] Typically, EMT occurs during implantation, embryogenesis, and organ development. There is increasing evidence that suggests that EMT is associated with cancer progression (metastasis), suggesting that epithelial cancer cells activate EMT while becoming more malignant.[54]

Hepatic IGF-1 production is under the control of GH, other hormones, including insulin, and nutritional status.[55] Mice with higher circulating levels of IGF-1 demonstrate morphologic changes to the mammary epithelial cells and have a higher frequency of breast cancers.[55] Overexpression of IGF-1 under the control of the bovine keratin 5 promoter allowed for the expression of the IGF-1 transgene in the myoepithelial cells of the mouse mammary gland.[56] The mammary epithelial cells were exposed to high levels of IGF-1 by paracrine signaling, which is believed to model the local production of IGF-1 and paracrine signaling that occurs in human breast cancers.[56] Local IGF-1 production in this model promoted mammary gland hyperplasia, spontaneous mammary tumorigenesis, and increased susceptibility to chemical carcinogens.[56] A reduction of circulating IGF-1 levels can prolong tumor latency and reduce tumor size.[57] However, studies inhibiting IGF-1R signaling have not shown the predicted beneficial effects on tumor growth. A study by Konijeti and colleagues[58] combined dietary fat reduction with an IGF-1R blocking antibody to examine the effects on prostate cancer progression in a mouse model. Although, previous in vitro studies by this group and others found that blocking the IGF-1R inhibited cell growth and induced apoptosis, neither the dietary fat reduction nor the IGF-1R blocking therapy separately, or in combination, affected the tumor weight or volume.[58] These results suggest that in prostate cancer there may be other pathways that support tumor growth and progression. Furthermore, clinical trials using specific anti-IGF-1R antibodies have been relatively unsuccessful in reducing cancer growth.[59–61] Phase II studies on patients with squamous cell carcinoma of the head and neck (SCCHN) found that there was no clinically significant benefit of the anti-IGF-1R antibody.[60] The treatment was tolerated but resulted in hyperglycemia in 41% of the patients.[60] This may have been through the resultant increase of circulating GH that is known to have anti-insulin activity through the suppression of glucose uptake in tissues and enhancement of glucose synthesis in the liver. The trial also showed that the anti-IGF-1R antibody was unable to significantly inhibit the PI3K/Akt and MAPK signaling pathways in patients with SCCHN.[60] A phase I/II trial in patients with advanced non–small cell lung cancer also demonstrated little benefit.[61] Moreover, a similar negative result was seen in patients with metastatic refractory colorectal cancer.[59] These clinical trials, as well as other unsuccessful lung, hepatocellular carcinoma, and colorectal cancer trials, indicate that blocking the IGF-1R is not enough to achieve clinical response. Therefore, it is possible that only a specific subset of cancers are responsive to IGF-1R targeted therapy or that other receptors and signaling pathways, such as the insulin receptor signaling pathway, may be compensating for the inhibition of IGF-1R signaling.

Insulin Resistance and Hyperinsulinemia

Insulin resistance and hyperinsulinemia characterize prediabetes and early T2D. Insulin is a well-recognized growth factor. Various meta-analyses have shown that high levels of serum insulin and C-Peptide (a marker of insulin secretion) have correlated with increased risks of colorectal, pancreas, breast, and endometrial cancers in individuals without diabetes.[62] Hyperinsulinemia has also been associated with decreased breast cancer survival and recurrence-free survival.[63,64] Therefore, it is possible that hyperinsulinemia can promote the progression of breast cancer in patients, especially because it has been reported that insulin receptor (IR) expression is elevated in various breast cancer tissues and cancer cell lines.[65] The IR receptor is an RTK that typically signals through the PI3K/Akt pathway.[48] Active phosphorylated forms of the IR, along with phosphorylated insulin receptor substrate-1, trigger phosphorylation and activation of the PI3K catalytic subunit.[66] Downstream of PI3K is a serine/threonine kinase, Akt. It has been noted that Akt activation promotes cell-cycle progression, cell survival, and tumor cell invasion.[67] Furthermore, Akt can induce EMT by repressing the transcription of E-cadherin.[67,68] It is possible that in hyperinsulinemic patients, insulin may act through the IR on breast cancer cells and may promote downstream signaling and more growth of these cells. There are 2 isoforms of the insulin receptor: IR-A and IR-B. IR-B has 22 exons and is mostly expressed in metabolic tissues, including adipose tissue, muscle, and liver.[69] IR-A, which lacks exon 11, is believed to lead to more mitogenic signaling and is expressed normally in the placenta and fetal tissues, as well as cancer tissues.[69] Studies on human breast cancer have shown that greater IR-A to IR-B expression in breast cancer specimens correlated with resistance to hormone-targeted therapy.[70] Insulin may signal through IR-B or IR-A and, thus, in the setting of endogenous hyperinsulinemia, increased mitogenic signaling may occur via IR-A on the cancer cells. Hyperinsulinemia may also exert indirect effects on tumor growth through IGF-1. As noted previously, insulin increases circulating IGF-1 levels.[71] Additionally, insulin decreases insulin-like growth factor binding protein-1 (IGFBP-1), which may lead to an increase in local "free" IGF-1 in the tissues.[62] Through this potential mechanism, hyperinsulinemia may be able to drive tumor growth by acting directly on its cognate IR, likely the IR-A isoform, or by acting indirectly on the IGF-1R or the hybrid IR/IGF-1Rs.[62]

Hyperinsulinemia in a nonobese mouse model (MKR mouse) has been linked to an increase in mammary tumor growth.[72] These MKR mice were generated by the overexpression of the kinase dead IGF-1R, through a point mutation of a lysine-to-arginine residue introduced in the ATP-binding domain, in skeletal muscle under control of the creatine kinase promoter.[73] The overexpression of this dominant negative IGF-1R inhibited both the IGF-1R and IR in skeletal muscle through hybrids formed with the endogenous receptors. The MKR mice showed significant insulin resistance, hyperinsulinemia, and the male mice became hyperglycemic, however the female mice demonstrated only insulin resistance, hyperinsulinemia, and reduced body fat without hyperglycemia and hyperlipidemia, representing a prediabetic condition.[72] The female MKR mice had increased tumor growth following carcinogen, transgenic, or orthotopic induction of mammary tumors.[72] Ferguson and colleagues[74] found an increase in tumor metastases from c-Myc/VEGF overexpressing tumors in MKR mice, the increase in pulmonary metastases was observed even after intravenous injection of tumor cells. These findings suggest that hyperinsulinemia promotes increased survival and/or proliferation of circulating tumor cells that arrest in the lung. The study also demonstrated elevated levels of c-Myc, matrix metalloproteinase 9, IR, IGF-1R, and vascular endothelial growth factor (VEGF) in tumors from the hyperinsulinemic mice.[74] Reducing insulin levels in the MKR mice using an insulin-sensitizing agent resulted in reduced primary tumor growth and metastasis.[74]

Downregulation of the IR has been shown to inhibit anchorage-independent growth in the metastatic human estrogen receptor–negative LCC6 breast cancer cells, and the estrogen receptor–positive human T47D breast cancer cells.[75] In the LCC6, downregulation of the IR inhibited xenograft tumor growth in athymic mice.[75] In this study, Zhang and colleagues[75] investigated the proliferative, angiogenic, lymphangiogenic, and metastatic properties of these 2 breast cancer cells lines during IR downregulation. The reduction of IR expression led to a decrease of VEGF-A production, which is associated with angiogenesis. The group studied lymphangiogenic markers and found that xenografts with decreased IR expression had significantly reduced lymphatic and blood vessel development.[75] Furthermore, they noted that tail vein injections of IR-downregulated tumor cells caused significantly fewer lung metastases.[75] This suggests that by blocking insulin signaling, it is possible to inhibit or reduce the metastatic characteristics of malignant cancer cells.

Therefore, from human and animal studies, hyperinsulinemia, IR expression, and IR signaling are associated with increased tumor growth and metastasis. Potential targets for therapy could be aimed at reducing insulin levels, or blocking IR signaling alone or in addition to blocking IGF-1R signaling.

Hyperglycemia

Chronic hyperglycemia is a characteristic of diabetes. Studies have linked hyperglycemia to promoting tumor cell proliferation and metastasis in cancers associated with T2D.[76] Various epidemiologic studies have shown that elevated blood glucose has a direct association with an increase in breast cancer risk.[77]

Hyperglycemia has been linked to the Warburg Effect, where cancer cells shift to obtaining energy from glycolysis rather than the TCA cycle.[78] Cancer cells have been characterized by high rates of glucose uptake and glucose metabolism. Therefore, a hyperglycemic environment may provide the necessary conditions for these cancer cells to survive and proliferate. Glucose is also a substrate for fatty acid synthase (FAS), an enzyme that allows for the synthesis of fatty acids.[79] The increase of FAS in malignant breast cancer cell lines promoted survival in these cells.[79] Furthermore, FAS also conferred resistance to chemotherapeutic agents in MCF-7 and T47D cells, by preventing apoptosis.[79] This link between hyperglycemia and chemotherapy resistance may contribute to the poor prognosis and increase in cancer mortality that is seen in patients with T2D and breast cancer.[37]

Studies have also found that hyperglycemia induces EMT in various cell lines.[80] In rat renal proximal tubular epithelial (NRK-52E) cells, expressions of alpha-smooth muscle actin and vimentin, which are mesenchymal markers, were increased, whereas these cells lost the expression of the epithelial cell marker E-cadherin after exposure to high glucose.[80] Furthermore, TGF-β levels were also increased in cells exposed to high glucose levels.[80] In many carcinomas, growth factors, such as TGF-β or epidermal growth factor, can lead to the induction of EMT by increasing the expression various EMT-inducing transcription factors, most commonly Snail, Slug, zinc finger E-box binding homeobox 1 (ZEB1), and Twist.[81–83] Hyperglycemia may also promote metastatic spread by increasing angiogenesis. An increase of microRNA 467 (miRNA467) has been found with hyperglycemia. miR467 inhibits thrombospondin-1, an important antiangiogenic protein.[84] This mechanism of silencing thrombospondin-1 can provide insight into how exposure to hyperglycemia can induce angiogenesis and promote tumor progression.

These studies suggest that the hyperglycemia of T2D can contribute to the development and progression of cancers by promoting transformation of cancer cells, providing the necessary energy source and allowing for cell survival and resistance to chemotherapy.

CYTOKINES AND ADIPOKINES
Inflammation

T2D is strongly associated with obesity, which can promote systemic inflammation and insulin resistance in adipose tissues. Epidemiologic studies have linked elevated levels of the inflammatory markers C-reactive protein (CRP) and interleukin 6 (IL-6) with the development of T2D.[85] It has been noted that overeating can result in cytokine hypersecretion, which can promote the development of insulin resistance.[85] Cytokines are signaling molecules, within the immune response system, that are secreted in response to injury from infection, inflammation, and chemicals.[86] Cytokines are known to regulate growth, signaling, and differentiation in stromal and tumor cells. Prolonged exposure and production of these cytokines has been associated with tumor formation and progression. Various cytokines have been associated with tumor development, however IL-1β, IL-6, and tumor necrosis factor-alpha (TNF-α) have been cited as the major cytokines linking T2D to cancer progression.[85]

TNF-α activates the TNF receptors (TNFR) that promote a series of signal transduction pathways and regulate genes involved in inflammation, cell survival and cell death. TNFR activation can lead to the activation of pathways, such as the FAS-associated signal via death domain/caspase 8/caspase 3, MAPK, Jun Kinase, and nuclear factor (NF)-kB pathway.[86] NF-kB activation is known to have antiapoptotic effects through negative regulation of proapoptotic factors.[86] Animal models have shown that constitutive production of TNF-α promotes the growth and metastasis of tumors.[87]

TNF-α homozygous knockout mice on a high-fat, high-caloric diet demonstrated better sensitivity to insulin when compared with the TNF-α wild-type mice on the same diet.[88] Furthermore, these TNF-α–deficient obese mice had lower levels of circulating free fatty acids and higher levels of Glut4 protein in muscle, and mice lacking TNF-α or TNFR demonstrated improved insulin sensitivity.[88] This suggests that TNF-α can promote obesity-related insulin resistance. Furthermore, TNF-α production has been associated with poor prognosis in human cancers.[89] TNF-α has been shown to upregulate the expression of C-X-C chemokine receptor type 4.[86] This chemokine receptor has been associated with an increase in metastasis and tumor cell survival in various cancers.[86] These studies demonstrate that TNF-α can promote the progression of cancer in the setting of inflammation. These studies also suggest that TNF-α/TNFR signaling may be important for therapeutics.

Another group of cytokines important in T2D and cancer are the interleukins, such as IL-1β and IL-6. Studies have shown that patients with high IL-1β–producing tumors generally have a worse prognosis than patients with tumors that do not produce high levels of IL-1β.[86] IL-1β is known to upregulate the inflammatory response and is overexpressed in breast carcinoma cells.[90] Human breast carcinoma samples were assayed for IL-1β levels and the higher levels of IL-1β were correlated with an increased invasion and a more aggressive phenotype of the breast carcinoma cells.[91] Local IL-1β production by cancer cells can, through autocrine signaling, stimulate the tumor cells to proliferate and invade. MCF-7 cells treated with IL-1β showed significantly increased cell proliferation.[92] Furthermore, studies have found that IL-1β can induce the expression of matrix metalloproteinases and stimulate neighboring cells to produce VEGF, IL-6, TNF-α, and TGF-β.[93] This suggests that in the setting of chronic inflammation, such as in obesity, increased levels of circulating IL-1β can promote the proliferation and invasion of tumor cells. Furthermore, autocrine and paracrine IL-1β can provide the tumor with the necessary environment to grow.

IL-6 is also negatively correlated with cancer survival, with high IL-6 levels being associated with worse progression-free and overall survival.[94] IL-6 has pro-tumorigenic effects on cancer cells by increasing the survival and the proliferation of the cells.[95] IL-6 binds to the IL-6R on the cell surface and activates Janus Kinase 1 (JAK1), which has tyrosine kinase activity.[95] JAK1 activates signal transducer and activator of transcription 3 (STAT3), a transcription factor that can lead to the increase of cell growth, differentiation, and inhibition of apoptosis.[95] Constitutive STAT3 expression enhanced breast cancer cell migration. It was shown that constitutive activation of STAT3 in mice did not induce tumor growth alone.[96] However, constitutive activation of STAT3 in a transgenic MMTV-Neu oncogene mouse model of breast cancer showed that there was cooperation between the Neu oncogene and STAT3 to promote tumorigenesis.[96] This suggests that IL-6 does not drive the formation of the tumors, but instead provides an environment in which these malignant cancer cells can grow. In human malignant kidney cells, a short hairpin RNA knockdown of IL-6 resulted in a reduction of tumor growth.[97] Furthermore, IL-6 knockout mice were resistant to carcinogen-induced tumors.[97]

Epidemiologic data indicated that many cancers are related to chronic infections or inflammation.[98] It is believed that obesity is associated with an accumulation of macrophages that aggregate and surround the mammary gland.[99] In obese mice, the macrophages were associated with increased levels of TNF-α and IL-1β.[99] Moreover, the proinflammatory cytokines have been associated with increasing the transcription of aromatase, which converts androgens to estrogens.[99] Obese mice produced higher levels of TNF-α and IL-1β, and had more induction of aromatase activity than lean mice.[99] This is also consistent with the findings that aromatase levels are increased in the breast tissue of obese women compared with healthy individuals.[100] This suggests that inflammation caused by obesity produces an environment that is rich in the proinflammatory markers that allow for increased aromatase expression. This in turn can contribute to the increased risk of cancer in obese patients.

Inflammation is now considered to be one of the key hallmarks of cancer that allows for a permissive tumor-growing microenvironment.[101] These studies show that there is clearly interplay between the inflammatory markers and cancer cell progression. In patients with obesity, the metabolic syndrome, and T2D, these cytokines are increased and can contribute to deregulation of the cell cycle and in turn promote tumorigenesis. In the setting of obesity, the metabolic syndrome, and T2D, decreasing inflammatory cytokines, such as TNF-α, IL-1β, and IL-6, may improve insulin sensitivity and reduce tumor progression.

Adipokines

The adipose tissue produces hormones and cytokine-like factors. Two such adipokines (cytokines produced by the adipose tissue), leptin and adiponectin, are related to obesity, T2D, and breast cancer.

Leptin is a proinflammatory adipokine that is expressed by the Ob gene and regulates food intake, inflammation, immunity, cell proliferation, and differentiation of different cell types.[102] Leptin has been shown to increase proliferation, migration, and invasion of cancer cells. In some cases, it has been reported to increase levels of VEGF.[43] Leptin receptor expression has been reported to be higher in many human breast cancers compared with normal breast epithelial cells.[103] Furthermore, patients who demonstrated higher leptin and leptin receptor levels showed an increase in metastases.[43] In MCF-7 cells, a knockdown of the leptin receptor resulted in a decrease of tumor volume in a mouse xenograft model.[102] About 60% of ovarian cancers have an overexpression of the leptin receptor.[102] In a cell culture model of human ovarian cancer, it was discovered that leptin stimulated the expression of an antiapoptotic protein.[104] Furthermore, leptin was able to induce growth in the ovarian cancer cell line by activating JAK, MAPK, and PI3K/Akt pathways.[104] In a mouse MMTV-TGF-α model with leptin receptor deficiency, mammary tumors failed to form.[105]

Adiponectin is an anti-inflammatory adipokine secreted by adipose tissues. It has been found to possess a protective role against obesity and T2D.[106] Adiponectin binds to its adiponectin receptors 1 and 2 (AdipoR1 and AdipoR2).[106] These receptors then activate various signaling pathways, such as adenosine monophosphate-activated kinase (AMPK) and p38 MAPK.[106] There is an inverse relationship between adiponectin plasma concentrations and BMI.[107] A prospective study found that patients with high adiponectin levels had a 40% lower risk of developing T2D than patients with low adiponectin concentrations.[108] Furthermore, epidemiologic studies have found that low adiponectin levels are associated with an increased risk of breast cancer.[107] In women, low serum adiponectin concentrations correlated with larger tumors and a worse prognosis.[109] Obese and diabetic mice administered adiponectin had a reduction in hyperglycemia, improved insulin sensitivity, and increased fatty acid oxidation in muscle tissue.[43] Therefore, adiponectin may reduce tumor growth by reducing insulin and glucose levels. Moreover, in MDA-MB-231 breast cancer cells, it was discovered that adiponectin activated AMPK, leading to reduced invasion of the cells.[110] Activated AMPK promoted the increase of protein phosphatase 2A (PP2A), a tumor suppressor typically lost or decreased in patients with breast cancer, which dephosphorylates AKT.[110] Furthermore, the reduction of tumor growth and volume in mice with increased adiponectin concentrations demonstrated the protective effect of adiponectin in vivo.[111] These data suggest that adiponectin levels may be used as an additional screen to predict the risk of breast cancer, especially in patients with T2D and obesity. Furthermore, increasing adiponectin concentrations and adiponectin-induced reactivation of PP2A may be a therapeutic target for breast cancer.

This section focused on the potential roles of adipokines and cytokines in promoting cancer growth and metastases in the setting of obesity, the metabolic syndrome, and T2D. Reducing inflammatory cytokines, decreasing leptin levels, or increasing adiponectin may have beneficial effects on tumors by directly influencing the signaling pathways in tumors and by indirectly improving glycemia and insulin resistance.

SUMMARY

There have been numerous epidemiologic studies connecting T2D, the metabolic syndrome, and obesity with increased risk of developing and dying from many different cancers. As discussed in this review, there are various mechanisms that may contribute to the progression of cancer in insulin-resistant, diabetic, or obese individuals. It is hypothesized that normal cells obtain oncogenic mutations that transform the cells into cancer cells, the growth and metastases of which are then propagated in the setting of T2D. Studies are currently ongoing to uncover the precise mechanisms that link T2D, obesity, and the metabolic syndrome with cancer. By understanding the mechanisms that are involved in the link between T2D and cancer, targeted screening could be performed to prevent tumor development, and better therapeutic strategies could be designed to target specific pathways and reduce mortality in individuals with T2D and cancer.

REFERENCES

1. Kaplan MA, Pekkolay Z, Kucukoner M, et al. Type 2 diabetes mellitus and prognosis in early stage breast cancer women. Med Oncol 2012;29(3):1576–80.
2. Liu X, Ji J, Sundquist K, et al. The impact of type 2 diabetes mellitus on cancer-specific survival: a follow-up study in Sweden. Cancer 2012;118(5):1353–61.
3. Campbell PT, Newton CC, Patel AV, et al. Diabetes and cause-specific mortality in a prospective cohort of one million U.S adults. Diabetes Care 2012;35(9):1835–44.
4. Calle EE, Rodriguez C, Walker-Thurmond K, et al. Overweight, obesity, and mortality from cancer in a prospectively studied cohort of U.S adults. N Engl J Med 2003;348(17):1625–38.
5. DeFronzo RA. Pathogenesis of type 2 diabetes mellitus. Med Clin North Am 2004;88(4):787–835, ix.
6. LeRoith D, Gavrilova O. Mouse models created to study the pathophysiology of type 2 diabetes. Int J Biochem Cell Biol 2006;38(5–6):904–12.
7. Onitilo AA, Engel JM, Glurich I, et al. Diabetes and cancer I: risk, survival, and implications for screening. Cancer Causes Control 2012;23(6):967–81.
8. Gordon-Dseagu VL, Shelton N, Mindell JS. Epidemiological evidence of a relationship between type-1 diabetes mellitus and cancer: a review of the existing literature. Int J Cancer 2013;132(3):501–8.
9. Shu X, Ji J, Li X, et al. Cancer risk among patients hospitalized for Type 1 diabetes mellitus: a population-based cohort study in Sweden. Diabet Med 2010;27(7):791–7.
10. Hemminki K, Houlston R, Sundquist J, et al. Co-morbidity between early-onset leukemia and type 1 diabetes—suggestive of a shared viral etiology? PLoS One 2012;7(6):e39523.
11. Gallagher EJ, Leroith D, Karnieli E. The metabolic syndrome—from insulin resistance to obesity and diabetes. Med Clin North Am 2011;95(5):855–73.
12. Haggstrom C, Stocks T, Rapp K, et al. Metabolic syndrome and risk of bladder cancer: prospective cohort study in the metabolic syndrome and cancer project (Me-Can). Int J Cancer 2011;128(8):1890–8.
13. Bjorge T, Lukanova A, Jonsson H, et al. Metabolic syndrome and breast cancer in the me-can (metabolic syndrome and cancer) project. Cancer Epidemiol Biomarkers Prev 2010;19(7):1737–45.
14. Borena W, Strohmaier S, Lukanova A, et al. Metabolic risk factors and primary liver cancer in a prospective study of 578,700 adults. Int J Cancer 2012;131(1):193–200.
15. Stocks T, Rapp K, Bjorge T, et al. Blood glucose and risk of incident and fatal cancer in the metabolic syndrome and cancer project (me-can): analysis of six prospective cohorts. PLoS Med 2009;6(12):e1000201.
16. Borena W, Stocks T, Jonsson H, et al. Serum triglycerides and cancer risk in the metabolic syndrome and cancer (Me-Can) collaborative study. Cancer Causes Control 2011;22(2):291–9.
17. Stocks T, Van Hemelrijck M, Manjer J, et al. Blood pressure and risk of cancer incidence and mortality in the metabolic syndrome and cancer project. Hypertension 2012;59(4):802–10.

18. Grundy SM, Cleeman JI, Daniels SR, et al. Diagnosis and management of the metabolic syndrome: an American Heart Association/National Heart, Lung, and Blood Institute Scientific Statement. Circulation 2005;112(17):2735–52.
19. Renehan AG, Tyson M, Egger M, et al. Body-mass index and incidence of cancer: a systematic review and meta-analysis of prospective observational studies. Lancet 2008;371(9612):569–78.
20. Adami HO, McLaughlin J, Ekbom A, et al. Cancer risk in patients with diabetes mellitus. Cancer Causes Control 1991;2(5):307–14.
21. Chari ST, Leibson CL, Rabe KG, et al. Probability of pancreatic cancer following diabetes: a population-based study. Gastroenterology 2005;129(2):504–11.
22. Zhang PH, Chen ZW, Lv D, et al. Increased risk of cancer in patients with type 2 diabetes mellitus: a retrospective cohort study in China. BMC Public Health 2012;12(1):567.
23. Haslam DW, James WP. Obesity. Lancet 2005;366(9492):1197–209.
24. Vigneri P, Frasca F, Sciacca L, et al. Diabetes and cancer. Endocr Relat Cancer 2009;16(4):1103–23.
25. Boyle P, Boniol M, Koechlin A, et al. Diabetes and breast cancer risk: a meta-analysis. Br J Cancer 2012;107(9):1608–17.
26. El-Serag HB. Hepatocellular carcinoma. N Engl J Med 2011;365(12):1118–27.
27. Arase Y, Kobayashi M, Suzuki F, et al. Effect of type 2 diabetes on risk for malignancies includes hepatocellular carcinoma in chronic hepatitis C. Hepatology 2013;57(3):964–73.
28. Hsing AW, Tsao L, Devesa SS. International trends and patterns of prostate cancer incidence and mortality. Int J Cancer 2000;85(1):60–7.
29. Cheng KC, Chen YL, Lai SW, et al. Risk of esophagus cancer in diabetes mellitus: a population-based case-control study in Taiwan. BMC Gastroenterol 2012;12:177.
30. Wang JY, Chao TT, Lai CC, et al. Risk of colorectal cancer in type 2 diabetic patients: a population-based cohort study. Jpn J Clin Oncol 2013;43(3):258–63.
31. Pan A, Malik VS, Hu FB. Exporting diabetes mellitus to Asia: the impact of western-style fast food. Circulation 2012;126(2):163–5.
32. Zimmet P, Alberti KG, Shaw J. Global and societal implications of the diabetes epidemic. Nature 2001;414(6865):782–7.
33. Seshasai SR, Kaptoge S, Thompson A, et al. Diabetes mellitus, fasting glucose, and risk of cause-specific death. N Engl J Med 2011;364(9):829–41.
34. Zanders MM, Boll D, van Steenbergen LN, et al. Effect of diabetes on endometrial cancer recurrence and survival. Maturitas 2013;74(1):37–43.
35. Hwang A, Narayan V, Yang YX. Type 2 diabetes mellitus and survival in pancreatic adenocarcinoma: a retrospective cohort study. Cancer 2013;119(2):404–10.
36. Redaniel MT, Jeffreys M, May MT, et al. Associations of type 2 diabetes and diabetes treatment with breast cancer risk and mortality: a population-based cohort study among British women. Cancer Causes Control 2012;23(11):1785–95.
37. Peairs KS, Barone BB, Snyder CF, et al. Diabetes mellitus and breast cancer outcomes: a systematic review and meta-analysis. J Clin Oncol 2011;29(1):40–6.
38. Mitin T, Chen MH, Zhang Y, et al. Diabetes mellitus, race and the odds of high grade prostate cancer in men treated with radiation therapy. J Urol 2011;186(6):2233–7.
39. Yeh HC, Platz EA, Wang NY, et al. A prospective study of the associations between treated diabetes and cancer outcomes. Diabetes Care 2012;35(1):113–8.

40. D'Amico AV, Braccioforte MH, Moran BJ, et al. Causes of death in men with prevalent diabetes and newly diagnosed high- versus favorable-risk prostate cancer. Int J Radiat Oncol Biol Phys 2010;77(5):1329–37.

41. Snyder CF, Stein KB, Barone BB, et al. Does pre-existing diabetes affect prostate cancer prognosis? A systematic review. Prostate Cancer Prostatic Dis 2010; 13(1):58–64.

42. Lawlor DA, Smith GD, Ebrahim S. Hyperinsulinaemia and increased risk of breast cancer: findings from the British Women's Heart and Health Study. Cancer Causes Control 2004;15(3):267–75.

43. Ouchi N, Parker JL, Lugus JJ, et al. Adipokines in inflammation and metabolic disease. Nat Rev Immunol 2011;11(2):85–97.

44. Giovannucci E, Harlan DM, Archer MC, et al. Diabetes and cancer: a consensus report. Diabetes Care 2010;33(7):1674–85.

45. Yang Y, Mauldin PD, Ebeling M, et al. Effect of metabolic syndrome and its components on recurrence and survival in colon cancer patients. Cancer 2012; 119(8):1512–20.

46. Hankinson SE, Willett WC, Colditz GA, et al. Circulating concentrations of insulin-like growth factor-I and risk of breast cancer. Lancet 1998;351(9113):1393–6.

47. Yee D, Paik S, Lebovic GS, et al. Analysis of insulin-like growth factor I gene expression in malignancy: evidence for a paracrine role in human breast cancer. Mol Endocrinol 1989;3(3):509–17.

48. Ikushima H, Miyazono K. TGFbeta signalling: a complex web in cancer progression. Nat Rev Cancer 2010;10(6):415–24.

49. Samani AA, Yakar S, LeRoith D, et al. The role of the IGF system in cancer growth and metastasis: overview and recent insights. Endocr Rev 2007;28(1): 20–47.

50. Creighton CJ, Casa A, Lazard Z, et al. Insulin-like growth factor-I activates gene transcription programs strongly associated with poor breast cancer prognosis. J Clin Oncol 2008;26(25):4078–85.

51. Walsh LA, Damjanovski S. IGF-1 increases invasive potential of MCF 7 breast cancer cells and induces activation of latent TGF-beta1 resulting in epithelial to mesenchymal transition. Cell Commun Signal 2011;9(1):10.

52. Kim HJ, Litzenburger BC, Cui X, et al. Constitutively active type I insulin-like growth factor receptor causes transformation and xenograft growth of immortalized mammary epithelial cells and is accompanied by an epithelial-to-mesenchymal transition mediated by NF-kappaB and snail. Mol Cell Biol 2007; 27(8):3165–75.

53. Huber MA, Kraut N, Beug H. Molecular requirements for epithelial-mesenchymal transition during tumor progression. Curr Opin Cell Biol 2005;17(5):548–58.

54. Kalluri R, Weinberg RA. The basics of epithelial-mesenchymal transition. J Clin Invest 2009;119(6):1420–8.

55. Tornell J, Carlsson B, Pohjanen P, et al. High frequency of mammary adenocarcinomas in metallothionein promoter-human growth hormone transgenic mice created from two different strains of mice. J Steroid Biochem Mol Biol 1992; 43(1–3):237–42.

56. de Ostrovich KK, Lambertz I, Colby JK, et al. Paracrine overexpression of insulin-like growth factor-1 enhances mammary tumorigenesis in vivo. Am J Pathol 2008;173(3):824–34.

57. Wu Y, Cui K, Miyoshi K, et al. Reduced circulating insulin-like growth factor I levels delay the onset of chemically and genetically induced mammary tumors. Cancer Res 2003;63(15):4384–8.

58. Konijeti R, Koyama S, Gray A, et al. Effect of a low-fat diet combined with IGF-1 receptor blockade on 22Rv1 prostate cancer xenografts. Mol Cancer Ther 2012; 11(7):1539–46.
59. Reidy DL, Vakiani E, Fakih MG, et al. Randomized, phase II study of the insulin-like growth factor-1 receptor inhibitor IMC-A12, with or without cetuximab, in patients with cetuximab- or panitumumab-refractory metastatic colorectal cancer. J Clin Oncol 2010;28(27):4240–6.
60. Schmitz S, Kaminsky-Forrett MC, Henry S, et al. Phase II study of figitumumab in patients with recurrent and/or metastatic squamous cell carcinoma of the head and neck: clinical activity and molecular response (GORTEC 2008-02). Ann Oncol 2012;23(8):2153–61.
61. Weickhardt A, Doebele R, Oton A, et al. A phase I/II study of erlotinib in combination with the anti-insulin-like growth factor-1 receptor monoclonal antibody IMC-A12 (cixutumumab) in patients with advanced non-small cell lung cancer. J Thorac Oncol 2012;7(2):419–26.
62. Becker S, Dossus L, Kaaks R. Obesity related hyperinsulinaemia and hyperglycaemia and cancer development. Arch Physiol Biochem 2009;115(2):86–96.
63. Goodwin PJ, Ennis M, Pritchard KI, et al. Fasting insulin and outcome in early-stage breast cancer: results of a prospective cohort study. J Clin Oncol 2002; 20(1):42–51.
64. Lipscombe LL, Goodwin PJ, Zinman B, et al. The impact of diabetes on survival following breast cancer. Breast Cancer Res Treat 2008;109(2):389–95.
65. Mauro L, Bartucci M, Morelli C, et al. IGF-I receptor-induced cell-cell adhesion of MCF-7 breast cancer cells requires the expression of junction protein ZO-1. J Biol Chem 2001;276(43):39892–7.
66. Rodriguez-Viciana P, Warne PH, Vanhaesebroeck B, et al. Activation of phosphoinositide 3-kinase by interaction with Ras and by point mutation. EMBO J 1996;15(10):2442–51.
67. Larue L, Bellacosa A. Epithelial-mesenchymal transition in development and cancer: role of phosphatidylinositol 3' kinase/AKT pathways. Oncogene 2005; 24(50):7443–54.
68. Grille SJ, Bellacosa A, Upson J, et al. The protein kinase Akt induces epithelial mesenchymal transition and promotes enhanced motility and invasiveness of squamous cell carcinoma lines. Cancer Res 2003;63(9):2172–8.
69. Frasca F, Pandini G, Scalia P, et al. Insulin receptor isoform A, a newly recognized, high-affinity insulin-like growth factor II receptor in fetal and cancer cells. Mol Cell Biol 1999;19(5):3278–88.
70. Harrington SC, Weroha SJ, Reynolds C, et al. Quantifying insulin receptor isoform expression in FFPE breast tumors. Growth Horm IGF Res 2012;22(3–4): 108–15.
71. Thissen JP, Ketelslegers JM, Underwood LE. Nutritional regulation of the insulin-like growth factors. Endocr Rev 1994;15(1):80–101.
72. Novosyadlyy R, Lann DE, Vijayakumar A, et al. Insulin-mediated acceleration of breast cancer development and progression in a nonobese model of type 2 diabetes. Cancer Res 2010;70(2):741–51.
73. Fernandez AM, Kim JK, Yakar S, et al. Functional inactivation of the IGF-I and insulin receptors in skeletal muscle causes type 2 diabetes. Genes Dev 2001; 15(15):1926–34.
74. Ferguson RD, Novosyadlyy R, Fierz Y, et al. Hyperinsulinemia enhances c-Myc-mediated mammary tumor development and advances metastatic progression to the lung in a mouse model of type 2 diabetes. Breast Cancer Res 2012;14(1):R8.

75. Zhang H, Fagan DH, Zeng X, et al. Inhibition of cancer cell proliferation and metastasis by insulin receptor downregulation. Oncogene 2010;29(17): 2517–27.

76. Shikata K, Ninomiya T, Kiyohara Y. Diabetes mellitus and cancer risk: review of the epidemiological evidence. Cancer Sci 2013;104(1):9–14.

77. Sieri S, Muti P, Claudia A, et al. Prospective study on the role of glucose metabolism in breast cancer occurrence. Int J Cancer 2012;130(4):921–9.

78. Garber K. Energy boost: the Warburg effect returns in a new theory of cancer. J Natl Cancer Inst 2004;96(24):1805–6.

79. Zeng L, Biernacka KM, Holly JM, et al. Hyperglycaemia confers resistance to chemotherapy on breast cancer cells: the role of fatty acid synthase. Endocr Relat Cancer 2010;17(2):539–51.

80. Zhou L, Xue H, Yuan P, et al. Angiotensin AT1 receptor activation mediates high glucose-induced epithelial-mesenchymal transition in renal proximal tubular cells. Clin Exp Pharmacol Physiol 2010;37(9):e152–7.

81. Pan B, Ren H, He Y, et al. HDL of patients with type 2 diabetes mellitus elevates the capability of promoting breast cancer metastasis. Clin Cancer Res 2012; 18(5):1246–56.

82. Shi Y, Massague J. Mechanisms of TGF-beta signaling from cell membrane to the nucleus. Cell 2003;113(6):685–700.

83. Al Moustafa AE, Achkhar A. Yasmeen A: EGF-receptor signaling and epithelial-mesenchymal transition in human carcinomas. Front Biosci (Schol Ed) 2012;4: 671–84.

84. Bhattacharyya S, Sul K, Krukovets I, et al. Novel tissue-specific mechanism of regulation of angiogenesis and cancer growth in response to hyperglycemia. J Am Heart Assoc 2012;1(6):e005967.

85. Haffner SM. Insulin resistance, inflammation, and the prediabetic state. Am J Cardiol 2003;92(4A):18J–26J.

86. Vendramini-Costa DB, Carvalho JE. Molecular link mechanisms between inflammation and cancer. Curr Pharm Des 2012;18(26):3831–52.

87. Hotamisligil GS, Shargill NS, Spiegelman BM. Adipose expression of tumor necrosis factor-alpha: direct role in obesity-linked insulin resistance. Science 1993; 259(5091):87–91.

88. Uysal KT, Wiesbrock SM, Marino MW, et al. Protection from obesity-induced insulin resistance in mice lacking TNF-alpha function. Nature 1997;389(6651): 610–4.

89. Aggarwal BB, Shishodia S, Sandur SK, et al. Inflammation and cancer: how hot is the link? Biochem Pharmacol 2006;72(11):1605–21.

90. Chavey C, Bibeau F, Gourgou-Bourgade S, et al. Oestrogen receptor negative breast cancers exhibit high cytokine content. Breast Cancer Res 2007;9(1):R15.

91. Jin L, Yuan RQ, Fuchs A, et al. Expression of interleukin-1beta in human breast carcinoma. Cancer 1997;80(3):421–34.

92. Honma S, Shimodaira K, Shimizu Y, et al. The influence of inflammatory cytokines on estrogen production and cell proliferation in human breast cancer cells. Endocr J 2002;49(3):371–7.

93. Lewis AM, Varghese S, Xu H, et al. Interleukin-1 and cancer progression: the emerging role of interleukin-1 receptor antagonist as a novel therapeutic agent in cancer treatment. J Transl Med 2006;4:48.

94. Bozcuk H, Uslu G, Samur M, et al. Tumour necrosis factor-alpha, interleukin-6, and fasting serum insulin correlate with clinical outcome in metastatic breast cancer patients treated with chemotherapy. Cytokine 2004;27(2–3):58–65.

95. Ghosh S, Ashcraft K. An IL-6 link between obesity and cancer. Front Biosci (Elite Ed) 2013;5:461–78.
96. Barbieri I, Pensa S, Pannellini T, et al. Constitutively active Stat3 enhances neu-mediated migration and metastasis in mammary tumors via upregulation of Cten. Cancer Res 2010;70(6):2558–67.
97. Ancrile B, Lim KH, Counter CM. Oncogenic Ras-induced secretion of IL6 is required for tumorigenesis. Genes Dev 2007;21(14):1714–9.
98. Schetter AJ, Heegaard NH, Harris CC. Inflammation and cancer: interweaving microRNA, free radical, cytokine and p53 pathways. Carcinogenesis 2010; 31(1):37–49.
99. Subbaramaiah K, Howe LR, Bhardwaj P, et al. Obesity is associated with inflammation and elevated aromatase expression in the mouse mammary gland. Cancer Prev Res (Phila) 2011;4(3):329–46.
100. Morris PG, Hudis CA, Giri D, et al. Inflammation and increased aromatase expression occur in the breast tissue of obese women with breast cancer. Cancer Prev Res (Phila) 2011;4(7):1021–9.
101. Hanahan D, Weinberg RA. Hallmarks of cancer: the next generation. Cell 2011; 144(5):646–74.
102. Vansaun MN. Molecular pathways: adiponectin and leptin signaling in cancer. Clin Cancer Res 2013;19(8):1926–32.
103. Giordano C, Vizza D, Panza S, et al. Leptin increases HER2 protein levels through a STAT3-mediated up-regulation of Hsp90 in breast cancer cells. Mol Oncol 2012;7(3):379–91.
104. Chen C, Chang YC, Lan MS, et al. Leptin stimulates ovarian cancer cell growth and inhibits apoptosis by increasing cyclin D1 and Mcl-1 expression via the activation of the MEK/ERK1/2 and PI3K/Akt signaling pathways. Int J Oncol 2013; 42(3):1113–9.
105. Cleary MP, Juneja SC, Phillips FC, et al. Leptin receptor-deficient MMTV-TGF-alpha/Lepr(db)Lepr(db) female mice do not develop oncogene-induced mammary tumors. Exp Biol Med (Maywood) 2004;229(2):182–93.
106. Duan XF, Tang P, Li Q, et al. Obesity, adipokines, and hepatocellular carcinoma. Int J Cancer 2013;133(8):1776–83.
107. Vona-Davis L, Howard-McNatt M, Rose DP. Adiposity, type 2 diabetes and the metabolic syndrome in breast cancer. Obes Rev 2007;8(5):395–408.
108. Duncan BB, Schmidt MI, Pankow JS, et al. Adiponectin and the development of type 2 diabetes: the atherosclerosis risk in communities study. Diabetes 2004; 53(9):2473–8.
109. Miyoshi Y, Funahashi T, Kihara S, et al. Association of serum adiponectin levels with breast cancer risk. Clin Cancer Res 2003;9(15):5699–704.
110. Kim KY, Baek A, Hwang JE, et al. Adiponectin-activated AMPK stimulates dephosphorylation of AKT through protein phosphatase 2A activation. Cancer Res 2009;69(9):4018–26.
111. Wang Y, Lam JB, Lam KS, et al. Adiponectin modulates the glycogen synthase kinase-3beta/beta-catenin signaling pathway and attenuates mammary tumorigenesis of MDA-MB-231 cells in nude mice. Cancer Res 2006;66(23):11462–70.

Obstructive Sleep Apnea

An Unexpected Cause of Insulin Resistance and Diabetes

Michael Morgenstern, MD, Janice Wang, MD, Norman Beatty, BS,
Tom Batemarco, BS, Anthony L. Sica, PhD, Harly Greenberg, MD*

KEYWORDS

- Obstructive sleep apnea • OSA • CPAP • Diabetes • Insulin resistance
- Metabolic syndrome • Cardiometabolic risk

KEY POINTS

- Obstructive sleep apnea (OSA) is independently associated with cardiovascular and cerebrovascular risk.
- OSA and its pathophysiologic features, including intermittent hypoxia and sleep fragmentation, are associated with insulin resistance and diabetes.
- Treatment of OSA with continuous positive airway pressure may reduce cardiometabolic risk.

INTRODUCTION

Obstructive sleep apnea (OSA), which results from upper airway occlusion during sleep, affects at least 4% of men and 2% of women.[1] In addition to excessive daytime somnolence with impairment in cognitive and other functional domains, a substantial body of evidence from large-scale epidemiologic, cross-sectional, and prospective studies demonstrates that OSA is an independent risk factor for cardiovascular and cerebrovascular morbidity and mortality. The Sleep Heart Health Study (SHHS), which included more than 6000 subjects, and the Wisconsin Sleep Cohort study, which followed more than 1500 subjects, established associations of OSA with all-cause mortality, as well as with cardiovascular mortality, that were independent of confounding factors such as age, sex, and obesity. Independent associations of OSA with hypertension, congestive heart failure, coronary artery disease, cerebrovascular disease,

Division of Pulmonary, Critical Care and Sleep Medicine, Department of Medicine, Hofstra-North Shore LIJ School of Medicine, 410 Lakeville Road, Suite 107, New Hyde Park, NY 11042, USA
* Corresponding author.
E-mail address: hgreenbe@nshs.edu

Endocrinol Metab Clin N Am 43 (2014) 187–204
http://dx.doi.org/10.1016/j.ecl.2013.09.002
0889-8529/14/$ – see front matter © 2014 Elsevier Inc. All rights reserved.

and cardiac arrhythmias have also been reported.[2–4] However, the specific mechanisms whereby OSA leads to these adverse cardiovascular and cerebrovascular outcomes have not been definitively delineated. Candidate mechanisms include apnea-induced sympathetic nervous system activation, endothelial dysfunction, systemic inflammation, oxidative stress, increased coagulability, and metabolic dysfunction leading to insulin resistance, diabetes, and the metabolic syndrome (MS). This article focuses on the association of OSA, and its component physiologic perturbations, with abnormalities in insulin and glucose metabolism as a potential mechanism linking OSA with type 2 diabetes and cardiometabolic disorders.

OBSERVATIONAL STUDIES LINKING OSA WITH ABNORMALITIES OF INSULIN AND GLUCOSE METABOLISM AND TYPE 2 DIABETES

Collective evidence from cross-sectional studies over the last two decades has linked OSA with glucose intolerance, insulin resistance, and type 2 diabetes. However, because risk factors for OSA and metabolic dysfunction overlap, it has been difficult to definitively identify an independent impact of OSA.

As a symptom suggestive but not diagnostic of OSA, self-reported snoring has been used as a limited surrogate marker for OSA in population-based studies. In a 10-year prospective study of 2668 Swedish males between the ages of 30 and 69, subjects were surveyed regarding the presence of habitual snoring and a self-reported diagnosis of diabetes.[5] The aim of the study was to determine if a relationship exists between diabetes and habitual snoring relative to obesity. The self-reported incidence of diabetes over 10 years was higher in habitual snorers (5.4%) compared with those without habitual snoring (2.4%) (P<.001). Considering obesity, 13.5% of obese snorers developed diabetes compared with 8.6% of obese nonsnorers, although this did not reach significance (P = .17). However, after adjustment for potential confounders including age, weight, smoking, alcohol dependence, and physical inactivity, the odds ratio (OR) for development of self-reported diabetes was higher in obese snorers, 7.0 (95% CI 2.9, 16.9), than in obese nonsnorers, 5.1 (95% CI 2.7, 9.5). The investigators concluded that habitual snoring increases the risk for developing diabetes in obese males; however, without objective measures of OSA and diabetes. These results are intriguing but not definitive.

The SHHS is a prospective cohort study comprised of subjects initially recruited from nine ongoing epidemiologic investigations of cardiovascular disease. Subjects were recruited without regard to signs or symptoms of OSA. Full ambulatory polysomnographic testing to assess for the presence and severity of OSA was performed in each of the 6441 participants at entry to the SHHS. Fasting insulin and glucose levels, as well as oral glucose tolerance tests (OGTTs), were performed in 2656 of the SHHS subjects within a year of enrollment. Impaired glucose tolerance was defined as a fasting plasma glucose level of 110 to 125 mg/dl and a 2-hour OGTT glucose level greater than or equal to 140 mg/dl but less than 200 mg/dl. Diabetes was diagnosed based on a fasting plasma glucose greater than or equal to 126 mg/dl or 2-hour OGTT greater than or equal to 200 mg/dl. The presence and severity of OSA was measured by the apnea-hypopnea index (AHI; number of apneas and hypopneas per hour of sleep: normal <5/h, mild 5–14/h, moderate >15–29/h, severe ≥30/h). Subjects with an AHI in the moderate or severe ranges had an increased prevalence of impaired fasting and 2-hour OGTT glucose levels compared with subjects with a normal AHI (17.5% and 8.8% of the cohort, respectively, in subjects with AHIs ≥15/h compared with 8.7% and 4.0% in subjects with AHIs <5/h). After adjusting for potential confounders, including age, gender, smoking status, body mass index

(BMI), waist circumference, and self-reported sleep duration, subjects with mild or moderate-to-severe OSA had ORs of 1.27 (95% CI 0.98, 1.64) and 1.46 (95% CI 1.09, 1.97), respectively, for glucose intolerance compared with subjects with AHIs less than five events per hour of sleep. Severity of nocturnal hypoxemia, measured by the average oxyhemoglobin saturation during sleep and percentage of sleep time with oxyhemoglobin saturation below 90%, was independently associated with glucose intolerance, even after adjustment for confounding covariates. As a marker of insulin resistance, the homeostasis model assessment (HOMA-IR) index was calculated. Higher AHI, in the moderate-to-severe range, as well as greater severity of nocturnal hypoxemia, were associated with increased HOMA-IR values, providing evidence for an association of OSA severity with insulin resistance.[6]

Another landmark study is the Wisconsin Sleep Cohort, a population-based longitudinal study established in 1988 that followed middle-aged subjects for 20 years, all of whom had polysomnographic testing at entry. Cross-sectional and prospective data from this cohort were analyzed to determine the prevalence and incidence of type 2 diabetes and if there is evidence for an independent association between diabetes and OSA. Diabetes was defined by a physician diagnosis of diabetes or a fasting glucose of greater than or equal to 126 mg/dl. Polysomnographic testing, followed by a fasting plasma glucose determination, was performed in 1387 participants at entry into the Wisconsin Sleep Cohort. Similar to observations from the SHHS, severity of OSA, as defined by the AHI, was correlated with the prevalence of diabetes: 2.8% of subjects with an AHI of less than five per hour had a diagnosis of diabetes compared with 14.7% of subjects with an AHI of greater than or equal to 15 per hour. The OR for having a diabetes diagnosis was 2.30 (95% CI 1.28, 4.11; $P = .005$) in subjects with an AHI of greater than or equal to 15 per hour compared with subjects with an AHI of less than five per hour, after adjustment for age, sex, and body habitus. However, a-4 year longitudinal analysis of 978 participants without diabetes at entry did not demonstrate a statistically significant association of diabetes incidence with severity of OSA at baseline after adjustment for age, gender, and waist circumference.[7]

In the Australian community of Busselton, Marshall and colleagues[8] studied a sample of 399 participants (294 male subjects) who had OSA assessed by overnight home sleep respiratory monitoring followed by determination of fasting blood glucose. Moderate-to-severe OSA was a univariate risk factor for prevalent diabetes (OR = 4.37, 95% confidence limit [CL] = 1.12, 17.12) and, longitudinally, an independent risk factor for a 4-year incident diabetes (OR = 13.45, 95% CL = 1.59, 114.11) after adjustment for age, gender, BMI, waist circumference, high-density lipoprotein (HDL) cholesterol, and mean arterial pressure. Mild OSA, as in the Wisconsin Sleep cohort, was not associated with an increased risk of incident diabetes compared with subjects without OSA.

Evidence for an association between OSA and the development of diabetes was also demonstrated in another community-based study with a longer follow-up of an average of 11.3 years.[9] Initially, 141 men without diabetes underwent overnight respiratory monitoring at baseline and then followed for 11 years with plasma glucose and serum insulin sampling. Twenty-three subjects developed diabetes at the end of the follow-up period. Nocturnal hypoxemia, as defined by an oxygen desaturation index (ODI, number of oxygen desaturation events per hour) greater than five per hour was associated with an OR of 4.4 (95% CI 1.1–18.1) for development of diabetes, after adjusting for age, BMI, and hypertension at baseline. The HOMA-IR index was used as a measure of insulin resistance. An abnormal HOMA-IR was significantly associated with metrics describing OSA severity, including an AHI greater than five per hour, ODI greater than five per hour, and low minimum nocturnal arterial oxygen saturation. Nine of the subjects diagnosed with OSA were treated with continuous positive airway pressure (CPAP) therapy for a mean of 9.3 years by the end of the follow-up period. The incidence of diabetes was lower in subjects with OSA who were treated with CPAP therapy compared with those who were untreated. These findings add to the evidence linking OSA with incident insulin resistance and diabetes. Although the numbers are small and observational, results of this study also suggest a potential role for CPAP therapy in mitigating the adverse effects of OSA on glycemic control.

PREVALENCE OF OSA IN SUBJECTS WITH TYPE 2 DIABETES

Several, but not all, of the population-based studies previously described demonstrated an independent association of OSA with both prevalent and incident insulin resistance, and type 2 diabetes. Conversely, other studies have assessed the prevalence of OSA in patients with type 2 diabetes and have found remarkably high prevalence rates of OSA. In the SHHS, 58% of subjects with type 2 diabetes had an abnormal AHI.[10–12] The prevalence of OSA in obese subjects with type 2 diabetes was also assessed with ambulatory nocturnal respiratory monitoring in the Sleep AHEAD study, a four-site ancillary study of the Look AHEAD Trial (Action for Health in Diabetes). Look AHEAD is a 16-center trial investigating the long-term health impact of lifestyle intervention designed to achieve and maintain weight loss in more than 5000 obese adults with type 2 diabetes. Sleep testing was performed in 306 participants in the Sleep AHEAD study. Remarkably, 86.6% of obese subjects with type 2 diabetes in this study had an abnormal AHI indicating sleep apnea. The mean AHI in this cohort was 20.5 plus or minus 16.8 per hour, which indicates moderate OSA.[10]

INSULIN AND GLUCOSE HOMEOSTASIS ASSESSMENT IN PATIENTS WITH OSA

Observational data linking OSA with impairment of insulin sensitivity, independent of obesity, have been evident for more than a decade. Using an OGTT with calculation of composite and hepatic insulin sensitivity indices, Tassone and colleagues[13] demonstrated reduced insulin sensitivity in obese OSA patients compared with BMI-matched obese controls without OSA. Insulin sensitivity indices were impaired in both of these groups compared with normal BMI subjects without OSA. These findings imply that, although obesity impairs insulin sensitivity, further impairment is induced by an independent effect of OSA. In another investigation, Ip and colleagues[14] used the HOMA to evaluate the association of OSA with insulin resistance. Although obesity was a major determinant of insulin resistance, metrics describing the severity of OSA, including the AHI and minimum oxygen saturation during sleep were independent determinants of insulin resistance. The association between OSA and insulin resistance was evident in both obese and nonobese OSA subjects. A subsequent study using the frequently sampled intravenous glucose tolerance test with minimal model analysis, which assessed various parameters describing insulin sensitivity, glucose effectiveness (ie, the ability of glucose to influence its own production and use, independent of insulin), and pancreatic β-cell function, was performed in nondiabetic subjects with OSA. Dual energy x-ray absorptiometry (DEXA) scans were used to assess body fat composition. OSA was associated with reduced insulin sensitivity independent of percent body fat, age, and sex. Measures of pancreatic β-cell function were also reduced in moderate-to-severe OSA. This study provides further evidence that OSA impairs insulin sensitivity, glucose effectiveness, and pancreatic β-cell function independent of the effects of obesity.[15]

IMPACT OF OSA ON GLYCEMIC CONTROL IN TYPE 2 DIABETES

The impact of OSA on insulin and glucose metabolism should be evident in patients with type 2 diabetes and OSA. Aronsohn and colleagues[16] studied 60 type 2 diabetic subjects consecutively recruited from outpatient primary care and endocrinology clinics. Overnight polysomnography (PSG) was performed to assess for OSA and a hemoglobin A1c (HbA1c) level was obtained in all subjects. Again, a remarkably high prevalence of OSA was demonstrated in this diabetic cohort with 77% of subjects having an abnormal AHI greater than or equal to five per hour. Increasing severity of OSA was significantly correlated with worsening glycemic control, assessed by higher HbA1c. This finding was independent of age, sex, race, BMI, number of diabetes medications, and years of diabetes. Compared with patients without OSA, the adjusted mean HbA1c was increased by 1.49% in mild OSA, 1.93% in moderate OSA, and 3.69% in severe OSA compared with subjects without OSA.

INDEPENDENT ASSOCIATION OF OSA WITH THE METABOLIC SYNDROME

Another important link between OSA and the development of diabetes and cardiovascular disease is syndrome Z, a term developed to describe the association of OSA with the metabolic syndrome, which is a combination of obesity, insulin resistance, hypertension, and dyslipidemia. The OR for metabolic syndrome in OSA has been documented to range from fivefold to as high as ninefold, compared with subjects without OSA, independent of age and BMI.[17–19] In a Chinese community-based study of 255 subjects, severity of OSA correlated with an increasing prevalence of the metabolic syndrome.[19] A Japanese case-control study analyzed lean men with an average BMI of 23 kg/m^2 with and without OSA and demonstrated an association of OSA with three components of the metabolic syndrome: insulin resistance, hypertension, and dyslipidemia.[20] This study suggested that, although OSA and the metabolic syndrome are closely linked to obesity, OSA may be an independent risk factor for the metabolic syndrome.

PATHOPHYSIOLOGY OF OSA AND POTENTIAL LINKS TO INSULIN RESISTANCE AND TYPE 2 DIABETES

OSA results from upper airway occlusion during sleep, usually in the velopharyngeal and retroglossal regions. Both anatomic factors, including enlarged soft tissues of the upper airway and narrowed craniofacial skeletal structure, as well as insufficient neural drive to the upper airway dilator muscles during sleep, contribute to OSA. Upper airway occlusion can be partial, resulting in hypopneas, or complete, resulting in apneas. These disordered breathing events may cause several pathophysiologic perturbations. First, some degree of arousal from sleep occurs at the termination of obstructive apneic events, which is necessary to reactivate inspiratory drive to the upper airway dilator muscles that reopens the closed upper airway. These arousals, which are often observed on the cortical electroencephalogram (EEG), result in fragmentation of sleep and contribute to daytime somnolence, which is a characteristic clinical feature of OSA (**Fig. 1**). In addition, activation of the autonomic nervous system occurs in association with obstructive apneas and hypopneas, with parasympathetic activity predominating during apneas and sympathetic tone increasing at the termination of apneic events. In addition, elevated levels of circulating and urinary catecholamines have been observed in OSA. Interestingly, elevated sympathetic tone is not only evident during sleep; it also has been demonstrated to persist during the day, when breathing is normal in OSA patients.[21,22]

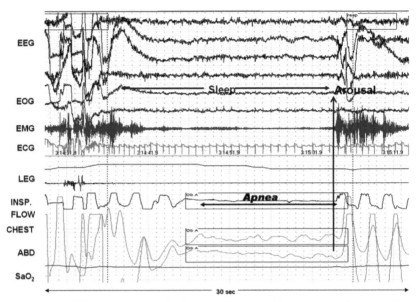

Fig. 1. An epoch (30-second segment) of a polysomnographic recording demonstrating an obstructive apnea. Note that the termination of the apnea is associated with an arousal from sleep, indicated by an increase in EEG frequency and submental EMG tone. Note the decrease in heart rate during the apnea with an increase after apnea termination. ABD, abdomen; EEG, electroencephalogram; EMG, submental electromyogram; EOG, electrooculogram; INSP. FLOW, inspiratory flow; LEG, anterior tibialis electromyogram; SaO₂, saturation level of oxygen.

Another significant pathophysiologic feature of OSA is intermittent hypoxia (IH) and reoxygenation that accompanies apneic events (**Fig. 2**). IH has physiologic consequences that differ from those of chronic hypoxia. Repetitive decreases and increases in oxygen saturation contribute to formation of reactive oxygen and nitrogen species that increase oxidative stress and can activate redox-sensitive cellular signaling pathways.[23–27]

CHRONIC IH AND INSULIN RESISTANCE

Although some investigators contend that obesity is the main risk factor responsible for the association of OSA with diabetes, a large body of evidence is accumulating that links the pathophysiologic perturbations of OSA, independent of the effects of

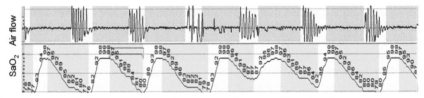

Fig. 2. Five-minute segment of a polysomnographic recording showing recurrent apneas and intermittent episodes of oxygen desaturation followed by reoxygenation (intermittent hypoxemia and reoxygenation) characteristic of severe OSA. SaO₂, saturation level of oxygen.

obesity, with alterations of insulin and glucose metabolism. Animal and human data indicate that long-term exposure to IH, such as that occurring in association with OSA, can alter glucose homeostasis and insulin resistance. Exposure of lean mice to IH during their sleep period was accomplished by placing animals in chambers in which the fraction of inspired oxygen (F_{IO_2}) was decreased from 21% to between 5% and 6% with a return to 21% once each minute during their sleep period, thereby mimicking the IH associated with severe OSA. Exposure protocols ranged from several hours to several months. Insulin sensitivity was assessed during exposure to IH using the hyperinsulinemic-euglycemic clamp technique in chronically instrumented but unhandled mice. IH-induced insulin resistance was evidenced by a 21% reduction in the exogenous glucose necessary to maintain euglycemia during the hyperinsulinemic-euglycemic clamp. In addition, fasting hyperglycemia was observed because of IH. Thus, these data provide strong evidence for a causal relationship between exposure to IH and insulin resistance that is independent of obesity. Similar findings to those observed in lean mice were also seen in mice with diet-induced obesity and in genetically obese mice.[28,29]

Potential mechanisms that could explain these findings include an impact of IH on hepatic glucose output as well as on glucose uptake in skeletal muscle. In these studies, IH did not affect hepatic glucose output; however, IH significantly impaired glucose uptake by skeletal muscle. The impact of IH was most pronounced in oxidative muscle fibers, whereas glycolytic muscle fibers were unaffected. Thus, glucose disposition in oxidative muscle tissue is apparently impaired by IH in a manner that is independent of obesity.[28,30]

CHRONIC INTERMITTENT HYPOXIA, OXIDATIVE STRESS, AND SYSTEMIC INFLAMMATION

Oxidative stress and systemic inflammation induced by IH is another potential mechanism that may lead to insulin resistance and pancreatic β-cell dysfunction in OSA. IH has shown to increase generation of free radicals, including reactive oxygen species (ROS) and reactive nitrogen species. Mitochondrial dysfunction induced by hypoxia is an important source of these free radicals. Other sources of ROS resulting from IH include NADPH oxidase and xanthine oxidase. Overproduction of free radicals can damage macromolecules. Elevated markers of lipid peroxidation, a contributing factor to atherosclerosis, which has been reported in OSA patients, provides evidence that this effect may be clinically significant.[26]

In addition, activation of redox-sensitive nuclear transcription factors, such as nuclear factor kappa beta (NF-κβ) and hypoxia-inducible factor 1-α (HIF-1α), has also been observed because of IH in animal models and in humans with OSA.[25,31,32] In fact, in in vitro studies IH selectively induces NF-κβ expression, whereas continuous hypoxia does not. Furthermore, HIF-1α is better expressed following exposure to IH than with continuous hypoxic stimulation.[33] These transcription factors regulate expression of genes that encode proinflammatory cytokines, proteins important in adaptation to hypoxia, as well as proteins that regulate lipogenesis and lipolysis, among many other genes. Several animal models have demonstrated that long-term exposure to IH increases circulating proinflammatory cytokines, activates leukocytes, and causes endothelial dysfunction with accelerated atherosclerosis.[25–27] In subjects with OSA, the degree of NF-κβ expression in circulating neutrophils was highly correlated with indices of apnea severity. Furthermore, NF-κβ activity was reduced to baseline levels following 1 month of therapeutic CPAP.[25] Elevated circulating levels of tumor necrosis factor α (TNF-α), interleukin

(IL)-6, IL-8, IL-1β, adhesion molecules, and C-reactive protein (CRP) have all been observed in OSA, with decreases after CPAP therapy.[34] Evidence from human and animal studies suggests that TNF-α and IL-6 may contribute to insulin resistance.[35] Furthermore, elevated levels of some of these cytokines, including CRP, IL-6, and IL-1β independently predict an increased risk for type 2 diabetes.[36–38] Thus, systemic inflammation, induced by IH, which is characteristic of OSA, may represent another mechanism through which OSA may contribute to abnormal insulin and glucose metabolism and development of type 2 diabetes.

IMPACT OF IH ON PANCREATIC β-CELL FUNCTION

The development of insulin resistance is only one factor that can lead to development of clinical diabetes. Impaired pancreatic β-cell function may reduce compensatory increases in insulin secretion that are necessary to maintain normal blood glucose levels in the setting of insulin resistance. Diabetes can develop when β-cells are unable to compensate for insulin resistance. Recent data indicate that IH may also impair pancreatic β-cell function. Adult male lean mice were exposed to IH for 8 hours during their sleep period for 30 days. Exposed mice demonstrated elevated plasma fasting insulin without a change in glucose, indicating insulin resistance. However, no evidence for pancreatic β-cell proliferation or hypertrophy was observed. In fact, insulin content was decreased in pancreatic islets taken from animals exposed to IH. Furthermore, IH-exposed animals demonstrated severely impaired glucose-stimulated insulin secretion. Impairment of insulin synthesis and processing was subsequently demonstrated in these pancreatic β-cells. Additional experiments demonstrated that mitochondrial-derived ROS may play an important role in IH-induced pancreatic β-cell dysfunction.[39]

SYMPATHETIC NEURAL ACTIVATION

Another potential mechanism that might link IH with peripheral insulin resistance is an increase in sympathetic neural activity that occurs in response to IH in animal models and to OSA in humans.[22] Catecholamines increase insulin resistance and decrease insulin-mediated glucose uptake in the periphery.[40] Furthermore, activation of the hypothalamic pituitary adrenal axis is known to impair insulin sensitivity and increase mobilization of glucose. The impact of activation of the sympathetic nervous system resulting from IH on insulin resistance was assessed in animal studies that used the ganglionic blocker hexamethonium to prevent autonomic activation. Blockade of autonomic activity had no impact on development of insulin resistance in response to IH. Therefore, at least in animal models of IH, mechanisms other than sympathetic neural activation are responsible for development of insulin resistance. Nevertheless, in the clinical setting, overactivation of the sympathetic nervous system and the hypothalamic pituitary adrenal axis (due to sleep apnea and its associated sleep fragmentation) may contribute to insulin resistance in OSA.

ADIPOSE TISSUE HYPOXIA AND SYSTEMIC INFLAMMATION

There has been a remarkable evolution in contemporary understanding of the role of white adipose tissue (WAT) in normal physiologic function and in response to endogenous stressors.[41–44] The traditional view of WAT as a reservoir of stored energy in the form of triacylglycerols has been replaced by a more expansive concept of WAT as an endocrine organ involved in different metabolic activities as well as the site of a major group of secretory cells, the adipocytes. Such a conceptual change in the functional status of WAT was motivated by the discovery of the hormone leptin that was coded for by the ob gene in the obese (ob/ob) mouse.[45] Interestingly, leptin affects central neural structure via the melanocortin system of the hypothalamus (arcuate nucleus) and is associated with cessation of feeding and with energy expenditure, whereas, in the periphery, it increases hepatic lipid oxidation and lipolysis in skeletal muscle and adipocytes.[41] Equally important, adipocytes are also known to secrete other hormones and cytokines (adipokines) that have important functions in health and disease, including (1) adiponectin and resistin for glucose metabolism, (2) cholesteryl ester transfer protein for lipid metabolism, (3) angiotensinogen and angiotensin II necessary for blood pressure homeostasis, and (4) plasminogen activator inhibitor-1 (PAI-1) for coagulation.[41,43,44] However, much recent work has focused on the inflammatory adipokines, which include cytokines, chemokines, and acute phase proteins (haptoglobin and PAI-1), and their roles in the development of obesity-related insulin resistance.[33,44] A large number of cytokines and chemokines are secreted by adipocytes; these include TNF-α, IL-1β, IL-6, IL-8, IL-10, monocyte chemoattractant protein-1 (MCP-1), macrophage migration inhibitory factor (MIF), and transforming growth factor β (TGF-β).[33,41,43,44] Proinflammatory secretory products of adipocytes are associated with obesity-induced proinflammatory states as they are elevated in the circulation of obese subjects with insulin resistance, whereas the antiinflammatory adipokine, adiponectin, is diminished in the circulation of obese subjects with insulin resistance.[44]

Our understanding of the link between disease and obesity was advanced considerably by the recognition that visceral obesity represented a state of chronic mild inflammation due to secreted adipokines.[46] Additionally, because adipose tissue increases in size, macrophages are attracted and retained within adipose tissue by the actions of the chemokines MCP-1 and MIF, respectively.[44] Consequently, a massive infiltration of type M1-macrophages occurs and these secrete the proinflammatory adipokines IL-6 and TNF-α.[47] Hence, the effect of M1-macrophage arrival in adipose tissues is to increase the degree of inflammation in already inflamed tissues. Such inflammatory processes play a significant role in the cause of insulin resistance via inhibition of adipocyte storage of lipids, secretions of adipokines, enhanced lipolysis, and reduced reesterification of free fatty acids (FFAs) resulting in elevation of FFAs in the circulation.[48]

Although several hypotheses have been raised to explain the cause of inflammation in adipose tissue,[33,47,48] there is mounting evidence that hypoxia occurs within enlarged regions of visceral adipose tissue.[33,44] As adipose hypertrophy ensues, a reduction in adipose tissue blood flow occurs.[48] Further complicating perfusion of adipose tissue is the increase in dimensions of adipocytes (some exceeding 150 μm in diameter); hence, limited or no perfusion occurs due to the diffusion limitation of oxygen ($\sim$ 100 μm).[49] As previously discussed, hypoxic stress is associated with activation of inflammatory signaling pathways, including the transcription factors hypoxia-inducible factor 1α (HIF-1α) and NF-$\kappa\beta$.[33] OSA prevalence in the obese population has generated the hypothesis that OSA may exacerbate adipose tissue hypoxia, thus contributing to adipose tissue inflammation and providing an additional pathway leading to insulin resistance with the clinical sequelae of cardiometabolic disorders.[36,50]

HUMAN STUDIES LINKING IH AND SLEEP FRAGMENTATION WITH INSULIN RESISTANCE AND PANCREATIC β-CELL DYSFUNCTION

The data linking insulin resistance and pancreatic β-cell dysfunction with IH have been observed in animal studies. However, recent experiments in healthy human volunteers have corroborated these findings. Louis and Punjabi[51] exposed 13 healthy subjects to

5 hours of IH by altering the inspired F_{IO_2} from room air to 5% oxygen approximately 25 times per hour during wakefulness, simulating the degree of IH observed in moderate OSA. A frequently sampled intravenous glucose tolerance test was performed with assessment of insulin-dependent and insulin independent measures of glucose disposal. Five hours of exposure to IH led to decreased insulin sensitivity that was not accompanied by a commensurate increase in insulin secretion. In addition, decreased glucose effectiveness, which indicates the ability of glucose to enhance its disposal independent of insulin, was observed. An increase in sympathetic nervous system activity, without a change in serum cortisol levels, also occurred.

Another physiologic perturbation of OSA is recurrent arousals from sleep that cause sleep fragmentation. Disturbed sleep may also lead to alterations in insulin and glucose metabolism. The impact of sleep fragmentation on glucose and insulin metabolism was similarly tested in healthy human volunteers with the frequently sampled intravenous glucose tolerance test. Sleep was fragmented by inducing microarousals on the cortical EEG with mechanical and auditory stimuli presented 30 times per hour during sleep, simulating the arousal frequency and sleep disruption observed in moderate-to-severe OSA. Results were compared with a night of undisturbed sleep. Insulin sensitivity and glucose effectiveness were reduced by 20% and 25%, respectively, after sleep fragmentation. In addition, an increase in sympathetic nervous system activity was observed with elevated morning serum cortisol levels. Thus, sleep fragmentation, such as that occurring in OSA, can also adversely affect glucose homeostasis independent of IH.

CPAP THERAPY IN OSA AND CHANGES IN INSULIN SENSITIVITY

Some observational studies have indicated that CPAP therapy for OSA not only relieves symptoms related to sleep apnea, it also improves insulin sensitivity. However, the reported impact of CPAP on insulin sensitivity is variable among studies, with some investigators demonstrating significant improvement either in all subjects or in a subset of subjects, whereas others note no change. This disparity may be related to differences in methods of assessment of insulin sensitivity, variation in study population characteristics, and variable adherence to CPAP therapy. For example, in subjects with moderate-to-severe OSA using CPAP therapy, an observational study demonstrated significant improvement in insulin sensitivity after 2 days and after 3 months using the hyperinsulinemic-euglycemic clamp technique. However, the improvement in insulin sensitivity was most pronounced in subjects with a BMI less than 30 kg/m^2.[52] A recent meta-analysis of 12 prospective observational studies of nondiabetic adults newly diagnosed with moderate-to-severe OSA demonstrated that 3 to 24 weeks of CPAP treatment resulted in a significant decrease in insulin resistance as assessed by the homeostasis model for insulin resistance (HOMA-IR).[53]

Several randomized, controlled trials have shown significant improvements in insulin sensitivity in OSA patients treated with CPAP, compared with sham-CPAP, as assessed by the Gutt index, quantitative insulin sensitivity check index (QUICKI), short insulin tolerance test, and the hyperinsulinemic-euglycemic clamp technique, as well as other metrics of insulin-glucose metabolism.[54–56] One study showed a trend toward improvement in insulin sensitivity after CPAP therapy using the hyperinsulinemic-euglycemic clamp (glucose clamp–derived index of insulin sensitivity [SIClamp]), although the degree of improvement did not reach statistical significance.[57] Mean nightly hours of CPAP use in that study were only 3.6, which might explain the failure to obtain a statistically significant result. In support of this contention, another randomized, placebo-controlled study demonstrated incremental improvement in the insulin sensitivity index with each additional hour of nightly CPAP use.[56] This finding highlights the importance of optimal nightly adherence to CPAP therapy to achieve beneficial outcomes. In that study, however, significant improvements in insulin sensitivity were only observed in subjects with severe OSA (AHI≥30 per hour). In another study, nightly CPAP therapy for OSA resulted in a significant increase in glucose disappearance rate (K_{itt}) in as little as 1 week.[55] Other placebo-controlled studies demonstrated a trend toward, but not statistically significant, improvement in insulin sensitivity with CPAP therapy for OSA as assessed by the HOMA-IR technique.[54,55,57–60]

Some of the variability in results of these outcome studies may reflect not only differences in patient characteristics and CPAP adherence rates; they may also reflect differing methodologies used to assess insulin sensitivity. For example, the QUICKI has a substantially better linear correlation with SIClamp than HOMA-IR and performs better in patients with insulin resistance. Likewise, HOMA-IR is a good surrogate for the effect of insulin on hepatic glucose production, but may not accurately represent other sites of insulin response and may be less accurate in the setting of severely impaired pancreatic β-cell function.[61] Furthermore, OSA, and its treatment with CPAP, may alter various aspects of insulin and glucose metabolism, including skeletal muscle insulin sensitivity and pancreatic β-cell function that may not be adequately assessed by these metrics.[55]

CPAP THERAPY IN OSA AND CHANGES IN GLYCOSYLATED HEMOGLOBIN

The percentage of HbA1c, a marker of long-term glucose control in diabetic individuals, has been positively correlated with severity of OSA in patients with type 2 diabetes. HbA1c increased by an average of 1.49%, 1.93%, and 3.69%, respectively, in patients with mild, moderate, and severe OSA, after adjusting for age, gender, BMI, race, number of antidiabetic medications, exercise, duration of diabetes, and total sleep time compared with patients without OSA.[16] Several studies have shown improvement in HbA1c after 3 months of CPAP therapy.[60,62–64] Predictably, the degree of improvement in HbA1c was related to the number of hours of nightly CPAP usage.[60,62] In one study, subjects who used CPAP for more than 4 hours per night (mean 6.6 hours per night) achieved the greatest improvement in HbA1c.[62] In contrast, in another investigation in which the mean duration of nightly CPAP use was only 3.6 hours per night (SD = 2.8), improvement in HbA1c was not observed.[57] These findings indicate that CPAP therapy may improve glucose control in type 2 diabetes, but adequate nightly adherence to CPAP is essential to achieve this beneficial outcome.

IMPACT OF CPAP THERAPY FOR OSA ON THE METABOLIC SYNDROME

Previous studies have shown that OSA may independently contribute to development of MS.[65] Components of MS include systemic arterial hypertension, hyperglycemia, hypercholesterolemia, hypertriglyceridemia, abdominal obesity, and insulin resistance. This constellation of conditions significantly increases risk for cardiovascular and cerebrovascular disease and diabetes.[65]

The effect of CPAP therapy for OSA on MS has been explored by several investigators.[54,58–60,66,67] In a randomized, placebo-controlled study, 20% of subjects with MS and OSA who were treated with CPAP for 3 months showed reversal of MS components and no longer met criteria for this condition after treatment of OSA.[60] In contrast, another randomized, controlled study, with a shorter duration of CPAP therapy (6 weeks), did not demonstrate a change in the portion of subjects meeting criteria for MS despite significant reductions in blood pressure.[58] Of all of the components of MS, CPAP therapy seems to have the greatest impact on systemic arterial pressure. The latter study, as well as several other randomized, placebo-controlled studies, demonstrated significant reduction in arterial blood pressure with CPAP therapy for OSA.[55,58,60] Further evidence for the impact of CPAP therapy on hypertension in OSA comes from a study that showed that when CPAP was withdrawn from previously treated OSA subjects, systemic arterial pressure significantly increased.[66]

Another component of MS, hyperlipidemia, may also be affected by OSA and may improve with CPAP therapy. Animal models have shown that IH increases serum triglyceride and low-density lipoprotein (LDL)-cholesterol levels, possibly by increasing activity of sterol regulatory element–binding protein-1 and sterol-coenzyme A desaturase-1, which enhances conversion of saturated to monounsaturated fatty acids, increases serum triglycerides, and promotes lipoprotein secretion.[68] In accord with these findings, lipid profiles in OSA patients have been shown to improve with CPAP therapy and include changes in serum triglycerides, LDL, non-HDL, total cholesterol, and HDL to total cholesterol ratio.[55,60]

Abdominal or visceral obesity is another feature of MS that has been associated with increased cardiovascular risk that may also be improved with CPAP therapy for OSA. In a randomized, controlled study, in which nearly half of the study participants had both OSA and type 2 diabetes, significant reduction in BMI, in addition to decreases in visceral and subcutaneous fat, was observed after 3 months of CPAP.[60] However, other randomized, controlled studies of nondiabetic OSA subjects failed to demonstrate an impact of CPAP therapy on visceral, subcutaneous, or hepatic fat distribution.[53,54,67]

Although some data remain conflicting, evidence is mounting that CPAP therapy for moderate-to-severe OSA may improve components of MS, which may ultimately reduce cardiovascular and cerebrovascular risks.

SCREENING FOR OSA IN PATIENTS WITH TYPE 2 DIABETES

Both type 2 diabetes and OSA are independently associated with increased cardiovascular and cerebrovascular risk.[69] Furthermore, the incidence of OSA in obese type 2 diabetic individuals has shown to be quite high.[10] Thus, identification and treatment of OSA in patients with type 2 diabetes may be of paramount importance for successful cardiometabolic risk reduction.

Classic symptoms of OSA include heavy snoring, witnessed pauses of breathing during sleep and daytime somnolence.[69] Anatomic factors such as obesity (BMI>30 kg/m^2), large neck circumference (>16 inches for women, >17 inches for men), a crowded oropharynx with a low lying soft palate, large base of tongue, and tonsillar hypertrophy, as well as craniofacial abnormalities such as retrognathia, increase the risk of OSA.[70] However, many patients with OSA may not volunteer OSA-related symptoms at routine office visits, necessitating active questioning or screening. Although questions regarding OSA symptoms should ideally be part of routine history and physical examinations, this may not always be practical. Thus, several self-administered screening tools have been developed that can facilitate identification of patients who may require referral for further assessment of OSA.

The Epworth Sleepiness Scale (ESS) measures subjectively reported tendency to doze off during a variety of situations. However, the ESS is only 39.0% sensitive for detection of moderate-to-severe OSA. The STOP-Bang questionnaire is an eight-item questionnaire that assesses risk factors for OSA. A STOP-Bang score greater than or equal to three has 87% sensitivity, but low specificity (43.3%), for identifying moderate-to-severe OSA. Increasing the cutoff score for the STOP-Bang to a range of five to eight increases specificity but reduces sensitivity.[71] The ten-question Berlin questionnaire is composed of three categories. A high risk of OSA is identified by positive answers in two or more categories, which yields 78.6% sensitivity, with 50.5% specificity, for detection of moderate-to-severe OSA.[72,73] The Sleep Apnea Clinical Score is a 36-item questionnaire that has been validated for calculation of likelihood ratios for the presence of OSA.[74] A score of greater than or equal to 15 yields a likelihood ratio of 4.45 of moderate-to-severe sleep apnea.[75] The sensitivities and specificities of these tools are listed in **Table 1**. The STOP-Bang questionnaire and the Berlin questionnaire can each be completed in less than 5 minutes, allowing them to be used as effective OSA screening tools in a busy clinical setting. Although the sensitivity of the ESS for OSA is relatively low, it can also provide useful data regarding the degree of daytime somnolence and its improvement with treatment.

DIAGNOSIS AND TREATMENT OF OSA

Once a patient is referred for further sleep evaluation, the diagnosis of OSA, and its severity, should be assessed by recording physiologic parameters during sleep. The gold standard is attended PSG performed in a sleep laboratory that comprehensively assesses sleep and breathing with recordings of the EEG, electromyogram, electrooculogram, ECG, nasal/oral airflow, thoracic and abdominal respiratory effort, oxygen saturation, and an audio recording of snoring throughout the night.[76] An alternative, more limited respiratory assessment, performed during home sleep testing (HST), has recently gained popularity and it may be useful in cases in which the pretest probability of moderate or severe OSA is high.[77] The main advantages of HST are reduced costs compared with PSG and a more familiar environment for the patient.[78] However, HST has many limitations that can reduce its usefulness because it usually only monitors airflow, respiratory effort, and oxygen saturation with no objective measure of sleep duration or sleep quality. This may lead to underestimation of the severity and impact of sleep-disordered breathing, particularly in patients with milder degrees of OSA. In addition, because sleep is not objectively recorded during most HSTs, false-negative results may occur in patients with coexisting insomnia. HSTs are also inadequate for assessment of other sleep disorders or for assessment of sleep-disordered breathing in patients with significant comorbid cardiopulmonary disease. Therefore, patients suspected of having OSA with negative HST results should usually be referred for confirmatory in-laboratory PSG.[76]

Various treatment modalities are available for OSA. Successful therapeutic outcome depends on tailoring treatment recommendations to patient-specific needs and

Table 1
Predictive parameters for the Epworth Sleepiness Scale, STOP-BANG questionnaire, and Berlin questionnaire for moderate-to-severe OSA

	Epworth Sleepiness Scale	STOP-BANG Questionnaire	Berlin Questionnaire
Sensitivity (%)	39.0	87.0	78.6
Specificity (%)	71.4	43.3	50.5
OR (95% CI)	1.6	5.1	3.7
Area under the receiver operating characteristic curve (95% CI)	0.53	0.64	0.67

expectations, with strong consideration given to comorbidities such as cardiac, pulmonary, and cerebrovascular disease, as well as to coexisting sleep disorders such as insomnia. CPAP therapy is the mainstay of treatment of OSA, with randomized, placebo-controlled trials clearly demonstrating improvement in quality of life metrics, daytime somnolence, and neurobehavioral performance, not only in subjects with moderate-to-severe OSA, but also in subjects with milder sleep apnea.[79,80] Several alternatives to CPAP therapy that also have demonstrated efficacy include mandibular advancement oral appliance therapy, surgical approaches to the upper airway, and bariatric surgery in appropriately selected patients. Because OSA is a chronic condition, long-term disease management to assure compliance with effective therapy is essential to achieve optimal functional outcomes as well as cardiovascular risk reduction.[81]

SUMMARY

Epidemiologic studies demonstrated a high prevalence of insulin resistance and type 2 diabetes in patients with OSA. Furthermore, an extremely high prevalence of OSA has been documented in obese patients with type 2 diabetes. The pathophysiology of OSA, which includes sleep fragmentation, activation of the sympathetic nervous system, and IH resulting from recurrent apneas, may contribute to abnormal glucose and insulin metabolism. Both animal and human studies demonstrated that IH, with its associated systemic inflammation and oxidative stress, contributes to hepatic and peripheral insulin resistance as well as to pancreatic β-cell dysfunction, independent of obesity. Recognition of OSA in patients with type 2 diabetes is important because effective treatment with CPAP may improve insulin sensitivity, HbA1C, systemic hypertension, and other components of MS that contribute to long-term cardiovascular and cerebrovascular risk.

REFERENCES

1. Young T, Palta M, Dempsey J, et al. The occurrence of sleep-disordered breathing among middle-aged adults. N Engl J Med 1993;328:1230–5.
2. Peppard PE, Young T, Palta M, et al. Prospective study of the association between sleep-disordered breathing and hypertension. N Engl J Med 2000; 342:1378–84.
3. Punjabi NM, Caffo BS, Goodwin JL, et al. Sleep-disordered breathing and mortality: a prospective cohort study. PLoS Med 2009;6:e1000132.
4. Young T, Finn L, Peppard PE, et al. Sleep disordered breathing and mortality: eighteen-year follow-up of the Wisconsin sleep cohort. Sleep 2008;31:1071–8.
5. Elmasry A, Janson C, Lindberg E, et al. The role of habitual snoring and obesity in the development of diabetes: a 10-year follow-up study in a male population. J Intern Med 2000;248:13–20.
6. Punjabi NM, Shahar E, Redline S, et al. Sleep-disordered breathing, glucose intolerance, and insulin resistance: the Sleep Heart Health Study. Am J Epidemiol 2004;160:521–30.
7. Reichmuth KJ, Austin D, Skatrud JB, et al. Association of sleep apnea and type II diabetes: a population-based study. Am J Respir Crit Care Med 2005;172: 1590–5.
8. Marshall NS, Wong KK, Phillips CL, et al. Is sleep apnea an independent risk factor for prevalent and incident diabetes in the Busselton Health Study? J Clin Sleep Med 2009;5:15–20.

9. Lindberg E, Theorell-Haglow J, Svensson M, et al. Sleep apnea and glucose metabolism: a long-term follow-up in a community-based sample. Chest 2012; 142:935–42.

10. Foster GD, Sanders MH, Millman R, et al. Obstructive sleep apnea among obese patients with type 2 diabetes. Diabetes Care 2009;32:1017–9.

11. Pamidi S, Tasali E. Obstructive sleep apnea and type 2 diabetes: is there a link? Front Neurol 2012;3:126.

12. Resnick HE, Redline S, Shahar E, et al. Diabetes and sleep disturbances: findings from the Sleep Heart Health Study. Diabetes Care 2003;26:702–9.

13. Tassone F, Lanfranco F, Gianotti L, et al. Obstructive sleep apnoea syndrome impairs insulin sensitivity independently of anthropometric variables. Clin Endocrinol (Oxf) 2003;59:374–9.

14. Ip MS, Lam B, Ng MM, et al. Obstructive sleep apnea is independently associated with insulin resistance. Am J Respir Crit Care Med 2002;165: 670–6.

15. Punjabi NM, Beamer BA. Alterations in Glucose Disposal in Sleep-disordered Breathing. Am J Respir Crit Care Med 2009;179:235–40.

16. Aronsohn RS, Whitmore H, Van Cauter E, et al. Impact of untreated obstructive sleep apnea on glucose control in type 2 diabetes. Am J Respir Crit Care Med 2010;181:507–13.

17. Coughlin SR, Mawdsley L, Mugarza JA, et al. Obstructive sleep apnoea is independently associated with an increased prevalence of metabolic syndrome. Eur Heart J 2004;25:735–41.

18. Gruber A, Horwood F, Sithole J, et al. Obstructive sleep apnoea is independently associated with the metabolic syndrome but not insulin resistance state. Cardiovasc Diabetol 2006;5:22.

19. Lam JC, Lam B, Lam CL, et al. Obstructive sleep apnea and the metabolic syndrome in community-based Chinese adults in Hong Kong. Respir Med 2006; 100:980–7.

20. Kono M, Tatsumi K, Saibara T, et al. Obstructive sleep apnea syndrome is associated with some components of metabolic syndrome. Chest 2007;131: 1387–92.

21. Chandra S, Sica AL, Wang J, et al. Respiratory effort-related arousals contribute to sympathetic modulation of heart rate variability. Sleep Breath 2013. [Epub ahead of print].

22. Narkiewicz K, Somers VK. Sympathetic nerve activity in obstructive sleep apnoea. Acta Physiol Scand 2003;177:385–90.

23. Arnaud C, Poulain L, Levy P, et al. Inflammation contributes to the atherogenic role of intermittent hypoxia in apolipoprotein-E knock out mice. Atherosclerosis 2011;219:425–31.

24. Drager LF, Yao Q, Hernandez KL, et al. Chronic Intermittent Hypoxia Induces Atherosclerosis via Activation of Adipose Angiopoietin-like 4. Am J Respir Crit Care Med 2013;188:240–8.

25. Htoo AK, Greenberg H, Tongia S, et al. Activation of nuclear factor kappaB in obstructive sleep apnea: a pathway leading to systemic inflammation. Sleep Breath 2006;10:43–50.

26. Lavie L. Intermittent hypoxia: the culprit of oxidative stress, vascular inflammation and dyslipidemia in obstructive sleep apnea. Expert Rev Respir Med 2008; 2:75–84.

27. Savransky V, Nanayakkara A, Li J, et al. Chronic intermittent hypoxia induces atherosclerosis. Am J Respir Crit Care Med 2007;175:1290–7.

28. Drager LF, Li J, Reinke C, et al. Intermittent hypoxia exacerbates metabolic effects of diet-induced obesity. Obesity (Silver Spring) 2011;19:2167–74.

29. O'Donnell CP. Metabolic consequences of intermittent hypoxia. Adv Exp Med Biol 2007;618:41–9.

30. Polotsky VY, Li J, Punjabi NM, et al. Intermittent hypoxia increases insulin resistance in genetically obese mice. J Physiol 2003;552:253–64.

31. Greenberg H, Ye X, Wilson D, et al. Chronic intermittent hypoxia activates nuclear factor-kappaB in cardiovascular tissues in vivo. Biochem Biophys Res Commun 2006;343:591–6.

32. Jelic S, Lederer DJ, Adams T, et al. Vascular inflammation in obesity and sleep apnea. Circulation 2010;121:1014–21.

33. Trayhurn P, Wang B, Wood IS. Hypoxia and the endocrine and signalling role of white adipose tissue. Arch Physiol Biochem 2008;114:267–76.

34. Lavie L. Oxidative stress inflammation and endothelial dysfunction in obstructive sleep apnea. Front Biosci (Elite Ed) 2012;4:1391–403.

35. Alam I, Lewis K, Stephens JW, et al. Obesity, metabolic syndrome and sleep apnoea: all pro-inflammatory states. Obes Rev 2007;8:119–27.

36. Calvin AD, Albuquerque FN, Lopez-Jimenez F, et al. Obstructive sleep apnea, inflammation, and the metabolic syndrome. Metab Syndr Relat Disord 2009;7: 271–8.

37. Pradhan AD, Manson JE, Rifai N, et al. C-reactive protein, interleukin 6, and risk of developing type 2 diabetes mellitus. JAMA 2001;286:327–34.

38. Spranger J, Kroke A, Mohlig M, et al. Inflammatory cytokines and the risk to develop type 2 diabetes: results of the prospective population-based European Prospective Investigation into Cancer and Nutrition (EPIC)-Potsdam Study. Diabetes 2003;52:812–7.

39. Wang N, Khan SA, Prabhakar NR, et al. Impairment of pancreatic beta-cell function by chronic intermittent hypoxia. Exp Physiol 2013;98(9):1376–85.

40. Deibert DC, DeFronzo RA. Epinephrine-induced insulin resistance in man. J Clin Invest 1980;65:717–21.

41. Hajer GR, van Haeften TW, Visseren FL. Adipose tissue dysfunction in obesity, diabetes, and vascular diseases. Eur Heart J 2008;29:2959–71.

42. Kershaw EE, Flier JS. Adipose tissue as an endocrine organ. J Clin Endocrinol Metab 2004;89:2548–56.

43. Kwon H, Pessin JE. Adipokines mediate inflammation and insulin resistance. Front Endocrinol (Lausanne) 2013;4:71.

44. Trayhurn P. Endocrine and signalling role of adipose tissue: new perspectives on fat. Acta Physiol Scand 2005;184:285–93.

45. Zhang Y, Proenca R, Maffei M, et al. Positional cloning of the mouse obese gene and its human homologue. Nature 1994;372:425–32.

46. Ross R. Atherosclerosis is an inflammatory disease. Am Heart J 1999;138: S419–20.

47. Gordon S, Taylor PR. Monocyte and macrophage heterogeneity. Nat Rev Immunol 2005;5:953–64.

48. Ye J. Adipose tissue vascularization: its role in chronic inflammation. Curr Diab Rep 2011;11:203–10.

49. Brahimi-Horn MC, Pouyssegur J. Oxygen, a source of life and stress. FEBS Lett 2007;581:3582–91.

50. Arnardottir ES, Mackiewicz M, Gislason T, et al. Molecular signatures of obstructive sleep apnea in adults: a review and perspective. Sleep 2009; 32:447–70.

51. Louis M, Punjabi NM. Effects of acute intermittent hypoxia on glucose metabolism in awake healthy volunteers. J Appl Physiol 2009;106:1538–44.

52. Harsch IA, Schahin SP, Radespiel-Troger M, et al. Continuous positive airway pressure treatment rapidly improves insulin sensitivity in patients with obstructive sleep apnea syndrome. Am J Respir Crit Care Med 2004;169: 156–62.

53. Yang D, Liu Z, Yang H, et al. Effects of continuous positive airway pressure on glycemic control and insulin resistance in patients with obstructive sleep apnea: a meta-analysis. Sleep Breath 2013;17:33–8.

54. Hoyos CM, Killick R, Yee BJ, et al. Cardiometabolic changes after continuous positive airway pressure for obstructive sleep apnoea: a randomised sham-controlled study. Thorax 2012;67:1081–9.

55. Lam JC, Lam B, Yao TJ, et al. A randomised controlled trial of nasal continuous positive airway pressure on insulin sensitivity in obstructive sleep apnoea. Eur Respir J 2010;35:138–45.

56. Weinstock TG, Wang X, Rueschman M, et al. A controlled trial of CPAP therapy on metabolic control in individuals with impaired glucose tolerance and sleep apnea. Sleep 2012;35:617–625B.

57. West SD, Nicoll DJ, Wallace TM, et al. Effect of CPAP on insulin resistance and HbA1c in men with obstructive sleep apnoea and type 2 diabetes. Thorax 2007; 62:969–74.

58. Coughlin SR, Mawdsley L, Mugarza JA, et al. Cardiovascular and metabolic effects of CPAP in obese males with OSA. Eur Respir J 2007;29:720–7.

59. Kritikou I, Basta M, Vgontzas AN, et al. Sleep Apnea, Sleepiness, Inflammation and Insulin Resistance in middle-aged Men and Women. Eur Respir J 2013. [Epub ahead of print].

60. Sharma SK, Agrawal S, Damodaran D, et al. CPAP for the metabolic syndrome in patients with obstructive sleep apnea. N Engl J Med 2011;365:2277–86.

61. Muniyappa R, Lee S, Chen H, et al. Current approaches for assessing insulin sensitivity and resistance in vivo: advantages, limitations, and appropriate usage. Am J Physiol Endocrinol Metab 2008;294:E15–26.

62. Babu AR, Herdegen J, Fogelfeld L, et al. Type 2 diabetes, glycemic control, and continuous positive airway pressure in obstructive sleep apnea. Arch Intern Med 2005;165:447–52.

63. Hassaballa HA, Tulaimat A, Herdegen JJ, et al. The effect of continuous positive airway pressure on glucose control in diabetic patients with severe obstructive sleep apnea. Sleep Breath 2005;9:176–80.

64. Shpirer I, Rapoport MJ, Stav D, et al. Normal and elevated HbA1C levels correlate with severity of hypoxemia in patients with obstructive sleep apnea and decrease following CPAP treatment. Sleep Breath 2012;16:461–6.

65. Tasali E, Ip MS. Obstructive sleep apnea and metabolic syndrome: alterations in glucose metabolism and inflammation. Proc Am Thorac Soc 2008;5:207–17.

66. Kohler M, Stoewhas AC, Ayers L, et al. Effects of continuous positive airway pressure therapy withdrawal in patients with obstructive sleep apnea: a randomized controlled trial. Am J Respir Crit Care Med 2011;184:1192–9.

67. Sivam S, Phillips CL, Trenell MI, et al. Effects of 8 weeks of continuous positive airway pressure on abdominal adiposity in obstructive sleep apnoea. Eur Respir J 2012;40:913–8.

68. Savransky V, Jun J, Li J, et al. Dyslipidemia and atherosclerosis induced by chronic intermittent hypoxia are attenuated by deficiency of stearoyl coenzyme A desaturase. Circ Res 2008;103:1173–80.

69. Punjabi NM. The epidemiology of adult obstructive sleep apnea. Proc Am Thorac Soc 2008;5:136–43.
70. Gami AS, Caples SM, Somers VK. Obesity and obstructive sleep apnea. Endocrinol Metab Clin North Am 2003;32:869–94.
71. Chung F, Subramanyam R, Liao P, et al. High STOP-Bang score indicates a high probability of obstructive sleep apnoea. Br J Anaesth 2012;108:768–75.
72. Chung F, Yegneswaran B, Liao P, et al. Validation of the Berlin questionnaire and American Society of Anesthesiologists checklist as screening tools for obstructive sleep apnea in surgical patients. Anesthesiology 2008;108:822–30.
73. Silva GE, Vana KD, Goodwin JL, et al. Identification of patients with sleep disordered breathing: comparing the four-variable screening tool, STOP, STOP-Bang, and Epworth Sleepiness Scales. J Clin Sleep Med 2011;7:467–72.
74. Flemons WW, Whitelaw WA, Brant R, et al. Likelihood ratios for a sleep apnea clinical prediction rule. Am J Respir Crit Care Med 1994;150:1279–85.
75. Mulgrew AT, Fox N, Ayas NT, et al. Diagnosis and initial management of obstructive sleep apnea without polysomnography: a randomized validation study. Ann Intern Med 2007;146:157–66.
76. Kirsch DB. In-home testing for obstructive sleep apnea. Continuum (Minneap Minn) 2013;19:223–8.
77. Collop NA, Anderson WM, Boehlecke B, et al. Clinical guidelines for the use of unattended portable monitors in the diagnosis of obstructive sleep apnea in adult patients. Portable Monitoring Task Force of the American Academy of Sleep Medicine. J Clin Sleep Med 2007;3:737–47.
78. Gay PC, Selecky PA. Are sleep studies appropriately done in the home? Respir Care 2010;55:66–75.
79. Gay P, Weaver T, Loube D, et al. Evaluation of positive airway pressure treatment of sleep related breathing disorders in adults. Sleep 2006;29:381–401.
80. Weaver TE, Mancini C, Maislin G, et al. Continuous positive airway pressure treatment of sleepy patients with milder obstructive sleep apnea: results of the CPAP Apnea Trial North American Program (CATNAP) randomized clinical trial. Am J Respir Crit Care Med 2012;186:677–83.
81. Epstein LJ, Kristo D, Strollo PJ Jr, et al. Clinical guideline for the evaluation, management and long-term care of obstructive sleep apnea in adults. J Clin Sleep Med 2009;5:263–76.

Vitamin D and Diabetes

Joanna Mitri, MD, MS[a],*, Anastassios G. Pittas, MD, MS[b]

KEYWORDS

- Vitamin D • Type 2 diabetes • Insulin resistance • Insulin sensitivity
- 25-hydroxyvitamin D

KEY POINTS

- Observational studies suggest a link between vitamin D and diabetes.
- The potential effect of vitamin D appears to be more prominent among persons at risk for diabetes.
- The optimal blood 25-hydroxyvitamin D concentration associated with reduced risk of type 2 diabetes is not clear.
- The evidence from randomized controlled trials to support the hypothesis that vitamin D supplementation prevents type 2 diabetes is lacking.

INTRODUCTION

Type 2 diabetes mellitus is a significant global health care problem, and pharmacotherapies to treat the disease continue to emerge. However, the increasing burden of type 2 diabetes calls for an urgent need for innovative approaches to prevent its development. Recently, vitamin D has risen as a potential diabetes risk modifier.

The potentially significant extraskeletal role of vitamin D is highlighted in several recently published studies, including the demonstration of the expression of the vitamin D receptor in a large number of nonskeletal cells, including pancreatic beta cells. Additional evidence has strongly suggested that vitamin D plays an important role in modifying the risk of type 2 diabetes, an effect that is likely mediated by an effect of vitamin D on beta cell function, insulin sensitivity, and systemic inflammation. The evidence comes primarily from cross-sectional and longitudinal observational studies reporting on the association between vitamin D status and risk of type 2 diabetes or glycemia among patients with established type 2 diabetes.

Source of Funding: By research grants R01DK76092, U34DK091958 and U01DK098245 (to A.G. Pittas) from the National Institute of Diabetes and Digestive and Kidney Disease, the Office of the Director, National Institutes of Health, and the National Institutes of Health Office of Dietary Supplements.
[a] Division of Endocrinology, Diabetes and Metabolism, Prima CARE Medical Center, 277 Pleasant Street, Fall River, MA 02721, USA; [b] Division of Endocrinology, Diabetes and Metabolism, Tufts Medical Center, 800 Washington Street, Boston, MA 02111, USA
* Corresponding author.
E-mail address: joannamitri@hotmail.com

More recently, short-term, small randomized trials have reported the effect of vitamin D supplementation with or without calcium on diabetes risk and glycemia with mixed results.

The aims of the review are to (1) describe the biologic plausibility behind the potential association between vitamin D and diabetes, with emphasis on type 2 diabetes where most of the evidence exists and (2) summarize and synthesize the evidence from observational studies that report on the association of vitamin D status and risk of diabetes and from randomized trials that report on the effect of vitamin D supplementation on glycemia in patients with diabetes or at risk for diabetes.

REVIEW OF VITAMIN D PHYSIOLOGY

Vitamin D exists in 2 forms: cholecalciferol (vitamin D3) and ergocalciferol (vitamin D2). Vitamin D3 is synthesized in the skin on exposure to solar ultraviolet B (UVB) radiation. During exposure to solar UVB radiation, 7-dehydrocholesterol in the skin is converted to previtamin D3, which is immediately converted to vitamin D3 in a heat-dependent nonenzymatic process. Excessive exposure to sunlight degrades previtamin D3 and vitamin D3 into inactive phyto-products (photo-degradation), avoiding vitamin D toxicity in the setting of excess sunlight. Vitamin D3 is also found is certain foods, such as fatty fish. Vitamin D2 is synthesized by plants and is found mostly in nutrients supplemented with vitamin D (eg, milk) or dietary supplements. Whether endogenously synthesized or ingested through diet or supplements, vitamin D in the circulation is bound to the vitamin D-binding protein (DBP), which transports it to the liver, where vitamin D is converted by vitamin 25-hydroxylase to 25-hydroxyvitamin D (25OHD). This form of vitamin D is biologically inactive and must be converted primarily in the kidneys by 25-hydroxyvitamin D-1alpha-hydroxylase (CYP27B1) to the biologically active form, 1,25-dihydroxyvitamin D $(1,25[OH]_2D)$. The presence of CYP27B1 in extra-renal tissues suggests that vitamin D may have an important role beyond the musculoskeletal system. The 25-hydroxyvitamin D is the major circulating form of vitamin D and is an excellent biomarker of exposure, either from cutaneous synthesis or dietary intake.

CLASSIFICATION OF VITAMIN D STATUS

Clinicians and researchers use blood concentration of 25OHD as a biomarker to determine vitamin D status. However, there is no consensus on the 25OHD thresholds for vitamin D deficiency or insufficiency. The main guidelines by the Institute of Medicine (IOM) and the Endocrine Society differ on classification of vitamin D status, as shown in **Table 1**.[1,2] The differences are explained by what populations were targeted by the guidelines and how the evidence was synthesized. The IOM guidelines concentrated

Table 1		
Guidelines for vitamin D status by blood 25-hydroxyvitamin D concentration		
Cutoff, ng/mL[a]	**Institute of Medicine**	**Endocrine Society**
<12	Deficiency	Deficiency
12–19	Inadequacy	Deficiency
20–29	Sufficiency	Insufficiency
30–49	Sufficiency	Sufficiency
>50	Reason for concern	Sufficiency

[a] To convert 25(OH)D concentration from ng/mL to nmol/L multiply by 2.459.

on the general healthy population and placed emphasis on intervention studies. The IOM found no convincing evidence to link vitamin D with benefits for nonskeletal outcomes, such as diabetes. The IOM concluded that blood concentration of 25OHD higher than 20 ng/mL is consistent with favorable skeletal outcomes, whereas there are only sparse data to support a higher level. The IOM also concluded that a level higher than 50 ng/mL should be a cause of concern about potential adverse events. In contrast, the Endocrine Society clinical practice guidelines concentrate on people at high risk for vitamin D deficiency and placed more emphasis on observational (epidemiologic) studies. Endocrine Society guidelines concluded that blood concentration of 25OHD higher than 30 ng/mL is desirable for optimal skeletal outcomes without any upper limit that would be concerning for safety. However, the Endocrine Society guidelines have been criticized by incorrectly characterizing several large population subgroups as at high risk and recommending widespread screening for vitamin D deficiency.[3] Both guidelines agreed that recommendations will require reconsideration in the future as additional data from on-going randomized trials become available.

VITAMIN D INTAKE REQUIREMENTS

The IOM report on dietary reference intakes for calcium and vitamin D recommends 600 international units (IU) per day of vitamin D for individuals 9 to 70 years and 800 international units for those older than 70 years as the recommended dietary allowance (RDA) (**Table 2**),[2] which is defined as the intake that meets the needs of 97.5% of the healthy population. The IOM report also concluded that the tolerable upper intake level (UL), above which the potential for adverse effects may increase with chronic use, is 4000 IU per day. It is important to note that the UL amount is not intended as a target intake, rather, it is the upper limit for chronic intake of vitamin D above which toxicity may increase. In contrast, Endocrine Society clinical practice guidelines conclude that to raise the blood level of 25OHD consistently above 30 ng/mL, intakes of 1500 to 2000 IU per day may be required. The recommended intakes by the 2 guidelines differ for the same reasons as the recommendations for 25OHD levels. The IOM report clearly recognized the lack of long-term trials with vitamin D supplementation for nonskeletal outcomes as a major hurdle in establishing its recommendations, whereas the Endocrine Society guidelines applied evidence from observational studies to develop its recommendations and considered blood level of 25OHD as a clinically important surrogate outcome that correlates with health and disease. The latter assumption should be approached with caution because, although 25OHD is an

Table 2				
Vitamin D recommended intake[a]				
	Institute of Medicine		Endocrine Society	
	RDA,[b] IU	UL,[c] IU	Daily Requirement, IU	UL, IU
14–18 y	600	4000	600–1000	4000
19–70 y	600	4000	1500–2000	10,000
>70 y	800	4000	1500–2000	10,000

Abbreviations: RDA, recommended dietary allowance; UL, upper intake level.
[a] RDA for skeletal outcomes (fractures and falls) only under conditions of minimal sun exposure. Applicable to normal healthy population groups.
[b] RDA intake that meets needs of 97.5% of healthy population.
[c] Tolerable UL, above which potential risk of adverse effects may increase with chronic use.

excellent biomarker of exposure and correlates with outcomes, it is not a validated biomarker of effect that is causally related to health outcomes of interest. The evidence to support a causal association comes from long-term adequately powered randomized trials, which are lacking in relation to vitamin D and type 2 diabetes, as described in the following section.

BIOLOGIC PLAUSIBILITY OF AN ASSOCIATION BETWEEN VITAMIN D AND TYPE 2 DIABETES

Type 2 diabetes results from impaired beta cell function, increased insulin resistance, and systemic inflammation, and there is evidence that vitamin D affects these pathways, as described next.

Vitamin D and Insulin Secretion

Based on preclinical studies, vitamin D seems to play a regulatory role in insulin secretion, beta cell survival, and calcium flux within beta cells. A series of studies have shown that vitamin D deficiency impairs glucose-mediated insulin secretion in rat pancreatic beta cells,[4–8] whereas vitamin D supplementation seems to restore such glucose-stimulated insulin secretion.[4,7–11] Vitamin D may also have a direct effect on beta cell function, which seems to be exerted by binding of its circulating active form to the vitamin D receptor (VDR) that is expressed in pancreatic beta cells (Fig. 1).[12] Interestingly, mice lacking a functional VDR show impaired insulin secretion following a glucose load. Such impairment appears associated with a decrease in insulin synthesis by the beta cell, resulting in a reduction in the amount of stored insulin.[13] Activation of vitamin D mediated by the CYP27B1 also occurs within the pancreatic beta cell, allowing for an important paracrine effect of circulating 25-hydroxyvitamin D.[14] An additional effect of vitamin D on the pancreatic beta cell is the regulation of extracellular calcium concentration and flux through the beta cell.[15] Insulin secretion is a calcium-dependent process[16]; therefore, alterations in calcium flux could have an effect on insulin secretion.[17–19] Vitamin D also regulates the function of calbindin, a cytosolic calcium-binding protein found in pancreatic beta cells,[12,20] and acts as a modulator of depolarization-stimulated insulin release via regulation of intracellular calcium.[21]

Vitamin D and Insulin Sensitivity

There are several ways in which vitamin D could affect insulin sensitivity. $1,25(OH)_2D$ appears to stimulate the expression of insulin receptors, which in turn will affect insulin sensitivity.[22–25] The $1,25(OH)_2D$ enters insulin-responsive cells and interacts with the VDR, activating the VDR-retinoic acid X-receptor complex which binds to a vitamin D response element found in the human insulin receptor gene promoter region (Fig. 2). The result is an enhanced transcriptional activation of the insulin receptor gene increasing the total number of insulin receptors without altering their affinity. The $1,25(OH)_2D$ may also enhance insulin sensitivity by activating peroxisome proliferator-activated receptor delta (PPAR-δ), which is a transcription factor that regulates the metabolism of fatty acids in skeletal muscle and adipose tissue.[26] Vitamin D also has been found to improve muscle oxidative phosphorylation after exercise. Another potential effect of $1,25(OH)_2D$ on insulin sensitivity might be exerted via its regulatory role in extracellular calcium concentration and flux through cell membranes. Calcium is essential for insulin-mediated intracellular processes in insulin-responsive tissues, such as muscle and fat,[27,28] with a narrow range of intracellular calcium needed for optimal insulin-mediated functions.[29] Changes in intracellular calcium in

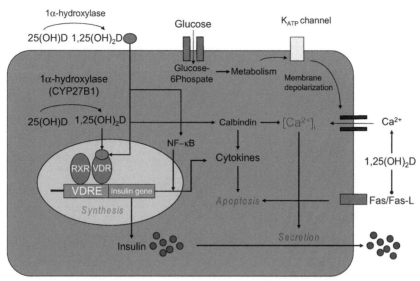

Fig. 1. Vitamin D and insulin secretion. Vitamin D can promote pancreatic beta cell function in several ways. The active form of vitamin D (1,25(OH)$_2$D), enters the beta cell from the circulation and interacts with the vitamin D receptor-retinoic acid x-receptor complex (VDR-RXR), which binds to the vitamin D response element (VDRE) found in the human insulin gene promoter, to enhance the transcriptional activation of the insulin gene and increase the synthesis of insulin. Vitamin D may promote beta cell survival by modulating the generation (through inactivation of NF-kB) and effects of cytokines. The antiapoptotic effect of vitamin D may also be mediated by downregulating the Fas-related pathways (Fas/Fas-L). Activation of vitamin D also occurs intracellularly by 1-alpha hydroxylase, which is expressed in pancreatic beta cells. Vitamin D also regulates calbindin, a cytosolic calcium-binding protein found in beta cells, which acts as a modulator of depolarization-stimulated insulin release via regulation of intracellular calcium. Calbindin may also protect against apoptotic cell death via its ability to buffer intracellular calcium. The effects of vitamin D may be mediated indirectly via its important and well-recognized role in regulating extracellular calcium (Ca^{2+}), calcium flux through the beta cell and intracellular calcium ([Ca^{2+}]$_i$). Alterations in calcium flux can directly influence insulin secretion, which is a calcium-dependent process. (*From* Eliades M, Pittas AG. Vitamin D and type 2 diabetes. In: Holick M, editor. Vitamin D: Physiology, molecular biology, and clinical applications. New York: Humana Press, 2010; with kind permission from Springer Science and Business Media.)

insulin target tissues may contribute to peripheral insulin resistance[29–36] via an impaired insulin signal transduction,[36,37] leading to decreased glucose transporter activity.[36–38] Hypovitaminosis D also leads to an increase in the levels of parathyroid hormone, which has been associated with insulin resistance.[39,40] Vitamin D also may affect insulin resistance indirectly through the renin-angiotensin-aldosterone system. Finally, vitamin D insufficiency has been associated with increased fat infiltration in skeletal muscle, which appears independent of body mass and is thought to contribute to a decreased insulin action.[41]

Vitamin D and Systemic Inflammation

Vitamin D could directly and/or indirectly lessen the effects of systemic inflammation in patients with type 2 diabetes in several ways. For example, 1,25(OH)$_2$D may protect against beta cell cytokine-induced apoptosis by directly modulating the expression

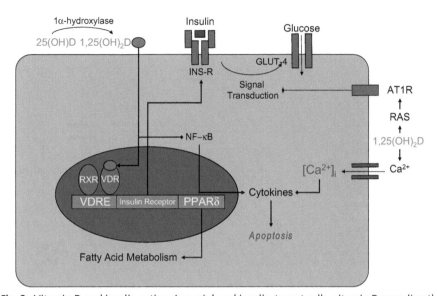

Fig. 2. Vitamin D and insulin action. In peripheral insulin-target cells, vitamin D may directly enhance insulin sensitivity by stimulating the expression of insulin receptors (INS-R), leading to activation of GLUT4 glucose transporters and/or by activating peroxisome proliferator-activated receptor (PPAR-δ), a transcription factor, which is implicated in the regulation of fatty acid metabolism in skeletal muscle and adipose tissue. The effects of vitamin D may be mediated indirectly via its important and well-recognized role in regulating extracellular calcium ([Ca^{2+}]i), calcium flux through the cell and intracellular calcium ([Ca^{2+}]i). Vitamin D may promote beta-cell survival by modulating the generation (through inactivation of NF-kB) and effects of cytokines. Vitamin D may also affect insulin resistance indirectly through the renin-angiotensin aldosterone system (RAS). AT1R, angiotensin II receptor 1; RXR-VDR, vitamin D receptor-retinoic acid x-receptor complex; VDRE, vitamin D response element. (*From* Eliades M, Pittas AG. Vitamin D and type 2 diabetes. In: Holick M, editor. Vitamin D: Physiology, molecular biology, and clinical applications. New York: Humana Press, 2010; with kind permission from Springer Science and Business Media.)

and activity of cytokines, hence improving insulin sensitivity.[42–45] One such pathway may be through the downregulation of nuclear factor (NF)-kB, a major transcription factor for tumor necrosis factor-alpha and other proinflammatory molecules.[46] Another pathway that may mediate the effect of 1,25(OH)$_2$D on beta cell function is through counteracting cytokine-induced Fas expression, which in turn will have anti-apoptotic effects.[47] Several other immune-modulating effects of 1,25(OH)$_2$D, such as blockade of dendritic cell differentiation, inhibition of lymphocyte proliferation, inhibition of foam cell formation, and cholesterol uptake by macrophages and enhanced regulatory T-lymphocyte development,[43,48] may provide additional protective pathways against beta cell destruction mediated by the systemic inflammation caused by type 2 diabetes.

ASSOCIATION BETWEEN VITAMIN D STATUS AND TYPE 2 DIABETES
Cross-Sectional Studies

There are many cross-sectional observational studies that have examined the association between vitamin D and type 2 diabetes and most have reported an inverse association between vitamin D status (25OHD concentration) and prevalent diabetes.

One of the largest such cohorts is the National Health and Nutrition Examination Survey in United States, which reported an inverse association between 25OHD concentration and prevalence of diabetes in non-Hispanic white and Mexican-American individuals, but not African American individuals.[49] Similarly, this inverse association was seen in other large cohorts from the United States,[40] Europe[50] and China.[51] The major limitation of cross-sectional studies is the potential of reverse causation; therefore, causality cannot be established.

Longitudinal Studies

Longitudinal studies, where vitamin D status is assessed before the outcome (type 2 diabetes) is ascertained, have nearly universally shown an inverse association of vitamin D status and incident type 2 diabetes (**Table 3**).[52–67] In these studies, vitamin D status was assessed by self-reported vitamin D intake, predicted 25OHD concentration, or measured plasma or serum 25OHD concentration.

In one of the largest studies to date in which vitamin D intake was the measure to assess vitamin D status, the Nurses' Health Study, after multivariate adjustment for age, BMI, and nondietary covariates, women who consumed more than 800 IU per day of vitamin D had a 23% lower risk for developing incident type 2 diabetes compared with women who consumed less than 200 IU per day (relative risk [RR] 0.77, 95% confidence interval [CI] 0.63–0.94; $P<.01$).[53] However, after adjusting for dietary factors, the association became nonsignificant. Similarly, in the Women's Health Study, an intake of 511 IU per day or more of vitamin D was associated with 27% lower risk of developing type 2 diabetes compared with an intake of 159 IU per day or less.[52] The Women's Health Study analysis is limited by the lack of adjustments for risk factors of type 2 diabetes other than age.

In a nested case-control study conducted in Finland, which included 2 cohorts, participants in the highest quartile of 25OHD (mean 25OHD 27.6 ng/mL) had a 40% lower risk of developing incident type 2 diabetes, compared with those in the lowest quartile (mean 25OHD 8.9 ng/mL), after multivariate adjustment. However, the lower risk was observed only in men.[54] On the other hand, in the Nurse's Health Study, the odds ratio for incident type 2 diabetes in the highest (mean 25OHD, 33.4 ng/mL) compared with the lowest quartile (mean 25OHD, 14.4 ng/mL) was 0.52 (95% CI 0.33–0.83) after multivariate adjustment. The inconsistency between the Finnish and the US female population could be secondary to different baseline mean 25OHD (15 ng/mL vs 23 ng/mL respectively), suggesting a threshold 25OHD concentration above which the risk of type 2 diabetes declines. In the Diabetes Prevention Program, which included a much larger number of participants at high risk for developing diabetes, those in the highest tertile of 25OHD (median concentration 30.1 ng/mL) had a hazard ratio of 0.72 (95% CI 0.56–0.90) for developing type 2 diabetes compared with participants in the lowest tertile (median concentration 12.8 ng/mL) after multivariate adjustment.[64]

Recently, 2 meta-analyses of longitudinal observational studies have been reported with nearly identical results. Song and colleagues[68] included 21 studies and a total of 76,000 participants and calculated the risk of developing type 2 diabetes, according to baseline 25OHD level. There was a 38% lower risk of developing type 2 diabetes in the highest tertile of 25OHD compared with the lowest tertile (RR 0.62, 95% CI 0.54–0.70, **Fig. 3**), with little heterogeneity between studies. The association was consistent regardless of diabetes diagnosis criteria, study size, or follow-up duration and remained significant after adjustment for BMI and intermediate biomarkers. A linear trend analysis showed that a 4 ng/mL increment in 25OHD levels was associated with a 4% lower risk of type 2 diabetes (95% CI 3–6; P for linear trend, 0.0001). In another meta-analysis of 16

Table 3

Observational longitudinal cohort studies of vitamin D status (plasma or serum 25[OH]D concentration, predicted 25[OH]D concentration or self-reported vitamin D intake) and incident type 2 diabetes

Study, Reference No., Year, Cohort [Country]	Male (%)	Mean Baseline Age (Range), y	White (%)	n[a]/N (Incidence)	Vitamin D Measure; Comparison[b]	Mean Follow-up, y (Start-End)	Results, Adjusted RR, OR, or HR (95% CI) P for Trend	Outcome (Ascertainment Method)	Adjustments
Liu et al,[52] 2005 Women's Health Study [US]	0	52 (45–75)	95	805/10,066 (8.0%)	Vitamin D intake (total); ≥511 vs ≤159 IU/d	9 (ND)	0.73 (0.54–0.99)[c] P = .02	Type 2 diabetes (validated self-report)	Age
Pittas et al,[53] 2006 [US]	0	46 (30–55)	98	4843/83,779 (5.8%)	Vitamin D intake (total); >800 vs ≤200 IU/d	20 (1980–2000)	0.87 (0.69–1.09) P = .67	Type 2 diabetes (validated self-report)	Age, BMI, exercise, residence, family history of diabetes, hypertension, calcium intake, smoking, alcohol, coffee, other diet
Knekt et al,[54] 2008 Finnish Mobile Clinic Health Examination Survey [Finland]	100	ND (40–74)	100	105/1628 (6.4%); nested case-control study with 206 control participants	25OHD concentration; 30 vs 10 ng/mL (means)	22 (1973–1994)	0.49 (0.15–1.64) P = .06	Type 2 diabetes (medication-treated, registry-based)	Age, BMI, exercise, season, smoking, education, medications
	0	ND (40–74)	100	125/1699 (7.4%); nested case-control study with 246 control participants	25OHD concentration; 25 vs 9 ng/mL (means)	—	0.91 (0.37–2.23) P = .66	—	Age, BMI, exercise, season, smoking, education, medications

Source	% Male	Mean age (range), y	% White (race)	Cases/N (%)	Exposure	Follow-up, y (years)	OR/RR (95% CI), P	Outcome	Adjustments
Knekt et al,[54] 2008 Mini-Finland Health Survey [Finland]	100	53 (40–69)	100	83/1948 (4.3%); nested case-control study with 245 control participants	25OHD concentration; 31 vs 9 ng/mL (means)	17 (1978–1994)	0.17 (0.05–0.52) P<.001	Type 2 diabetes (medication-treated, registry-based)	Age, BMI, exercise, season, smoking, education, medications
	0	ND (40–69)	100	99/2228 (4.4%); nested case-control study with 289 control participants	25OHD concentration; 25 vs 8 ng/mL (means)	—	1.45 (0.58–3.62) P = .83	—	Age, BMI, exercise, season, smoking, education, medications
Kirii et al,[55] 2009 Japan Public Health Center-based Prospective Study [Japan]	100	57 (40–69)	NR (~100% Japanese)	634/25,877 (2.4%)	Vitamin D intake (total); 720 vs 188 IU/d (means)	5 (1990–1998)	0.96 (0.74–1.23) P = .35	Type 2 diabetes (validated self-report)	Age, BMI, exercise, family history of diabetes, smoking, diet, hypertension
	0	57 (40–69)	NR (~100% Japanese)	480/33,919 (1.4%)	Vitamin D intake (total); 696 vs 192 IU/d (means)	5 (1990–1998)	0.88 (0.67–1.16) P = .67	Type 2 diabetes (validated self-report)	—
Liu et al,[56] 2010 Framingham Offspring Study [US]	54	60	~100	133/2956 (4.4%)	Predicted 25OHD score; 22 vs 17 ng/mL (medians)	7 (1991–2001)	0.60 (0.37–0.97) P = .03	Type 2 diabetes (medication-treated, laboratory-based)	Age, sex, waist circumference, family history of diabetes, hypertension, low HDL-cholesterol, high triglycerides, impaired fasting glucose, diet

(continued on next page)

Table 3
(continued)

Study, Reference No., Year, Cohort [Country]	Male (%)	Mean Baseline Age (Range), y	White (%)	n^a/N (Incidence)	Vitamin D Measure; Comparison^b	Mean Follow-up, y (Start–End)	Results, Adjusted RR, OR, or HR (95% CI) P for Trend	Outcome (Ascertainment Method)	Adjustments
Pittas et al,[57] 2010 Nurses' Health Study [US]	0	46 (30–55)	98	608/32,826 (1.8%); nested case-control study with 569 control participants	25OHD concentration; 33 vs 14 ng/mL (medians)	14 (1990–2004)	0.52 (0.33–0.83) P = .008	Type 2 diabetes (validated self-report)	Age, BMI, exercise, season, race, fasting status, latitude, hypercholesterolemia, hypertension, family history of diabetes, smoking, physical activity, alcohol, multivitamin use, diet
Anderson et al,[58] 2010 Intermountain Healthcare system [US]	25	55	NR	NR/41,497 (NR)	25OHD concentration; ≤15 vs >30 ng/mL	1.3 (2000–2009)	1.89 (1.54–2.33) P<.001	Diabetes (physician-diagnosed based on ICD-9 code)	Age, gender, hypertension, hyperlipidemia, heart failure, infection, depression, renal failure
Grimnes et al,[59] 2010 Tromso study [Norway]	NR	60 (Non smokers)	NR (majority Caucasians)	183/4157	25OHD concentration; 14 vs 29 ng/mL (means)	11 (1994–2005)	1.37 (0.89–2.10) P = NS	Type 2 diabetes (self-report verified by A1C and hospital discharge diagnosis)	Age, sex, BMI, physical activity, month (stratified by smoking status)
	NR	57 (smokers)	NR (majority Caucasians)	64/1962	25OHD concentration; 20 vs 39 ng/mL (means)	11 (1194–2005)	1.47 (0.62–3.48) P = NS	Type 2 diabetes (self-report verified by A1C and hospital discharge diagnosis)	Age, sex, BMI, physical activity, month (stratified by smoking status)

Study	%	Age		Cases/Total	Exposure	Duration (y)	OR (CI)	Outcome	Adjustments
Bolland et al,[60] 2010 Community dwelling women [Australia]	0	74 (>55)	100	15/1471	25OHD concentration; <20 vs ≥20 ng/mL	5 (1998–2003)	0.90 (0.4–1.9) P = NS	Type 2 diabetes (self-reported)	Age, weight, smoking, season, treatment allocation
Gagnon et al,[61] 2011 [Australia]	45	51	92	199/6537 (3.8%)	25OHD concentration; ≤19 vs ≥32 ng/mL	5 (1999–2005)	0.68 (0.43–1.07) P = .02	Type 2 diabetes (medication-treated, FPG or OGTT)	Age, gender, waist, exercise, race
Robinson et al,[62] 2011 WHI [US]	0	(50–79)	0	317/5140 (6.2%); nested case-control study	25OHD concentration; <20 vs ≥30 ng/mL	7.3	1.14 (0.68–1.90) P = .873	Diabetes (self-report, medication-treated)	Age, BMI, season, race, others
Thorand et al,[63] 2011 [Germany]	53	(35–74)	100	416/1683 (25%) case-control	25OHD concentration; 11 vs 68 ng/mL (median)	11	0.63 (0.44–0.90) P = .01	Type 2 diabetes (validated self-report)	Age, sex, survey, season, BMI, smoking, alcohol, physical activity, systolic blood pressure, total cholesterol/HDL cholesterol, parental history of DM
Pittas et al,[64] 2012 Diabetes Prevention Program [USA]	33	51	57	426/2040 (22%)	25OHD concentration; ≤13 vs ≥30 ng/mL	2.7 (1996–2001)	0.72 (0.56–0.90) P = .0054	Type 2 diabetes (OGTT)	Age, gender, body mass index, race, family history of diabetes, personal history of hypertension at baseline, smoking status at baseline, alcohol consumption, C-reactive protein, kidney function, self-reported physical activity, calcium intake, and treatment arm

(continued on next page)

Table 3
(continued)

Study, Reference No., Year, Cohort [Country]	Male (%)	Mean Baseline Age (Range), y	White (%)	nª/N (Incidence)	Vitamin D Measure; Comparisonᵇ	Mean Follow-up, y (Start–End)	Results, Adjusted RR, OR, or HR (95% CI) P for Trend	Outcome (Ascertainment Method)	Adjustments
Deleskog et al,[65] 2012 [Denmark]	100	(35–56)	100	145/1011	25OHD concentration; >28 vs <18 ng/mL	10	0.38 (0.21–0.71)	Type 2 diabetes (OGTT)	Age, gender, BMI, exercise, season, BP, family history of diabetes
Forouhi et al,[66] 2012 EPIC-Norfolk [Europe]	52	58	>90	621/826 nested case-control study	25OHD concentration; >32 vs <20 ng/mL	10	0.50 (0.32–0.76)	Type 2 diabetes (validated self-report)	Age, gender, BMI, exercise, season, family history of diabetes, cholesterol, alcohol, smoking, education, supplement use
Afzal et al,[67] 2013 Copenhagen City Heart Study [Europe]	43	56	100	810/9841	25OHD concentration; Quartiles value NR	29	1.35 (1.09–1.66)	Type 2 diabetes (self-report, medication treated, nonfasting glucose, registry based)	Sex, age, smoking status (never/ever), BMI, income, and duration and intensity of leisure time physical activities

To convert 25OHD concentration from ng/mL to nmol/L multiply by 2.459.

Abbreviations: 25OHD, plasma or serum 25-hydroxyvitamin D; BMI, body mass index; BP, blood pressure; CI, confidence interval; CVD, cardiovascular disease; DM, diabetes mellitus; FPG, fasting plasma glucose; HDL, high-density lipoprotein; HR, hazard ratio; ICD, International Classification of Diseases; IU, international units; ND, no data; NR, not reported; NS, not significant; OGTT, oral glucose tolerance test; OR, odds ratio; RR, relative risk.

ª Number of cases.

ᵇ Highest/lowest risk category versus reference category.

ᶜ Estimated from reported data.

Data from Refs.[52–67]

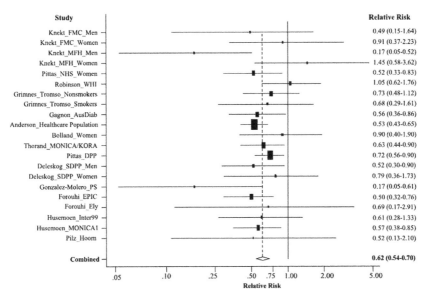

Fig. 3. A random-effects meta-analysis of 21 independent prospective studies with adjusted RR and 95% CI of type 2 diabetes in relation to serum 25(OH)D levels (the highest category vs the lowest category). (*From* Song Y, Wang L, Pittas AG, et al. Blood 25-hydroxy vitamin D levels and incident type 2 diabetes: a meta-analysis of prospective studies. Diabetes Care 2013;36:1422–8; with permission.)

studies, Afzal and colleagues[67] estimated the odds ratio for type 2 diabetes to be 1.5 (95% CI 1.33–1.70) for the bottom versus the top quartile of 25OHD concentration.

Despite the consistency of these results, the observational nature of these studies precludes an assessment of cause and effect because residual confounding cannot be excluded.

THE INFLUENCE OF VITAMIN D SUPPLEMENTATION ON TYPE 2 DIABETES

The effect of vitamin D supplementation on glycemia or incident type 2 diabetes has been reported in several trials with mixed results (**Table 4**).

In trials that included participants with normal glucose tolerance at baseline, vitamin D supplementation had a neutral effect on measures of glycemia, including fasting plasma glucose or hemoglobin A1c and insulin resistance measured by homeostasis model assessment (HOMA).[69–77] Similarly, vitamin D supplementation had no effect on incident type 2 diabetes in individuals with normal glucose tolerance at baseline.[71,72] The major limitation in interpreting these results is that most were designed for nonglycemic outcomes and the analyses on vitamin D and type 2 diabetes were post hoc.[69–72,75] In addition, all trials with the exception of the Women's Health Initiative trial[71] and the Randomized Evaluation of Calcium Or vitamin D (RECORD) trial[72] were underpowered for glycemic outcomes. It is also important to note that adherence to the intervention would have played a major role in interpreting the results. For example, in a post hoc analysis of the RECORD study, a community-based effectiveness trial designed for bone outcomes,[72] supplementation with 800 IU per day of vitamin D_3 (given in a 2 × 2 factorial design with calcium carbonate) did not change the risk of self-reported type 2 diabetes; however, among study participants who were highly compliant with

Table 4
Randomized controlled trials of the effect of vitamin D (cholecalciferol [D₃] or ergocalciferol [D₂]) supplementation (with or without calcium) on glycemic measures

Study, Reference No., Year [Country]	Men (%)	Mean Baseline Age and/or Range	BMI	Participants	Mean Baseline 25(OH)D Concentration, ng/mL Calcium Intake	Interventions (No. of Participants)	Study Duration	Effect of Vitamin D vs Placebo [P Value]
Nilas & Christiansen,[69] 1984 [Denmark]	0	45–54	ND	Postmenopausal healthy; n = 151	ND	D₃, 2000 IU/d (n = 25) vs 1(OH)₂D₃ 0.25 µg/d (n = 23) vs placebo (n = 103). All received calcium, 500 mg/d	2 y	↔ FPG 2.16 vs −5.94 vs 2.34 mg/dL
Pittas et al,[70] 2007 [US]	38	71 (≥65)	27	Normal fasting glucose; n = 222	30 Calcium intake, 750 mg/d	D₃, 700 IU/d plus calcium citrate, 500 mg/d (n = 108) vs placebo (n = 114)	3 y	↔ FPG change, 2.70 vs 2.16 mg/dL [P = .55] ↔ IR$_{HOMA}$
	52	71	—	Impaired fasting glucose; n = 92	30 Calcium intake, 680 mg/d	D₃, 700 IU/d plus calcium citrate 500 mg/d (n = 45) vs placebo (n = 47)	3 y	↓ FPG change, 0.36 vs 6.13 mg/dL [P = .042] ↓ IR$_{HOMA}$
De Boer et al,[71] 2008 [US]	0	62 (50–79)	—	Postmenopausal without diabetes	<32 (for 89% of participants)	D₃, 400 IU/d plus calcium carbonate 1000 mg/d (n = 16,999) vs placebo (n = 16,952)	7 y	↔ Incidence of Diabetes (self-reported), HR 1.01 (0.94–1.10) [P = .95] ↔ Insulin secretion ↔ IR$_{HOMA}$
	0	50–79	—	Normal fasting glucose; n = 1637	—	D₃, 400 IU/d plus calcium carbonate 1000 mg/d (n = 866) vs placebo (n = 771)	6 y	↔ FPG change, 3.80 vs 4.61 mg/dL [P = .32]
	0	50–79	—	Impaired fasting glucose; n = 1457	—	D₃, 400 IU/d plus calcium carbonate 1000 mg/d (n = 718) vs placebo (n = 739)	6 y	↔ FPG change, 3.93 vs 4.69 mg/dL [P = .79]

Avenell et al,[72] 2009 [UK]	15	77 (≥70)	ND	History of fracture	ND	D_3, 800 IU/d (n = 2649) vs placebo (n = 2643) (2 × 2 factorial design with calcium carbonate 1000 mg/d)	2–5 y	↔ Incidence of Diabetes (self-reported), intention-to-treat HR 1.11 (0.77–1.62) [P = .57] ↔ Incidence of Diabetes (self-reported), compliant HR 0.68 (0.40–1.16) [P = .16]
Zittermann et al,[73] 2009 [Germany]	33	48 (18–70)	33	Healthy; BMI >27 kg/m²; n = 200	12	D_3, 3332 IU/d (n = 82) vs placebo (n = 83). All received weight reduction advice for 24 wk	1 y	↔ Hemoglobin A1c change, −0.25% vs −0.25% [P = .96] ↔ FPG change, −0.21 vs −0.27 mmol/L (−3.8 vs −4.9 mg/dL) [P = .39]
von Hurst et al,[74] 2010 [New Zealand]	0 Indian (91%)	42 (23–68)	27.5	Insulin resistance, no diabetes; 25(OH)D <20 ng/mL; n = 81	8	D_3, 4000 IU/d (n = 42) vs placebo (n = 39)	26 wk	↔ FPG change, 0.1 vs 0.1 mmol/L (1.8 vs 1.8 mg/dL) [P = .82] ↓ IR_{HOMA} (change from baseline) −0.2 vs 0.2; P = .02; (highest effect seen when final 25OHD >80 nmol/L) ↓ Insulin ↔ HOMA2%B; C-peptide

(continued on next page)

Table 4
(continued)

Study, Reference No., Year [Country]	Men (%)	Mean Baseline Age and/or Range	BMI	Participants	Mean Baseline 25(OH)D Concentration, ng/mL Calcium Intake	Interventions (No. of Participants)	Study Duration	Effect of Vitamin D vs Placebo [P Value]
Jorde et al,[75] 2010 [Norway]	36	38 (21–70)	35	Overweight/Obese; no diabetes; n = 438	23	D$_3$, 40,000 IU/wk (equivalent to 5714 IU/d) (n = 150) vs D$_3$, 20,000 IU/wk (equivalent to 2857 IU/d) (n = 139) vs placebo (n = 149). All received calcium 500 mg/d	1 y	↔ Hemoglobin A1c change, 0.09% vs 0.11% vs 0.09% (0.4 vs 1.4 vs 1.4 mg/dL) [P = NS]; post hoc ↔ FPG change, 0.02 vs 0.08 vs 0.08 mmol/L [P = NS]; post hoc ↔ 2hPG change, 0.15 vs 0.36 vs −0.02 mmol/L (2.7 vs 6.5 vs −0.4 mg/d) [P = NS]; post hoc ↔ IR$_{HOMA}$ 0.23 vs −0.05 vs 0.36, P = NS ↔ QUICKI
Wood et al,[76] 2012 [UK]	0	64	26	Healthy (NGT) postmenopausal women; n = 305	13	D$_3$, 1000 IU/d orally (n = 101) vs D$_3$ 400 IU/d orally (n = 102) vs placebo (n = 102)	48 wk	↔ FPG change, −1.1 vs 0.9 vs −2.3 mg/dL [P = .23] ↔ HOMA-IR change
Nagpal et al,[77] 2009 [India]	100	43 (>35)	26	Healthy; Central obesity; n = 71	15	D$_3$, 120,000 IU 3 times (equivalent to 8571 IU/d) (n = 35) vs placebo (n = 36)	6 wk	↑ OGIS (change from baseline, ml/min*kg) 21.17 vs −8.89 P = .055 ↔ HOMA (change from baseline) 0.14 vs 0.16 P = .95 ↔ QUICKI 0 vs 0 P = .9

Mitri et al,[79] 2011 [US]	53	57	32	Prediabetes; n = 92	24	D3, 2000 IU/d vs placebo-vitamin D (n = 46); 2 × 2 factorial design with calcium 800 mg/d vs placebo-calcium (n = 46)	16 wk	↔ A1c change, 0.06 vs 0.14% [P = .08] ↔ FPG change, 2.4 vs 5.6 mg/dL [P = .172] ↔ 2hPG change, −7.2 vs 1.2 mg/dL [P = .22] ↑ DI change 300 vs −126 in D3 vs non D3, [P = .011] ↑ SI change −0.3 vs −0.9 in D3 vs non D3, [P = .16] ↑ AIR change, 34 vs −53 in D3 vs non D3 [P = .074]
Nazarian et al,[80] 2011 [US]	38	34-62	23-45	Pre-diabetes (FPG 100–125 mg/dL); 25OHD ≤30 ng/mL n = 8	20	D3, 10,000 IU/d for 4 wk (n = 8)	4 wk	No glycemic data ↔ DI (% from baseline) 21 [P = NS] ↑ SI (% from baseline) 42 [P = .012] ↓ AIRg (% from baseline) 20 [P = .011]
Davidson et al,[81] 2013 [US]	32	52 (ND)	32	Prediabetes (FPG 110–125 mg/dL; 2hPG 140–199 mg/dL); 25OHD <30 ng/mL; Latino and African American; n = 117	22	D3, orally weekly titrated to achieve 25OHD 65-90 ng/mL (mean dose required equivalent to 12,700 IU/d) (n = 56) vs Placebo (n = 53)	12 mo	↓ Hemoglobin A1c change, −0.1 vs 0.1% [P = .004] ↔ FPG change, 1 vs 4 mg/dL [P = .27] ↔ 2hPG change, −11 vs −9 mg/dL [P = .64] ↔ DI1 change, 0.2 vs 0 [P = .39] ↔ DI2 change, −0.1 vs 0 [P = .32] ↔ Proportion with diabetes [P = NA]

(continued on next page)

Table 4 (continued)								
Study, Reference No., Year [Country]	Men (%)	BMI	Mean Baseline Age and/or Range	Participants	Mean Baseline 25(OH)D Concentration, ng/mL Calcium Intake	Interventions (No. of Participants)	Study Duration	Effect of Vitamin D vs Placebo [P Value]
Harris et al,[100] 2012 [US]	35	32	56 (NR)	Pre-diabetes/early diabetes (FPG >100 mg/dL; A1c 5.8%–6.9%); Overweight; African American; n = 89	—	D$_3$, 4000 IU/d orally (n = 43) vs Placebo (n = 46)	12 wk	↔ Hemoglobin A1c change, −0.05 vs 0.05% [P = .97] ↔ FPG change, −0.18 vs −0.54 mg/dL [P = .81] ↔ 2hPG change, −7.2 vs −6.5 mg/dL [P = .98] ↓ Insulin sensitivity change (%), −4 vs 12 [P = .004] ↑ Insulin secretion change (%), 12 vs 2 mg/dL [P = .27] ↔ DI change, −11 vs −9 mg/dL [P = .64]
Witham et al,[84] 2010 [United Kingdom]	ND	31	65 (>18)	Type 2 diabetes; 25OHD <40 ng/mL; n = 61	18	D$_3$, 100,000 IU orally once (equivalent to 892 IU/d) (n = 19) vs D$_3$, 200,000 IU orally once (equivalent to 1785 IU/d) (n = 20) vs placebo (n = 22)	16 wk	↔ Hemoglobin A1c change, "no change" (data NR) ↔ FPG change, "no change" (data NR) ↔ IR$_{HOMA}$ change, "no change" (data NR)

Source				Population		Intervention	Duration	Results
Sugden et al,[82] 2008 [UK]	53	64	31	Stable type 2 diabetes; 25(OH)D <20 ng/mL; n = 34	15	D_2, 100,000 IU once (equivalent to 1785 IU/d) (n = 17) vs placebo (n = 17)	8 wk	↔ Hemoglobin A1c change, 0.01% vs −0.05% [P = .74]; ↔ IR_{HOMA} change, −39.7 vs −25.6 [P = .72]; IR_{HOMA} significantly improved if 25OHD rise >11 nmol/L
Jorde & Figenschau,[83] 2009 [Norway]	50	56 (21–75)	—	Stable type 2 diabetes; n = 32	24	D_3, 40,000 IU/wk (equivalent to 5714 IU/d) (n = 16) vs placebo (n = 16)	26 wk	↔ Hemoglobin A1c change, 0.2% vs −0.2% [P = .90]; ↔ FPG change, −0.2 vs 0.4 mmol/L (−3.6 vs 7.2 mg/dL) [P = .43]; ↔ IR_{HOMA} 0.3 vs −0.2, P = .58
Nikooyeh et al,[85] 2011 [Iran]	40	51	29	Type 2 diabetes (FPG ≥126 mg/dL)	12	D_3, 1000 IU/d in yogurt drink with 250 mg of calcium (n = 30) vs D_3, 1000 IU/d in yogurt drink with 500 mg of calcium (n = 30) vs placebo (plain yogurt drink; n = 30)	12 wk	↓ A1c change, −0.5 vs 1.2% [P<.01]; ↓ FPG change, −9 vs 16 mg/dL [P = .01]
Soric et al,[86] 2012 [Ohio, US]	45	54 (21–75)	ND	Type 2 diabetes (A1c >7%); n = 37	ND	D_3, 2000 IU/d orally (n = 19) vs Vitamin C, 500 mg/d orally (n = 18)	12 wk	↔ Hemoglobin A1c change, −0.4 vs 0.1% [P = .16]; ↓ Hemoglobin A1c change, −1.4% vs 0.2% [P = .013] when baseline A1c >9%

(continued on next page)

Table 4
(continued)

Study, Reference No., Year [Country]	Men (%)	Mean Baseline Age and/or Range	BMI	Participants	Mean Baseline 25(OH)D Concentration, ng/mL Calcium Intake	Interventions (No. of Participants)	Study Duration	Effect of Vitamin D vs Placebo [P Value]
Punthakee et al,[87] 2012 [33 countries]	60	66	—	Type 2 diabetes (A1c 7.4%) [TIDE study] n = 1221	ND	D₃, 1000 IU/d orally (n = 607) vs placebo (n = 614)	40 mo	↔ Hemoglobin A1c NR ↔ FPG change NR
Heshmat et al,[88] 2012 [Iran]	36	56 (37–79)	27.7	Type 2 diabetes on diet or oral agents (A1c <7.5%) n = 42	47	D₃, 300,000 IU/d orally ×1 dose (n = 21) vs placebo (n = 21)	3 mo	↔ Hemoglobin A1c −0.05% vs −0.2% P = .495 ↑ FPG 16.2 vs −9.7 (P = .007) ↑ HOMA 0.2 vs −0.9 P = .017

To convert 25(OH)D concentration from ng/mL to nmol/L multiply by 2.459; to convert FPG from mg/dL to nmol/L, multiply by 0.0555.

Abbreviations: ↓, decreased (statistically significant); ↑, increased (statistically significant); ↔, no difference (no statistical significance); 25(OH)D, plasma or serum 25-hydroxyvitamin D; 2hPG, plasma glucose 2 hours after 75 g glucose load; D₂, ergocalciferol; D₃, cholecalciferol; FPG, fasting plasma glucose; HR, hazard ratio; IR, insulin resistance; IR_HOMA, insulin resistance by homeostasis model assessment; ND, no data.

Data from Refs.[69–77,79–88,100]

supplementation, there was a notable trend toward reduction in type 2 diabetes risk with vitamin D_3 (odds ratio 0.68, 95% CI 0.40–1.16).

The potential effect of vitamin D supplementation appears to be more prominent among persons who are at high risk for diabetes (eg, prediabetes). In a post hoc subgroup analysis conducted using data from a completed trial designed for fractures, combined vitamin D_3 (700 IU/d) and calcium carbonate (500 mg/d) supplementation prevented the rise in insulin resistance (HOMA-IR) and fasting plasma glucose (FPG) in people with impaired fasting glucose, but not in individuals with normal fasting glucose at baseline,[70] suggesting that vitamin D may benefit only individuals at high risk for diabetes. In this study, the reduction in FPG over 3 years was similar to the reduction in FPG achieved with metformin or lifestyle, in the Diabetes Prevention Program, which was associated with a 31% to 58% decrease in incident diabetes.[78] In the Calcium and Vitamin D for type 2 Diabetes Mellitus study, vitamin D supplementation (2000 IU/d) in adults at risk for type 2 diabetes improved beta cell function and had a nearly statistically significant effect on the rise in A1c values.[79] Similarly, in another intervention study, where vitamin D was given without a placebo, insulin sensitivity improved after 4 weeks of vitamin D administration in persons with prediabetes.[80] However, Davidson and colleagues[81] found no effect of high-dose vitamin D supplementation on insulin secretion, insulin sensitivity, or incident diabetes in a population with impaired fasting glycemia or impaired glucose tolerance and low vitamin D levels. In this study, the average daily dose of vitamin D supplementation was close to 12,700 IU and the population was limited to non-Whites. According to the IOM, chronic administration of vitamin D in excess of 4000 IU per day may not be beneficial. Therefore, the supra-physiologic dose of vitamin D supplemented in the study by Davidson and colleagues[81] and the difference in ethnicity could explain the discrepancy with other studies in persons with prediabetes.

In most trials that included participants with established type 2 diabetes, vitamin D supplementation had no effect on glycemic outcome measures after a follow-up period of 8 to 26 weeks.[82–88] However, these studies were underpowered and the effect of concurrent diabetes pharmacotherapy on the outcome measured was not reported.

VITAMIN D AND TYPE 1 DIABETES

Type 1 diabetes is characterized by autoimmune destruction of pancreatic islet beta cells, leading to absolute insulin deficiency. Many effects of vitamin D on the pathophysiology of type 1 diabetes have been described, including changes in the immune-mediated destruction,[89] but also the beta cell itself. The latter effect may, at least in part, be mediated indirectly by the effect of vitamin D on calcium homeostasis. It also has been reported that specific vitamin D receptor polymorphisms interact with the HLADRB1 allele, which predisposes to type 1 diabetes.[90] Evidence from animal studies in nonobese diabetic mice, which undergo destruction of pancreatic beta cells that mimics the pathogenesis of type 1 diabetes in humans, suggests that vitamin D deficiency is associated with development of diabetes, whereas administration of $1,25(OH)_2D$ to these mice prevented the development of diabetes.[91]

In humans, the prevalence of type 1 diabetes has been inversely correlated with ultraviolet B radiation and altitude, suggesting that low vitamin D synthesis may be important in the pathogenesis of type 1 diabetes. Lack of vitamin D supplementation in infancy has been associated with increased risk of type 1 diabetes later in life. In the Finnish birth cohort study, children who regularly took the recommended dosage of 2000 IU per day of vitamin D had lower risk of developing diabetes compared with those who regularly received less than the recommended amount.[92] A meta-analysis based on 5 observational studies concluded that vitamin D supplementation in early childhood is associated with decreased diabetes risk.[93] Recently, Sorensen and colleagues[94] reported that lower maternal serum concentration of 25OHD during pregnancy was associated with an increased risk of childhood-onset type 1 diabetes, suggesting that in utero exposure to vitamin D may also be important. There are limited data from intervention studies with vitamin D in patients with type 1 diabetes. In patients with new-onset type 1 diabetes, Gabbay and colleagues[95] reported that supplementation with 2000 IU per day of cholecalciferol over 18 months resulted in a favorable immunologic effect and a slower decline of residual beta cell function but without any change in glycemia. Two earlier studies of calcitriol supplementation in type 1 diabetes did not show a positive effect on beta cell residual function.[96,97]

Although the data from animal and epidemiologic studies seem promising, large trials evaluating the efficacy and safety of vitamin D supplementation in prevention or treatment of type 1 diabetes are lacking.

SUMMARY

Findings from basic science suggest that vitamin D may play a significant role in both types of diabetes. In human studies, the evidence for a potential association is stronger for vitamin D and type 2 diabetes with much fewer data on type 1 diabetes. However, the evidence about type 2 diabetes in humans is derived almost exclusively from observational studies, which may be confounded by a variety of factors and, therefore, these studies preclude an assessment of cause and effect. There are no published trials specifically designed to test the safety and efficacy of long-term vitamin D administration to reduce the risk of developing type 2 diabetes; therefore, firm conclusions cannot be drawn regarding the role of vitamin D for prevention or treatment of diabetes. On numerous occasions, encouraging findings from observational studies were not confirmed by well-designed clinical trials (eg, hormone replacement therapy, vitamin E, and other supplements)[98,99] and prevailing clinical practice was overturned. Therefore, evidence from randomized controlled trials is needed to address the issue of causality and to rigorously assess the protective effect of vitamin D on type 2 diabetes.

There are several ongoing randomized trials to test the hypothesis that vitamin D supplementation lowers type 2 diabetes risk. The vitamin D and omega-3 trial (VITAL study, www.vitalstudy.org) is a large *community-based* 2 × 2 factorial trial that is testing the *effectiveness* of 2000 IU per day of vitamin D3 versus less than 800 IU per day (the other factor is omega-3 fatty acids vs placebo) in primary prevention of cancer, cardiovascular disease, and stroke. An ancillary study to VITAL will evaluate the effect of vitamin D supplementation on diabetes incidence, based on self-reported data among those with normal glucose tolerance at baseline. The vitamin D and type 2 diabetes study (D2d, www.d2dstudy.org) is a large multicenter clinical trial conducted in 20 cities around the United States, specifically designed to test whether vitamin D supplementation reduces risk of incident diabetes in patients with prediabetes. The D2d study will enroll approximately 2400 participants who will be followed for up to 4 years for development of diabetes.

If the results of these larger trials, and other ongoing studies, confirm a favorable benefit/harm ratio of vitamin D supplementation, vitamin D would likely be integrated into contemporary strategies for the prevention of type 2 diabetes in the more than 79 million Americans at risk of developing diabetes and to treatment in the more than 10 million Americans with established diabetes. Until then, vitamin D is a promising, yet unproven dietary intervention for type 2 diabetes.

REFERENCES

1. Holick MF, Binkley NC, Bischoff-Ferrari HA, et al. Evaluation, treatment, and prevention of vitamin D deficiency: an Endocrine Society clinical practice guideline. J Clin Endocrinol Metab 2011;96:1911–30.
2. Institute of Medicine. Dietary reference intakes for calcium and vitamin D. Washington, DC: The National Academies Press; 2011.
3. Rosen CJ, Abrams SA, Aloia JF, et al. IOM committee members respond to endocrine society vitamin D guideline. J Clin Endocrinol Metab 2012;97:1146–52.
4. Norman AW, Frankel JB, Heldt AM, et al. Vitamin D deficiency inhibits pancreatic secretion of insulin. Science 1980;209:823–5.
5. Chertow BS, Sivitz WI, Baranetsky NG, et al. Cellular mechanisms of insulin release: the effects of vitamin D deficiency and repletion on rat insulin secretion. Endocrinology 1983;113:1511–8.
6. Kadowaki S, Norman AW. Dietary vitamin D is essential for normal insulin secretion from the perfused rat pancreas. J Clin Invest 1984;73:759–66.
7. Tanaka Y, Seino Y, Ishida M, et al. Effect of vitamin D3 on the pancreatic secretion of insulin and somatostatin. Acta Endocrinol (Copenh) 1984;105:528–33.
8. Cade C, Norman AW. Vitamin D3 improves impaired glucose tolerance and insulin secretion in the vitamin D–deficient rat in vivo. Endocrinology 1986;119:84–90.
9. Bourlon PM, Faure-Dussert A, Billaudel B. The de novo synthesis of numerous proteins is decreased during vitamin D3 deficiency and is gradually restored by 1, 25-dihydroxyvitamin D3 repletion in the islets of langerhans of rats. J Endocrinol 1999;162:101–9.
10. Cade C, Norman AW. Rapid normalization/stimulation by 1,25-dihydroxyvitamin D3 of insulin secretion and glucose tolerance in the vitamin D-deficient rat. Endocrinology 1987;120:1490–7.
11. Clark SA, Stumpf WE, Sar M. Effect of 1,25 dihydroxyvitamin D3 on insulin secretion. Diabetes 1981;30:382–6.
12. Johnson JA, Grande JP, Roche PC, et al. Immunohistochemical localization of the 1,25(OH)2D3 receptor and calbindin D28k in human and rat pancreas. Am J Physiol 1994;267:E356–60.
13. Zeitz U, Weber K, Soegiarto DW, et al. Impaired insulin secretory capacity in mice lacking a functional vitamin D receptor. FASEB J 2003;17:509–11.
14. Bland R, Markovic D, Hills CE, et al. Expression of 25-hydroxyvitamin D3-1alpha-hydroxylase in pancreatic islets. J Steroid Biochem Mol Biol 2004; 89–90:121–5.
15. Sergeev IN, Rhoten WB. 1,25-Dihydroxyvitamin D3 evokes oscillations of intracellular calcium in a pancreatic beta-cell line. Endocrinology 1995;136:2852–61.
16. Milner RD, Hales CN. The role of calcium and magnesium in insulin secretion from rabbit pancreas studied in vitro. Diabetologia 1967;3:47–9.
17. Yasuda K, Hurukawa Y, Okuyama M, et al. Glucose tolerance and insulin secretion in patients with parathyroid disorders. Effect of serum calcium on insulin release. N Engl J Med 1975;292:501–4.
18. Gedik O, Zileli MS. Effects of hypocalcemia and theophylline on glucose tolerance and insulin release in human beings. Diabetes 1977;26:813–9.
19. Fujita T, Sakagami Y, Tomita T, et al. Insulin secretion after oral calcium load. Endocrinol Jpn 1978;25:645–8.

20. Kadowaki S, Norman AW. Pancreatic vitamin D–dependent calcium binding protein: biochemical properties and response to vitamin D. Arch Biochem Biophys 1984;233:228–36.

21. Sooy K, Schermerhorn T, Noda M, et al. Calbindin-D(28k) controls [Ca(2+)](i) and insulin release. Evidence obtained from calbindin-d(28k) knockout mice and beta cell lines. J Biol Chem 1999;274:34343–9.

22. Leal MA, Aller P, Mas A, et al. The effect of 1,25-dihydroxyvitamin D3 on insulin binding, insulin receptor mRNA levels, and isotype RNA pattern in U-937 human promonocytic cells. Exp Cell Res 1995;217:189–94.

23. Maestro B, Campion J, Davila N, et al. Stimulation by 1,25-dihydroxyvitamin D3 of insulin receptor expression and insulin responsiveness for glucose transport in U-937 human promonocytic cells. Endocr J 2000;47:383–91.

24. Maestro B, Molero S, Bajo S, et al. Transcriptional activation of the human insulin receptor gene by 1,25-dihydroxyvitamin D(3). Cell Biochem Funct 2002;20:227–32.

25. Maestro B, Davila N, Carranza MC, et al. Identification of a vitamin D response element in the human insulin receptor gene promoter. J Steroid Biochem Mol Biol 2003;84:223–30.

26. Dunlop TW, Vaisanen S, Frank C, et al. The human peroxisome proliferator-activated receptor delta gene is a primary target of 1alpha,25-dihydroxyvitamin D3 and its nuclear receptor. J Mol Biol 2005;349:248–60.

27. Ojuka EO. Role of calcium and AMP kinase in the regulation of mitochondrial biogenesis and GLUT4 levels in muscle. Proc Nutr Soc 2004;63:275–8.

28. Wright DC, Hucker KA, Holloszy JO, et al. Ca2+ and AMPK both mediate stimulation of glucose transport by muscle contractions. Diabetes 2004;53:330–5.

29. Draznin B, Sussman K, Kao M, et al. The existence of an optimal range of cytosolic free calcium for insulin-stimulated glucose transport in rat adipocytes. J Biol Chem 1987;262:14385–8.

30. Byyny RL, LoVerde M, Lloyd S, et al. Cytosolic calcium and insulin resistance in elderly patients with essential hypertension. Am J Hypertens 1992;5:459–64.

31. Draznin B, Lewis D, Houlder N, et al. Mechanism of insulin resistance induced by sustained levels of cytosolic free calcium in rat adipocytes. Endocrinology 1989;125:2341–9.

32. Draznin B, Sussman KE, Eckel RH, et al. Possible role of cytosolic free calcium concentrations in mediating insulin resistance of obesity and hyperinsulinemia. J Clin Invest 1988;82:1848–52.

33. Draznin B, Sussman KE, Kao M, et al. Relationship between cytosolic free calcium concentration and 2-deoxyglucose uptake in adipocytes isolated from 2- and 12-month-old rats. Endocrinology 1988;122:2578–83.

34. Ohno Y, Suzuki H, Yamakawa H, et al. Impaired insulin sensitivity in young, lean normotensive offspring of essential hypertensives: possible role of disturbed calcium metabolism. J Hypertens 1993;11:421–6.

35. Segal S, Lloyd S, Sherman N, et al. Postprandial changes in cytosolic free calcium and glucose uptake in adipocytes in obesity and non-insulin-dependent diabetes mellitus. Horm Res 1990;34:39–44.

36. Zemel MB. Nutritional and endocrine modulation of intracellular calcium: implications in obesity, insulin resistance and hypertension. Mol Cell Biochem 1998;188:129–36.

37. Williams PF, Caterson ID, Cooney GJ, et al. High affinity insulin binding and insulin receptor-effector coupling: modulation by Ca2+. Cell Calcium 1990;11:547–56.

38. Reusch JE, Begum N, Sussman KE, et al. Regulation of GLUT-4 phosphorylation by intracellular calcium in adipocytes. Endocrinology 1991;129:3269–73.
39. Chiu KC, Chuang LM, Lee NP, et al. Insulin sensitivity is inversely correlated with plasma intact parathyroid hormone level. Metabolism 2000;49:1501–5.
40. Reis JP, von Muhlen D, Kritz-Silverstein D, et al. Vitamin D, parathyroid hormone levels, and the prevalence of metabolic syndrome in community-dwelling older adults. Diabetes Care 2007;30:1549–55.
41. Gilsanz V, Kremer A, Mo AO, et al. Vitamin D status and its relation to muscle mass and muscle fat in young women. J Clin Endocrinol Metab 2010;95:1595–601.
42. Riachy R, Vandewalle B, Kerr Conte J, et al. 1,25-dihydroxyvitamin D3 protects RINm5F and human islet cells against cytokine-induced apoptosis: implication of the antiapoptotic protein A20. Endocrinology 2002;143:4809–19.
43. van Etten E, Mathieu C. Immunoregulation by 1,25-dihydroxyvitamin D3: basic concepts. J Steroid Biochem Mol Biol 2005;97:93–101.
44. Giulietti A, van Etten E, Overbergh L, et al. Monocytes from type 2 diabetic patients have a pro-inflammatory profile. 1,25-Dihydroxyvitamin D(3) works as anti-inflammatory. Diabetes Res Clin Pract 2007;77:47–57.
45. Gysemans CA, Cardozo AK, Callewaert H, et al. 1,25-Dihydroxyvitamin D3 modulates expression of chemokines and cytokines in pancreatic islets: implications for prevention of diabetes in nonobese diabetic mice. Endocrinology 2005;146: 1956–64.
46. Cohen-Lahav M, Douvdevani A, Chaimovitz C, et al. The anti-inflammatory activity of 1,25-dihydroxyvitamin D3 in macrophages. J Steroid Biochem Mol Biol 2007;103:558–62.
47. Riachy R, Vandewalle B, Moerman E, et al. 1,25-Dihydroxyvitamin D3 protects human pancreatic islets against cytokine-induced apoptosis via down-regulation of the Fas receptor. Apoptosis 2006;11:151–9.
48. Oh J, Weng S, Felton SK, et al. 1,25(OH)2 vitamin D inhibits foam cell formation and suppresses macrophage cholesterol uptake in patients with type 2 diabetes mellitus. Circulation 2009;120:687–98.
49. Scragg R, Sowers M, Bell C. Serum 25-hydroxyvitamin D, diabetes, and ethnicity in the Third National Health and Nutrition Examination Survey. Diabetes Care 2004;27:2813–8.
50. Hypponen E, Boucher BJ, Berry DJ, et al. 25-hydroxyvitamin D, IGF-1, and metabolic syndrome at 45 years of age: a cross-sectional study in the 1958 British Birth Cohort. Diabetes 2008;57:298–305.
51. Lu L, Yu Z, Pan A, et al. Plasma 25-hydroxyvitamin D concentration and metabolic syndrome among middle-aged and elderly Chinese individuals. Diabetes Care 2009;32:1278–83.
52. Liu S, Song Y, Ford ES, et al. Dietary calcium, vitamin D, and the prevalence of metabolic syndrome in middle-aged and older U.S. women. Diabetes Care 2005;28:2926–32.
53. Pittas AG, Dawson-Hughes B, Li T, et al. Vitamin D and calcium intake in relation to type 2 diabetes in women. Diabetes Care 2006;29:650–6.
54. Knekt P, Laaksonen M, Mattila C, et al. Serum vitamin D and subsequent occurrence of type 2 diabetes. Epidemiology 2008;19:666–71.
55. Kirii K, Mizoue T, Iso H, et al. Calcium, vitamin D and dairy intake in relation to type 2 diabetes risk in a Japanese cohort. Diabetologia 2009;52:2542–50.
56. Liu E, Meigs JB, Pittas AG, et al. Predicted 25-hydroxyvitamin D score and incident type 2 diabetes in the Framingham Offspring Study. Am J Clin Nutr 2010; 91:1627–33.

57. Pittas AG, Sun Q, Manson JE, et al. Plasma 25-hydroxyvitamin D concentration and risk of incident type 2 diabetes in women. Diabetes Care 2010;33: 2021–3.

58. Anderson JL, May HT, Horne BD, et al. Relation of vitamin D deficiency to cardiovascular risk factors, disease status, and incident events in a general healthcare population. Am J Cardiol 2010;106:963–8.

59. Grimnes G, Emaus N, Joakimsen RM, et al. Baseline serum 25-hydroxyvitamin D concentrations in the Tromso Study 1994-95 and risk of developing type 2 diabetes mellitus during 11 years of follow-up. Diabet Med 2010;27: 1107–15.

60. Bolland MJ, Bacon CJ, Horne AM, et al. Vitamin D insufficiency and health outcomes over 5 y in older women. Am J Clin Nutr 2010;91:82–9.

61. Gagnon C, Lu ZX, Magliano DJ, et al. Serum 25-hydroxyvitamin D, calcium intake, and risk of type 2 diabetes after 5 years: results from a national, population-based prospective study (the Australian Diabetes, Obesity and Lifestyle study). Diabetes Care 2011;34:1133–8.

62. Robinson JG, Manson JE, Larson J, et al. Lack of association between 25(OH)D levels and incident type 2 diabetes in older women. Diabetes Care 2011;34: 628–34.

63. Thorand B, Zierer A, Huth C, et al. Effect of serum 25-hydroxyvitamin D on risk for type 2 diabetes may be partially mediated by subclinical inflammation: results from the MONICA/KORA Augsburg study. Diabetes Care 2011; 34:2320–2.

64. Pittas AG, Nelson J, Mitri J, et al. Plasma 25-hydroxyvitamin D and progression to diabetes in patients at risk for diabetes: an ancillary analysis in the Diabetes Prevention Program. Diabetes Care 2012;35:565–73.

65. Deleskog A, Hilding A, Brismar K, et al. Low serum 25-hydroxyvitamin D level predicts progression to type 2 diabetes in individuals with prediabetes but not with normal glucose tolerance. Diabetologia 2012;55:1668–78.

66. Forouhi NG, Ye Z, Rickard AP, et al. Circulating 25-hydroxyvitamin D concentration and the risk of type 2 diabetes: results from the European Prospective Investigation into Cancer (EPIC)-Norfolk cohort and updated meta-analysis of prospective studies. Diabetologia 2012;55(8):2173–82.

67. Afzal S, Bojesen SE, Nordestgaard BG. Low 25-hydroxyvitamin D and risk of type 2 diabetes: a prospective cohort study and metaanalysis. Clin Chem 2013;59:381–91.

68. Song Y, Wang L, Pittas AG, et al. Blood 25-hydroxy vitamin D levels and incident type 2 diabetes: a meta-analysis of prospective studies. Diabetes Care 2013;36: 1422–8.

69. Nilas L, Christiansen C. Treatment with vitamin D or its analogues does not change body weight or blood glucose level in postmenopausal women. Int J Obes 1984;8:407–11.

70. Pittas AG, Harris SS, Stark PC, et al. The effects of calcium and vitamin D supplementation on blood glucose and markers of inflammation in nondiabetic adults. Diabetes Care 2007;30:980–6.

71. de Boer IH, Tinker LF, Connelly S, et al. Calcium plus vitamin D supplementation and the risk of incident diabetes in the Women's Health Initiative. Diabetes Care 2008;31:701–7.

72. Avenell A, Cook JA, MacLennan GS, et al. Vitamin D supplementation and type 2 diabetes: a substudy of a randomised placebo-controlled trial in older people (RECORD trial, ISRCTN 51647438). Age Ageing 2009;38:606–9.

73. Zittermann A, Frisch S, Berthold HK, et al. Vitamin D supplementation enhances the beneficial effects of weight loss on cardiovascular disease risk markers. Am J Clin Nutr 2009;89:1321–7.

74. von Hurst PR, Stonehouse W, Coad J. Vitamin D supplementation reduces insulin resistance in South Asian women living in New Zealand who are insulin resistant and vitamin D deficient—a randomised, placebo-controlled trial. Br J Nutr 2010;103:549–55.

75. Jorde R, Sneve M, Torjesen P, et al. No improvement in cardiovascular risk factors in overweight and obese subjects after supplementation with vitamin D3 for 1 year. J Intern Med 2010;267:462–72.

76. Wood AD, Secombes KR, Thies F, et al. Vitamin D3 supplementation has no effect on conventional cardiovascular risk factors: a parallel-group, double-blind, placebo-controlled RCT. J Clin Endocrinol Metab 2012;97:3557–68.

77. Nagpal J, Pande JN, Bhartia A. A double-blind, randomized, placebo-controlled trial of the short-term effect of vitamin D3 supplementation on insulin sensitivity in apparently healthy, middle-aged, centrally obese men. Diabet Med 2009;26:19–27.

78. Knowler WC, Barrett-Connor E, Fowler SE, et al. Reduction in the incidence of type 2 diabetes with lifestyle intervention or metformin. N Engl J Med 2002; 346:393–403.

79. Mitri J, Dawson-Hughes B, Hu FB, et al. Effects of vitamin D and calcium supplementation on pancreatic beta cell function, insulin sensitivity, and glycemia in adults at high risk of diabetes: the Calcium and Vitamin D for Diabetes Mellitus (CaDDM) randomized controlled trial. Am J Clin Nutr 2011;94:486–94.

80. Nazarian S, St Peter JV, Boston RC, et al. Vitamin D3 supplementation improves insulin sensitivity in subjects with impaired fasting glucose. Transl Res 2011;158: 276–81.

81. Davidson MB, Duran P, Lee ML, et al. High-dose vitamin D supplementation in people with prediabetes and hypovitaminosis D. Diabetes Care 2013;36:260–6.

82. Sugden JA, Davies JI, Witham MD, et al. Vitamin D improves endothelial function in patients with Type 2 diabetes mellitus and low vitamin D levels. Diabet Med 2008;25:320–5.

83. Jorde R, Figenschau Y. Supplementation with cholecalciferol does not improve glycaemic control in diabetic subjects with normal serum 25-hydroxyvitamin D levels. Eur J Nutr 2009;48:349–54.

84. Witham MD, Dove FJ, Dryburgh M, et al. The effect of different doses of vitamin D(3) on markers of vascular health in patients with type 2 diabetes: a randomised controlled trial. Diabetologia 2010;53(10):2112–9.

85. Nikooyeh B, Neyestani TR, Farvid M, et al. Daily consumption of vitamin D- or vitamin D + calcium-fortified yogurt drink improved glycemic control in patients with type 2 diabetes: a randomized clinical trial. Am J Clin Nutr 2011;93:764–71.

86. Soric MM, Renner ET, Smith SR. Effect of daily vitamin D supplementation on HbA1c in patients with uncontrolled type 2 diabetes mellitus: a pilot study. J Diabetes 2012;4:104–5.

87. Punthakee Z, Bosch J, Dagenais G, et al. Design, history and results of the Thiazolidinedione Intervention with vitamin D Evaluation (TIDE) randomised controlled trial. Diabetologia 2012;55:36–45.

88. Heshmat R, Tabatabaei-Malazy O, Abbaszadeh-Ahranjani S, et al. Effect of vitamin D on insulin resistance and anthropometric parameters in Type 2 diabetes; a randomized double-blind clinical trial. Daru 2012;20:10.

89. Takiishi T, Gysemans C, Bouillon R, et al. Vitamin D and diabetes. Rheum Dis Clin North Am 2012;38:179–206.

90. Israni N, Goswami R, Kumar A, et al. Interaction of vitamin D receptor with HLA DRB1 0301 in type 1 diabetes patients from North India. PLoS One 2009;4: e8023.
91. Mathieu C, Waer M, Laureys J, et al. Prevention of autoimmune diabetes in NOD mice by 1,25 dihydroxyvitamin D3. Diabetologia 1994;37:552–8.
92. Hypponen E, Laara E, Reunanen A, et al. Intake of vitamin D and risk of type 1 diabetes: a birth-cohort study. Lancet 2001;358:1500–3.
93. Zipitis CS, Akobeng AK. Vitamin D supplementation in early childhood and risk of type 1 diabetes: a systematic review and meta-analysis. Arch Dis Child 2008; 93:512–7.
94. Sorensen IM, Joner G, Jenum PA, et al. Maternal serum levels of 25-hydroxy-vitamin D during pregnancy and risk of type 1 diabetes in the offspring. Diabetes 2012;61:175–8.
95. Gabbay MA, Sato MN, Finazzo C, et al. Effect of cholecalciferol as adjunctive therapy with insulin on protective immunologic profile and decline of residual beta-cell function in new-onset type 1 diabetes mellitus. Arch Pediatr Adolesc Med 2012;166:601–7.
96. Walter M, Kaupper T, Adler K, et al. No effect of the 1alpha,25-dihydroxyvitamin D3 on beta-cell residual function and insulin requirement in adults with new-onset type 1 diabetes. Diabetes Care 2010;33:1443–8.
97. Bizzarri C, Pitocco D, Napoli N, et al. No protective effect of calcitriol on beta-cell function in recent-onset type 1 diabetes: the IMDIAB XIII trial. Diabetes Care 2010;33:1962–3.
98. Miller ER 3rd, Pastor-Barriuso R, Dalal D, et al. Meta-analysis: high-dosage vitamin E supplementation may increase all-cause mortality. Ann Intern Med 2005;142:37–46.
99. Anderson GL, Limacher M, Assaf AR, et al. Effects of conjugated equine estrogen in postmenopausal women with hysterectomy: the Women's Health Initiative randomized controlled trial. JAMA 2004;291:1701–12.
100. Harris SS, Pittas AG, Palermo NJ. A randomized, placebo-controlled trial of vitamin D supplementation to improve glycaemia in overweight and obese African Americans. Diabetes Obes Metab 2012;14:789–94.

Osteoporosis-associated Fracture and Diabetes

Salila Kurra, MD[a],*, Dorothy A. Fink, MD[b], Ethel S. Siris, MD[c]

KEYWORDS

- Bone • Osteoporosis • Diabetes • Diabetes complications • Fracture
- Skeletal disorder

KEY POINTS

- Because osteoporosis and diabetes mellitus are chronic diseases that are increasing in prevalence, understanding their complex interaction is integral to providing optimal care for patients.
- Osteoporosis-associated fracture is an important complication of diabetes to consider when evaluating patients with diabetes.
- Given the different causes of type 1 and type 2 diabetes, they have a unique relationship with bone but also have similar effects on bone when not treated adequately.
- Osteoporosis treatment options for diabetic patients are the same as for nondiabetic patients, including ensuring normal renal function before starting a bisphosphonate.

INTRODUCTION

Osteoporosis and diabetes mellitus (DM) are chronic diseases with increasing prevalence. Both have significant associated morbidity and mortality and may lead to severe debilitation if not treated adequately. Osteoporosis is a skeletal disorder characterized by reduced bone quantity and quality, which predisposes to fracture.[1,2] Fragility fractures, or low-trauma fractures, are common, affecting almost 1 in 2 older women and 1 in 3 older men.[3] The global burden of osteoporosis is significant, with approximately 9 million new osteoporotic fractures worldwide in the year 2000.[4] Diabetes is also increasing in prevalence. Prevalence of diabetes for all age groups is estimated to be 4.4% of the worldwide population by the year 2030.[5]

Disclosures: Dr E.S. Siris is a consultant for Amgen, Eli Lilly, Merck, Novartis, and Pfizer, and a speaker for Amgen, Eli Lilly.
a Metabolic Bone Diseases Unit, Department of Medicine, Toni Stabile Osteoporosis Center, Columbia University Medical Center, 180 Fort Washington Avenue, 9-904, New York, NY 10032, USA; b Division of Endocrinology, Department of Medicine, Columbia University Medical Center, 630 West 168th Street, PH8, New York, NY 10032, USA; c Metabolic Bone Diseases Unit, Department of Medicine, Toni Stabile Osteoporosis Center, Columbia University Medical Center, New York-Presbyterian Hospital, 180 Fort Washington Avenue, 9-904, New York, NY 10032, USA
* Corresponding author.
E-mail address: sk850@columbia.edu

Endocrinol Metab Clin N Am 43 (2014) 233–243
http://dx.doi.org/10.1016/j.ecl.2013.09.004
0889-8529/14/$ – see front matter © 2014 Elsevier Inc. All rights reserved.

endo.theclinics.com

Recent evidence shows that both type 1 and type 2 DM are associated with an increased fracture risk.[6] Although microvascular and macrovascular complications are the complications most commonly associated with diabetes, osteoporosis and risk of fracture must also be considered when treating patients with diabetes. Type 1 diabetes (T1D) is defined as a state of insulin deficiency, whereas type 2 diabetes (T2D) is characterized by insulin resistance with increased insulin levels. Given the different causes of T1D and T2D, they have unique interactions with bone. Skeletal disorders often associated with diabetes include osteoporosis-associated fracture, Charcot arthropathy, and renal osteodystrophy secondary to end-stage renal disease as a complication of diabetes.[7,8] Like others in the past,[9,10] this article focuses on osteoporosis-associated fracture as a metabolic complication of diabetes.

In recent years, osteoporosis-associated fracture has come to the forefront of complications associated with diabetes. Controversy exists over the exact mechanisms of bone loss in the setting of diabetes, but there is significant evidence to support that diabetes affects bone health. The meta-analysis by Vestergaard[11] showed that adults with T1D have a 6.9 relative risk of hip fracture and adults with T2D have a 1.3 relative risk of hip fracture. In addition, a meta-analysis by Janghorbani and colleagues[12] showed similar results with a 6.3 relative risk of hip fracture in adults with T1D and a 2.8 relative risk of hip fracture in adults with T2D. In the Vestergaard[11] study, patients with T1D had decreased bone mineral density (BMD) and increased fracture risk, but although the study noted a 6.9 relative risk of hip fracture, the BMD expected relative risk was only 1.4, suggesting that there are additional factors contributing to fracture risk. Another finding of the Vestergaard[11] study was that, despite an increased fracture risk, patients with T2D had higher than expected BMD. With data from the Health, Aging, and Body Composition (Health ABC) Study, Schwartz and colleagues[13] showed increased incidence of vertebral fracture in T2D despite increased BMD. The interaction between diabetes and bone health is complex and requires further exploration.

T1D VERSUS T2D AND BONE: SIMILARITIES

Despite their different underlying causes, without proper treatment or compliance with treatment both T1D and T2D can be complicated by hyperglycemia. Hyperglycemia in turn can be detrimental to bone; it has been shown that glucose can be toxic to osteoblasts, the cells associated with bone formation. High glucose concentrations impair the ability of osteoblastic cells to synthesize osteocalcin, which is a protein integral to bone formation.[14] Also serum osteocalcin levels seem to be suppressed by hyperglycemia in diabetic patients.[15] Bone biopsies done on individuals with diabetes have shown low bone formation on histomorphometry.[16] For a given BMD, diabetic bone seems to be less strong and therefore more likely to fracture.[17,18]

Chronic hyperglycemia also promotes advanced glycation and accumulation of advanced glycation end products (AGEs), which contribute to diabetes complications. Impaired renal function is also thought to lead to accumulation of AGEs. They are formed through a nonenzymatic reaction between reducing sugars and amine residues. AGEs act directly to induce cross-linking of long-lived proteins, resulting in alteration of vascular structure and function.[19] Accumulation of AGEs in bone collagen likely contributes to the reduction in bone strength for a given BMD.[20] The prime targets of AGE accumulation are the structural components of the connective tissue matrix. This accumulation can alter collagen function and thereby alter the function of bone.

Pentosidine is the most commonly measured AGE because of its intrinsic fluorescence.[19] Complications of diabetes including nephropathy, retinopathy, neuropathy, atherosclerotic disease, cardiomyopathy, and peripheral arterial disease have been studied extensively with regard to AGEs, and diabetes-associated bone disease has also come to the forefront of AGE-related complications.[13,21–23] Katayama and colleagues[24] showed that AGE modification of type 1 collagen impaired osteoblast cell differentiation and function in rodent models. AGEs may exert their effects on the receptor for advanced glycation end products (RAGE). Zhou and colleagues[25] showed that RAGE knockout mice had increased bone mass with decreased resorption ability, leading the investigators to conclude that RAGE enhances bone resorption through osteoclasts, the cells associated with bone resorption. In postmenopausal women with T2D and vertebral fractures, Yamamoto and colleagues[21] found that there were higher serum pentosidine levels compared with controls independently of BMD and osteoporosis risk factors and even after adjusting for diabetes duration, complications, and treatment with insulin or pioglitazone.

Studies examining glycemic control and its implications on the skeleton have not shown that tight control limits osteoporosis-related fracture.[26,27] However, in most studies, a single hemoglobin A_{1c} (HbA$_{1c}$) is the only measure of diabetes control and only represents glycemic control over a short period of time. Most postmenopausal women and men with T1D and T2D who develop fractures have had diabetes for decades and it is challenging to adequately assess an individual's lifetime diabetes control. Regardless, several studies have documented increased fracture rates associated with longer duration of diabetes in patients with both T1D and T2D.[28,29] Challenges to many of these studies include confounding factors such as other complications of diabetes, which may increase fracture risk as well. For example, the aforementioned study by Ivers and colleagues[29] showed that patients with both T1D and T2D who develop the visual complications of diabetes such as diabetic retinopathy and advanced cortical cataract are also at increased risk for fracture.

Based on prospective data on falls from the Study of Osteoporotic Fractures, Schwartz and colleagues[30] found an increased risk of falls in women older than 65 years with diabetes with a further increased risk in the setting of insulin use. This increased risk of falls likely contributes to the increased risk of fracture noted in this population. Although this increased fall risk is multifactorial, the complications commonly seen with diabetes, such as poor vision, peripheral neuropathy, reduced balance, and treatment-associated hypoglycemia, are themselves risk factors for falls. However, a case-control study by Vestergaard and colleagues[31] showed that both T1D and T2D confer an increased risk of fracture, but, except for diabetic kidney disease, the other complications associated with diabetes added little to the overall risk of fracture. The investigators concluded that the hyperglycemia likely contributes to decreases in bone strength.

Low states of bone turnover have been documented in both T1D and T2D, which may lead to lower mechanical strength and an increased risk of fracture.[16,32,33] Gennari and colleagues[33] recently showed that sclerostin, which is a protein that inhibits osteoblastic bone formation, is higher in T2D compared with T1D and controls, even after adjusting for age and body mass index (BMI). However, the negative association between sclerostin and parathyroid hormone (PTH) that is normally seen was not documented in patients with T1D or T2D, leading the investigators to conclude that PTH suppression of sclerostin may be impaired in both T1D and T2D. This mechanism may be another reason for bone loss in patients with diabetes.

T1D VERSUS T2D AND BONE: DIFFERENCES

Although T1D and T2D both result in states of chronic hyperglycemia, the underlying pathophysiology of T1D and T2D is different. The anabolic hormone insulin is absent in T1D and present (often increased) in T2D. However, given the changing milieu of diabetes, many patients with T1D who are insulin deficient have a BMI in the obese range and develop an insulin-resistant phenotype. In addition, many patients with T2D require insulin as their disease progresses, further complicating the effects that diabetes has on bone health.

Literature describing bone disease in patients with T1D dates to the 1920s.[34] Although there is controversy in the literature over the mechanisms of increased fracture risk, the occurrence of low BMD and fractures is well documented in patients with T1D.[35,36] Several studies have postulated that patients with T1D do not achieve peak bone mass during adolescence, which leads to a lower lifetime BMD and may ultimately increase risk of fracture.[37,38] Although T1D may be diagnosed after puberty, peak bone mass accrual continues into the early 20s and thus may be affected by hyperglycemia as well.

Insulinlike growth factor 1 (IGF-1), which is also a marker of bone formation, has been noted to be low in patients with uncomplicated insulin-dependent DM.[39] Kemink and colleagues[39] showed that, in diabetic patients with femoral neck osteopenia, the mean plasma IGF-I level was significantly lower ($P<.05$) than in those without osteopenia at this site. When they assessed only the male diabetic patients, significantly lower mean plasma IGF-I (−26%), serum alkaline phosphatase (−24%), and serum osteocalcin (−38%) levels were present in the patients with femoral neck osteopenia than in those without osteopenia at this site, suggesting reduced bone formation. They concluded that their data showed that, at least in male patients with insulin-dependent DM, osteopenia is the consequence of a reduced bone formation with a predominance of bone resorption rather than formation. This uncoupling of bone formation and resorption resembles the effects that glucocorticoids have on bone.

The most striking difference in patients with T2D compared with patients with T1D is not only their insulin resistance but that they paradoxically have an increased BMD compared with patients with T1D.[17,40–42] Despite this increased BMD, which seems to protect against fracture, patients with T2D have an increased risk of fracture, suggesting a bone quality defect given that they have a greater quantity of bone based on BMD. Lipscombe and colleagues[43] showed an increased risk of hip fracture in patients with T2D despite an increased BMD (hazard ratio [HR], 1.18 for men and 1.11 for women).

In the Women's Health Initiative Observational Study, postmenopausal women with diabetes were at increased risk of hip, foot, and spine fractures, and fractures overall, even after adjusting for falls.[41] Other studies that accounted for falls but still found an association of T2D with fracture risk are the Study of Osteoporotic Fractures; the Rotterdam Study; and the Health, Aging, and Body Composition Study.[17,42,44]

de Liefde and colleagues[42] showed that in the Rotterdam Study there was an increased nonvertebral fracture risk in patients with T2D even though they had higher BMDs in the femoral neck and lumbar spine (HR, 1.33 [1.00–1.77]). The study also performed a subset analysis comparing patients with treated T2D with patients with impaired glucose tolerance (IGT). The patients with treated T2D had an increased nonvertebral fracture risk compared with the patients with IGT, leading the investigators to conclude that duration of diabetes affects fracture risk. Using the Study of Osteoporotic Fractures, the Osteoporotic Fractures in Men Study, and the Health ABC study, Schwartz and colleagues[45] showed that patients with T2D had a higher risk of fracture for a given T score and age or fracture risk assessment tool (FRAX) score. The mean T-score difference for hip fracture was 0.59 and 0.38 for women and men, respectively.

Another difference between patients with T1D and T2D is that patients with T2D may be treated with thiazolidinediones. Using the data from A Diabetes Outcome Progression Trial, Kahn and colleagues[46,47] found that women randomized to rosiglitazone had an increased fracture risk. In addition, the Takeda Pharmaceutical Company issued a letter in 2007 that described an increased fracture risk in women receiving pioglitazone.[48]

Most recently, in a randomized, double-blind study in postmenopausal women with T2D, Bilezikian and colleagues[49] showed reductions in femoral neck, total hip, and lumbar spine BMD with daily use of rosiglitazone for 52 weeks compared with metformin. During the 24-week open-label phase when all patients received metformin, the BMD loss associated with rosiglitazone use was attenuated. In addition, both serum c-telopeptide, which is a marker of bone resorption, and procollagen type 1 N-terminal propeptide (P1NP), which is a marker of bone formation, increased in the patients randomized to rosiglitazone. In contrast, bone-specific alkaline phosphatase (BSAP), another marker of bone formation, decreased after treatment with rosiglitazone, which was similar to the results of the study by Berberoglu and colleagues.[50] The discordance between the bone turnover markers P1NP and BSAP is not fully understood, and Bilezikian and colleagues[49] postulated that impairment in mineralization processes may be required to increase BSAP.

QUANTIFYING RISK OF FRACTURE ASSOCIATED WITH DIABETES AND OSTEOPOROSIS

As detailed earlier, there is strong evidence to suggest that diabetes, regardless of the cause, and its associated complications can lead to bone loss and increased risk of fracture. Although both T1D and T2D are listed in the National Osteoporosis Foundation (NOF) guidelines as endocrine disorders that may cause or contribute to osteoporosis and fractures, there are currently no specific guidelines for screening for fracture risk in patients with diabetes.[51] It is also not currently part of the World Health Organization FRAX algorithm for assessing fracture risk.

Age, sex, BMI, prolonged glucocorticoid use, current smoking, 3 or more units per day of alcohol, secondary osteoporosis, rheumatoid arthritis, prior fragility fracture, parental history of hip fracture, and femoral neck BMD or T score are all included in the FRAX algorithm.[52] T1D is listed as a secondary cause of osteoporosis in FRAX, but is not included in the FRAX risk calculation if the femoral neck BMD is known. T2D is not formally part of FRAX. Schwartz and colleagues[45] estimated that the mean differences in T score for women and men with diabetes were 0.59 and 0.38, respectively. Giangregorio and colleagues[6] showed that, after adjusting for confounding factors, diabetes was a significant predictor of major osteoporotic fracture (HR, 1.61).

Apart from the inclusion of T1D as a secondary risk factor for osteoporosis in the FRAX algorithm, there are no guidelines that address screening for fracture risk for patients with T1D or T2D. The 2013 NOF Clinician's Guide to Prevention and Treatment of Osteoporosis recommends that women aged 65 years and older, and men aged 70 years and older, have BMD testing with dual-energy x-ray absorptiometry (DXA).[51] They also recommend that postmenopausal women and men aged 50 to 69 years have an osteoporosis evaluation based on risk factor profile, which includes T1D and T2D. The United States Preventive Service Task Force recommendations are in agreement with the NOF guidelines.[53]

MANAGEMENT

In the Ontario population-based study, Lipscombe and colleagues[43] found that, compared with individuals without diabetes, individuals with diabetes were less likely to have had a BMD test, and were more likely to be taking medications that increase risk of falling and decrease BMD. This finding underscores the importance of education regarding diabetes and associated osteoporosis and fractures. Health care providers must include bone health as part of routine clinical care for patients with diabetes in addition to addressing microvascular and macrovascular complications. Diabetes is associated with delayed fracture healing and therefore prevention is essential.[54,55] During clinical evaluations, dairy intake should be addressed. Given the concern of calcium deposition in blood vessels instead of bones in osteoporosis,[56] patients should be questioned regarding the amount of both dairy intake and calcium supplementation to ensure adequate, but not excessive, daily calcium intake.[51] In accordance with The Institute of Medicine (IOM), the NOF recommends that women older than 50 years and men older than 70 years have a calcium intake of 1200 mg per day. Men aged 50 to 70 years are recommended to take 1000 mg per day of calcium. In addition, for adults older than 50 years, the NOF recommends 800 to 1000 international units (IU) of vitamin D per day. They recommend that 25-hydroxy (OH) vitamin D levels be measured in patients at risk for deficiency with a goal 25-OH vitamin D level of 30 ng/mL.

Given the data showing a higher risk of fracture in women with T1D, it is reasonable to order a DXA scan on these patients at menopause instead of waiting until age 65 years. Although patients with T2D are also at increased risk of fracture, their BMD results may underestimate their relative risk for fracture, as discussed earlier. A diabetic patient compared with a nondiabetic patient with the same BMD and the same osteoporosis risk factors (other than diabetes) is at a higher risk of fracture. To account for this higher risk, using evidence from Schwartz and colleagues,[45] it may be prudent to adjust T scores in women with T2D by −0.6 and men with T2D by −0.4 to have a T score that more accurately identifies the level of fracture risk. Leslie and colleagues[9] concluded that it is also prudent to consider treating patients with T2D even if they are slightly below FRAX-based intervention thresholds given the challenges of interpreting BMD results and correctly determining fracture risk in patients with T2D. In the future, T2D may be included in fracture risk algorithms.

The Action to Control Cardiovascular Risk in Diabetes (ACCORD) randomized trial did not show any differences in fracture or fall risk between the intensive and standard glycemia groups.[26] However, the median HbA_{1c} in the intensive glycemic group was 6.4% and the median HbA_{1c} in the standard glycemic strategy was 7.5%. Most patients with uncontrolled diabetes do not have HbA_{1c} in the 7% range and thus more studies need to be completed to address uncontrolled, chronic hyperglycemia with fracture and fall risk. Regardless of the ACCORD data, patients with diabetes and osteoporosis need to have personalized diabetes plans to achieve glycemic control safely. Schwartz and colleagues[27] also showed in a substudy of the ACCORD trial using peripheral quantitative computed tomographic scans that bone strength at the radius and tibia was not improved with intensive glycemic control. When interpreting these data, it is important to take into account that the standard HbA_{1c} group is not representative of many patients who have chronic, uncontrolled hyperglycemia. It is well documented that achieving adequate glycemic control in patients with diabetes decreases the incidence of microvascular complications, such as retinopathy and neuropathy, which may lead to falls and subsequent fractures. Therefore, it is important to address fall prevention as well.[30]

The NOF recommends that postmenopausal women and men older than 50 years be considered for pharmacologic treatment in addition to calcium and vitamin D if they present with one of the following[51]:

1. A hip or vertebral fracture, which is a clinical diagnosis of osteoporosis
2. A T score of ≤2.5 at the femoral neck, total hip, or lumbar spine, which is the BMD-based diagnosis of osteoporosis
3. Low bone mass (T score between −1.0 and −2.5 at the hip or spine) and a 10-year absolute probability of fracture as assessed by FRAX of greater than or equal to 3% for hip fracture or greater than or equal to 20% for major osteoporotic fracture

TREATMENT

Osteoporosis treatment options for diabetic patients are the same as for nondiabetic patients. When a patient meets guidelines for treatment, there are several options including antiresorptive medications such as bisphosphonates and the anabolic agent teriparatide.

Diabetic nephropathy may limit use of bisphosphonates because they are contraindicated if estimated glomerular filtration rate is less than 30 to 35 mL/min because they are renally cleared. Potent antiresorptives such as bisphosphonates or denosumab are also a concern if patients have renal osteodystrophy in which potent antiresorptive treatment is contraindicated. The nature of the patient's bone disorder needs to be characterized before any pharmacologic treatment of osteoporosis can be initiated.

In postmenopausal women and older men with DM who do not have severe renal failure or renal bone disease and in whom there is an increase in bone resorption exceeding that of bone formation, an antiresorptive agent may be appropriate. Vestergaard and colleagues[57] showed that bisphosphonates and raloxifene exert bone-protective effects even in diabetic patients with states of low bone turnover. Keegan and colleagues[58] also showed that BMD in patients with T2D increased after treatment with alendronate. However, in both the Vestergaard and colleagues[57] and Giangregorio and colleagues[6] studies, patients with diabetes were less likely to receive osteoporosis treatment despite having a higher prevalence of fracture.

The uncoupling of bone resorption and bone formation that is seen in patients with DM resembles the effect of glucocorticoids on bone (namely some increase in bone resorption with a decrease in bone formation) so it is possible that the agents used to treat glucocorticoid-induced osteoporosis may be effective in the reduction in fracture risk in patients with DM. Both bisphosphonates and teriparatide are approved for the treatment of glucocorticoid-induced osteoporosis. One study in patients with glucocorticoid-induced osteoporosis found that the anabolic agent teriparatide led to a greater increase in total hip BMD and fewer vertebral fractures than alendronate.[59] Following a 2-year course of teriparatide, an antiresorptive is needed to preserve the increase in bone mass from the anabolic agent. Thus, until more data are available regarding the effectiveness and safety of antiresorptives such as bisphosphonates, raloxifene or denosumab, or the anabolic agent teriparatide in patients with diabetes, it is important to base decisions regarding treatment on the individual characteristics of patients and their absolute risk for fractures.

In conclusion, diabetes and osteoporosis are both chronic diseases that may lead to severe morbidity and mortality if not treated. Diabetes-associated osteoporosis and fracture are now at the forefront of diabetes complications and must be considered in evaluating, counseling, and treating patients with diabetes.

REFERENCES

1. NIH Consensus Development Panel on Osteoporosis Prevention, Diagnosis, and Therapy. Osteoporosis prevention, diagnosis, and therapy. JAMA 2001; 285(6):785–95 Epub 2001/02/15.
2. Bone health and osteoporosis: a report of the surgeon general. Rockville (MD): U.S. Department of Health and Human Services, Office of the Surgeon General; 2004.
3. Eisman JA, Bogoch ER, Dell R, et al. Making the first fracture the last fracture: ASBMR task force report on secondary fracture prevention. J Bone Miner Res 2012;27(10):2039–46 Epub 2012/07/28.
4. Johnell O, Kanis JA. An estimate of the worldwide prevalence and disability associated with osteoporotic fractures. Osteoporos Int 2006;17(12):1726–33 Epub 2006/09/20.
5. Wild S, Roglic G, Green A, et al. Global prevalence of diabetes: estimates for the year 2000 and projections for 2030. Diabetes Care 2004;27(5):1047–53 Epub 2004/04/28.
6. Giangregorio LM, Leslie WD, Lix LM, et al. FRAX underestimates fracture risk in patients with diabetes. J Bone Miner Res 2012;27(2):301–8 Epub 2011/11/05.
7. Pei Y, Hercz G, Greenwood C, et al. Renal osteodystrophy in diabetic patients. Kidney Int 1993;44(1):159–64 Epub 1993/07/01.
8. Schwartz AV. Diabetes mellitus: does it affect bone? Calcif Tissue Int 2003;73(6): 515–9 Epub 2003/10/01.
9. Leslie WD, Rubin MR, Schwartz AV, et al. Type 2 diabetes and bone. J Bone Miner Res 2012;27(11):2231–7 Epub 2012/10/02.
10. Kurra S, Siris E. Diabetes and bone health: the relationship between diabetes and osteoporosis-associated fractures. Diabetes Metab Res Rev 2011;27(5): 430–5 Epub 2011/03/25.
11. Vestergaard P. Discrepancies in bone mineral density and fracture risk in patients with type 1 and type 2 diabetes–a meta-analysis. Osteoporos Int 2007; 18(4):427–44 Epub 2006/10/28.
12. Janghorbani M, Van Dam RM, Willett WC, et al. Systematic review of type 1 and type 2 diabetes mellitus and risk of fracture. Am J Epidemiol 2007;166(5): 495–505 Epub 2007/06/19.
13. Schwartz AV, Garnero P, Hillier TA, et al. Pentosidine and increased fracture risk in older adults with type 2 diabetes. J Clin Endocrinol Metab 2009;94(7):2380–6 Epub 2009/04/23.
14. Inaba M, Terada M, Koyama H, et al. Influence of high glucose on 1,25-dihydroxyvitamin D3-induced effect on human osteoblast-like MG-63 cells. J Bone Miner Res 1995;10(7):1050–6 Epub 1995/07/01.
15. Kanazawa I, Yamaguchi T, Yamamoto M, et al. Serum osteocalcin level is associated with glucose metabolism and atherosclerosis parameters in type 2 diabetes mellitus. J Clin Endocrinol Metab 2009;94(1):45–9 Epub 2008/11/06.
16. Krakauer JC, McKenna MJ, Buderer NF, et al. Bone loss and bone turnover in diabetes. Diabetes 1995;44(7):775–82 Epub 1995/07/01.
17. Schwartz AV, Sellmeyer DE, Ensrud KE, et al. Older women with diabetes have an increased risk of fracture: a prospective study. J Clin Endocrinol Metab 2001; 86(1):32–8 Epub 2001/03/07.
18. Verhaeghe J, Suiker AM, Einhorn TA, et al. Brittle bones in spontaneously diabetic female rats cannot be predicted by bone mineral measurements: studies in diabetic and ovariectomized rats. J Bone Miner Res 1994;9(10):1657–67 Epub 1994/10/01.

19. Goh SY, Cooper ME. Clinical review: the role of advanced glycation end products in progression and complications of diabetes. J Clin Endocrinol Metab 2008;93(4):1143–52 Epub 2008/01/10.

20. Saito M, Fujii K, Mori Y, et al. Role of collagen enzymatic and glycation induced cross-links as a determinant of bone quality in spontaneously diabetic WBN/Kob rats. Osteoporos Int 2006;17(10):1514–23 Epub 2006/06/14.

21. Yamamoto M, Yamaguchi T, Yamauchi M, et al. Serum pentosidine levels are positively associated with the presence of vertebral fractures in postmenopausal women with type 2 diabetes. J Clin Endocrinol Metab 2008;93(3):1013–9 Epub 2007/12/28.

22. Tanaka S, Kuroda T, Saito M, et al. Urinary pentosidine improves risk classification using fracture risk assessment tools for postmenopausal women. J Bone Miner Res 2011;26(11):2778–84 Epub 2011/07/21.

23. Gineyts E, Munoz F, Bertholon C, et al. Urinary levels of pentosidine and the risk of fracture in postmenopausal women: the OFELY study. Osteoporos Int 2010;21(2):243–50 Epub 2009/05/08.

24. Katayama Y, Akatsu T, Yamamoto M, et al. Role of nonenzymatic glycosylation of type I collagen in diabetic osteopenia. J Bone Miner Res 1996;11(7):931–7 Epub 1996/07/01.

25. Zhou Z, Immel D, Xi CX, et al. Regulation of osteoclast function and bone mass by RAGE. J Exp Med 2006;203(4):1067–80 Epub 2006/04/12.

26. Schwartz AV, Margolis KL, Sellmeyer DE, et al. Intensive glycemic control is not associated with fractures or falls in the ACCORD randomized trial. Diabetes Care 2012;35(7):1525–31 Epub 2012/06/23.

27. Schwartz AV, Vittinghoff E, Margolis KL, et al. Intensive glycemic control and thiazolidinedione use: effects on cortical and trabecular bone at the radius and tibia. Calcif Tissue Int 2013;92(5):477–86 Epub 2013/02/05.

28. Forsen L, Meyer HE, Midthjell K, et al. Diabetes mellitus and the incidence of hip fracture: results from the Nord-Trondelag Health Survey. Diabetologia 1999;42(8):920–5 Epub 1999/09/24.

29. Ivers RQ, Cumming RG, Mitchell P, et al. Diabetes and risk of fracture: the Blue Mountains Eye Study. Diabetes Care 2001;24(7):1198–203 Epub 2001/06/26.

30. Schwartz AV, Hillier TA, Sellmeyer DE, et al. Older women with diabetes have a higher risk of falls: a prospective study. Diabetes Care 2002;25(10):1749–54 Epub 2002/09/28.

31. Vestergaard P, Rejnmark L, Mosekilde L. Diabetes and its complications and their relationship with risk of fractures in type 1 and 2 diabetes. Calcif Tissue Int 2009;84(1):45–55 Epub 2008/12/11.

32. Shu A, Yin MT, Stein E, et al. Bone structure and turnover in type 2 diabetes mellitus. Osteoporos Int 2012;23(2):635–41 Epub 2011/03/23.

33. Gennari L, Merlotti D, Valenti R, et al. Circulating sclerostin levels and bone turnover in type 1 and type 2 diabetes. J Clin Endocrinol Metab 2012;97(5):1737–44 Epub 2012/03/09.

34. Bouillon R. Diabetic bone disease. Calcif Tissue Int 1991;49(3):155–60 Epub 1991/09/01.

35. Miao J, Brismar K, Nyren O, et al. Elevated hip fracture risk in type 1 diabetic patients: a population-based cohort study in Sweden. Diabetes Care 2005;28(12):2850–5 Epub 2005/11/25.

36. Hadjidakis DJ, Raptis AE, Sfakianakis M, et al. Bone mineral density of both genders in type 1 diabetes according to bone composition. J Diabetes Complications 2006;20(5):302–7 Epub 2006/09/05.

37. Mastrandrea LD, Wactawski-Wende J, Donahue RP, et al. Young women with type 1 diabetes have lower bone mineral density that persists over time. Diabetes Care 2008;31(9):1729–35 Epub 2008/07/02.

38. Liu EY, Wactawski-Wende J, Donahue RP, et al. Does low bone mineral density start in post-teenage years in women with type 1 diabetes? Diabetes Care 2003; 26(8):2365–9 Epub 2003/07/29.

39. Kemink SA, Hermus AR, Swinkels LM, et al. Osteopenia in insulin-dependent diabetes mellitus; prevalence and aspects of pathophysiology. J Endocrinol Invest 2000;23(5):295–303 Epub 2000/07/06.

40. Melton LJ 3rd, Riggs BL, Leibson CL, et al. A bone structural basis for fracture risk in diabetes. J Clin Endocrinol Metab 2008;93(12):4804–9 Epub 2008/09/18.

41. Bonds DE, Larson JC, Schwartz AV, et al. Risk of fracture in women with type 2 diabetes: the Women's Health Initiative Observational Study. J Clin Endocrinol Metab 2006;91(9):3404–10 Epub 2006/06/29.

42. de Liefde II, van der Klift M, de Laet CE, et al. Bone mineral density and fracture risk in type-2 diabetes mellitus: the Rotterdam Study. Osteoporos Int 2005; 16(12):1713–20 Epub 2005/06/09.

43. Lipscombe LL, Jamal SA, Booth GL, et al. The risk of hip fractures in older individuals with diabetes: a population-based study. Diabetes Care 2007;30(4): 835–41 Epub 2007/03/30.

44. Strotmeyer ES, Cauley JA, Schwartz AV, et al. Nontraumatic fracture risk with diabetes mellitus and impaired fasting glucose in older white and black adults: the health, aging, and body composition study. Ann Intern Med 2005;165(14): 1612–7 Epub 2005/07/27.

45. Schwartz AV, Vittinghoff E, Bauer DC, et al. Association of BMD and FRAX score with risk of fracture in older adults with type 2 diabetes. JAMA 2011;305(21): 2184–92 Epub 2011/06/03.

46. Kahn SE, Zinman B, Lachin JM, et al. Rosiglitazone-associated fractures in type 2 diabetes: an Analysis from A Diabetes Outcome Progression Trial (ADOPT). Diabetes Care 2008;31(5):845–51 Epub 2008/01/29.

47. Kahn SE, Haffner SM, Heise MA, et al. Glycemic durability of rosiglitazone, metformin, or glyburide monotherapy. N Engl J Med 2006;355(23):2427–43 Epub 2006/12/06.

48. Takeda Pharmaceutical Company. Observation of an increased incidence of fractures in female patients who received long-term treatment with ACTOS (pioglitazone HCl) tablets for type 2 diabetes mellitus (letter to health care providers). Osaka (Japan): Takeda Pharmaceutical Company; 2007.

49. Bilezikian JP, Josse RG, Eastell R, et al. Rosiglitazone decreases bone mineral density and increases bone turnover in postmenopausal women with type 2 diabetes mellitus. J Clin Endocrinol Metab 2013;98(4):1519–28 Epub 2013/03/02.

50. Berberoglu Z, Gursoy A, Bayraktar N, et al. Rosiglitazone decreases serum bone-specific alkaline phosphatase activity in postmenopausal diabetic women. J Clin Endocrinol Metab 2007;92(9):3523–30 Epub 2007/06/28.

51. Cosman F, Lindsay R, LeBeur MS, et al. Clinician's guide to prevention and treatment of osteoporosis. Washington, DC: National Osteoporosis Foundation; 2013. p. 1–53.

52. Kanis JA, Johnell O, Oden A, et al. FRAX and the assessment of fracture probability in men and women from the UK. Osteoporos Int 2008;19(4):385–97 Epub 2008/02/23.

53. Nelson HD, Haney EM, Dana T, et al. Screening for osteoporosis: an update for the U.S. Preventive Services Task Force. Ann Intern Med 2010;153(2):99–111 Epub 2010/07/14.

54. Cozen L. Does diabetes delay fracture healing? Clin Orthop Relat Res 1972;82: 134–40 Epub 1972/01/01.

55. Chaudhary SB, Liporace FA, Gandhi A, et al. Complications of ankle fracture in patients with diabetes. J Am Acad Orthop Surg 2008;16(3):159–70 Epub 2008/03/05.

56. Vestergaard P. Acute myocardial infarction and atherosclerosis of the coronary arteries in patients treated with drugs against osteoporosis: calcium in the vessels and not the bones? Calcif Tissue Int 2012;90(1):22–9 Epub 2011/11/29.

57. Vestergaard P, Schwartz F, Rejnmark L, et al. Risk of femoral shaft and subtrochanteric fractures among users of bisphosphonates and raloxifene. Osteoporos Int 2011;22(3):993–1001 Epub 2010/12/18.

58. Keegan TH, Schwartz AV, Bauer DC, et al. Effect of alendronate on bone mineral density and biochemical markers of bone turnover in type 2 diabetic women: the fracture intervention trial. Diabetes Care 2004;27(7):1547–53 Epub 2004/06/29.

59. Saag KG, Shane E, Boonen S, et al. Teriparatide or alendronate in glucocorticoid-induced osteoporosis. N Engl J Med 2007;357(20):2028–39 Epub 2007/11/16.

Relationships Between Diabetes and Cognitive Impairment

Suzanne M. de la Monte, MD, MPH[a,b,c,d],*

KEYWORDS

- Diabetes • Insulin resistance • Cognitive impairment • Neurodegeneration
- Alzheimer disease • Insulin sensitizers • Obesity

KEY POINTS

- Alzheimer disease is a neurodegenerative disease associated with impairments in glucose metabolism and insulin resistance in the brain.
- Many of the molecular and biochemical defects in Alzheimer disease are identical to those in either type 1 or type 2 diabetes mellitus as well as other insulin-resistance disease states.
- Peripheral insulin-resistance disease states, including diabetes, obesity, and nonalcoholic fatty liver disease, are associated with cognitive impairment and can exacerbate Alzheimer disease, (ie, cause it to progress).
- Therapeutic measures used for diabetes show efficacy in the early and moderate stages of Alzheimer disease.
- Endocrinologists and diabetologists should play a larger role in the early detection and monitoring of cognitive impairment in obese and/or diabetic patients.

INTRODUCTION

Like most organ systems throughout the body, the brain requires insulin and insulinlike growth factors (IGFs) to maintain energy metabolism, cell survival, and homeostasis. In addition, insulin and IGFs support neuronal plasticity and cholinergic functions, which are needed for learning, memory, and myelin maintenance. Impairments in insulin and IGF signaling, caused by receptor resistance or ligand deficiency, disrupt

The author has no competing interests.

Funding sources are grants AA-11431 and AA-12908 from the National Institutes of Health.

[a] Department of Pathology (Neuropathology), Rhode Island Hospital, Warren Alpert Medical School of Brown University, Providence, RI, USA; [b] Department of Neurology, Rhode Island Hospital, Warren Alpert Medical School of Brown University, Providence, RI, USA; [c] Department of Neurosurgery, Rhode Island Hospital, Warren Alpert Medical School of Brown University, Providence, RI, USA; [d] Department of Medicine, Rhode Island Hospital, Warren Alpert Medical School of Brown University, Providence, RI, USA

* Pierre Galletti Research Building, Rhode Island Hospital, 55 Claverick Street, 4th Floor, Room 419, Providence, RI 02903.

E-mail address: Suzanne_DeLaMonte_MD@Brown.edu

Endocrinol Metab Clin N Am 43 (2014) 245–267

http://dx.doi.org/10.1016/j.ecl.2013.09.006
endo.theclinics.com

energy balance and disable networks that support a broad range of brain functions. Over the past several years, evidence that impairment in brain insulin and IGF signaling mediates cognitive impairment and neurodegeneration has grown, particularly in relation to mild cognitive impairment and Alzheimer disease (AD). Although amyloid deposits and phospho-tau–associated neuronal cytoskeletal lesions account for some AD-associated brain abnormalities, they do not explain the prominent and well-documented deficits in brain metabolism that begin very early in the course of the disease. Metabolic derangements in AD are similar to those in both type 1 type and 2 diabetes mellitus. However, the consequences of insulin/IGF receptor resistance and ligand deficiency include cognitive impairment and neurodegeneration caused by deficits in signaling through progrowth, proplasticity, and prosurvival pathways.

How brain insulin/IGF resistance and deficiency develop is not completely understood. Although a considerable number of studies have linked the recently increased rates of AD to other insulin resistance states, including obesity, type 2 diabetes mellitus (T2DM), nonalcoholic fatty liver disease (NAFLD), and metabolic syndrome, it is important to realize that most cases of sporadic (nonfamilial) AD arise with no evidence of peripheral insulin-resistance disease. This review focuses on how peripheral insulin-resistance diseases, including diabetes mellitus, contribute to cognitive impairment and neurodegeneration. The working hypothesis is that peripheral insulin resistance promotes or exacerbates cognitive impairment and neurodegeneration by causing brain insulin resistance. Mechanistically, insulin resistance with dysregulated lipid metabolism leads to increased inflammation, cytotoxic lipid production, oxidative and endoplasmic reticulum (ER) stress, and worsening of insulin resistance. Some investigators are researching the role of cytotoxic ceramides that can promote inflammation, oxidative stress, and insulin resistance. Ceramides generated in liver or visceral fat can leak into peripheral blood because of local cellular injury or death, cross the blood-brain barrier, and initiate or propagate a cascade of neurodegeneration mediated by brain insulin resistance, inflammation, stress, and cell death (**Fig. 1**). These concepts help delineate the strategies needed to detect, monitor, treat, and prevent AD as well as other major insulin-resistance diseases.

INSULIN SIGNALING
The Master Hormone

Insulin is a 5800 Da, 51 amino acid polypeptide, composed of A (21 residues) and B (30 residues) chains linked by disulfide bonds. Banting, Best and others are credited for discovering insulin in pancreatic secretions,[1,2] and later it was shown that it reversed hyperglycemia.[3] Nearly 30 years later, methods to stabilize insulin, prolong its actions, and delay its absorption emerged; 50 years after its discovery, 99% pure insulin, free of proinsulin and other islet polypeptides, was produced.[4] Genetic engineering and yeast fermentation technology have enabled human insulin to be efficiently produced on a large scale.[5] The field continues to evolve, with some of the latest advances directed toward replacing injectable insulin with an oral form[6] and optimizing approaches for intranasal delivery of insulin to treat diabetes or cognitive impairment (see later discussion).[7–9]

Insulin-Stimulated Effects

The main targets of insulin stimulation include skeletal muscle, adipose tissue, and liver, although virtually all organs, tissues, and cell types are responsive to insulin. Insulin regulates glucose uptake and utilization by cells and free fatty acid levels in peripheral blood. Free fatty acids are substrates for generating complex lipids. In skeletal

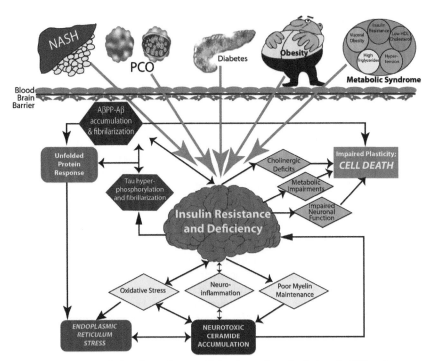

Fig. 1. Concept: Systemic insulin-resistance diseases mediate brain insulin/IGF resistance and neurodegeneration. In T2DM, nonalcoholic steatohepatitis (NASH), visceral obesity, and metabolic syndrome, dysregulated lipid metabolism causes oxidative stress and increased levels of toxic lipids, such as ceramides, which can cross the blood-brain barrier to promote brain insulin resistance. The molecular and biochemical consequences of brain insulin resistance are nearly identical to those in non–central nervous system organs and tissues (ie, oxidative stress, inflammation, ER stress, metabolic impairments, and local accumulations of neurotoxic lipids, [eg, ceramides]). However, the structural consequences are that the brain undergoes atrophy with progressive cell loss, white matter fiber and myelin degeneration, and synaptic disconnection, leading to impairments in learning and memory. Ultimately, a self-reinforcing cycle of neurodegeneration gets established, making it impossible to halt neurodegeneration by one mechanism. Instead, multipronged efforts must be used, including treatment of systemic insulin-resistance diseases. AβPP, amyloid-beta precursor protein; HDL, high-density lipoprotein; PCO, polycystic ovarian syndrome.

muscle, insulin stimulates glucose uptake by inducing translocation of the glucose transporter protein, GLUT4, from the Golgi to the plasma membrane.[10] In liver, insulin stimulates lipogenesis and triglyceride storage and inhibits gluconeogenesis. In adipose tissue, insulin decreases lipolysis and fatty acid efflux.[11] These prometabolic effects of insulin on glucose and free fatty acid disposal help to maintain energy balance.

IGFs

Insulin is closely related to IGF-1, which is also referred to as *somatomedin C* or *mechano growth factor*.[12,13] IGF-1 regulates growth during development and exerts anabolic effects on mature organs and tissues. IGF-1 contains 70 amino acids (7649 Da) in a single chain with 3 intramolecular disulfide bridges.[12,13] IGF-1 and IGF-2 are abundantly produced in liver and regulated by IGF-binding proteins.[14]

Insulin and IGF Signaling in the Brain

Within the last 15 to 20 years, information has steadily emerged about the expression and function of insulin and IGF polypeptides and receptors in the brain. It is now known that insulin and IGF signal to regulate a broad array of neuronal and glial activities, including growth, survival, metabolism, gene expression, protein synthesis, cytoskeletal assembly, synapse formation, neurotransmitter function, and plasticity,[15,16] which are needed to support cognitive function. Insulin, IGF-1, and IGF-2 polypeptide and receptor genes are expressed in neurons[15] and glial cells[17,18] throughout the brain; but their highest levels are within structures targeted by neurodegeneration.[15,19,20] Since genes that encode insulin, IGFs, and insulin-like peptides and their receptors have been identified in human, rodent, and drosophila brains,[21] related signaling networks allow for local control of diverse functions, including energy metabolism.

Insulin and IGF Signal Transduction

Brain insulin/IGF signaling mechanisms are virtually the same as in other organs. The networks are activated by ligand binding to specific receptors and subsequent activation of receptor tyrosine kinases and downstream signaling through insulin receptor substrate (IRS) proteins. The attendant activation of phosphoinositol-3-kinase (PI3K)-Akt and extracellular mitogen-activated protein kinase and the inhibition of glycogen synthase kinase 3β (GSK-3β) promote growth, survival, metabolism, and plasticity and inhibit apoptosis.[20]

INSULIN RESISTANCE AND NEURODEGENERATION
Insulin Resistance and its Consequences

Insulin resistance is classically defined as the state in which high levels of circulating insulin (hyperinsulinemia) are associated with hyperglycemia. The concept has broadened to include organ- and tissue-related impairments in insulin signaling associated with reduced activation of the pathways. As a result, progressively higher levels of ligand are needed to achieve normal insulin actions.[10] However, sustained high levels of insulin can cause insulin resistance,[22] thereby worsening and possibly broadening tissue involvement. Furthermore, hyperinsulinemia impairs insulin secretion from β cells in pancreatic islets, yielding hybrid states of both insulin resistance and insulin deficiency.[22]

Long-term consequences of insulin resistance include cellular energy failure (lack of fuel), elevated plasma lipids, and hypertension. In addition, chronic hyperinsulinemia vis-à-vis normoglycemia predicts future development of diabetes mellitus.[23] Insulin resistance is an independent predictor of serious diseases, including cerebrovascular and cardiovascular disease, hypertension, and malignancy.[24–28] Insulin resistance is now front and center stage because of its link to obesity, T2DM, NAFLD, metabolic syndrome, polycystic ovarian disease, age-related macular degeneration, and AD epidemics (**Fig. 2**).

AD Occurrence and Clinical Diagnosis

AD is the most common cause of dementia in North America. Sporadic AD has no clear genetic transmission and accounts for more than 90% of the cases. In contrast, familial (heritable) AD accounts for 5% to 10% of all cases. Over the past few decades, sporadic AD has become epidemic, raising questions about environmental and lifestyle mediators of cognitive impairment and neurodegeneration.[29] Although the clinical diagnosis of AD is based on criteria set by the National Institute of Neurologic

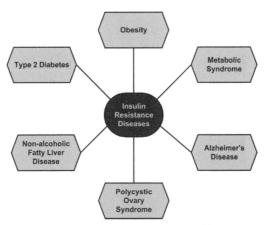

Fig. 2. Spectrum of insulin-resistance diseases affecting different primary target organs. Overlap among these diseases occurs frequently, and rates have increased with the obesity epidemic.

and Communicative Disorders and Stroke, the Alzheimer's Disease and Related Disorders Association, and the *Diagnostic and Statistical Manual of Mental Disorders* (Fourth Edition),[30] neuroimaging and a few biomarker panels have facilitated the detection of early brain metabolic derangements in AD.[31]

AD Neuropathology

Neuropathologic hallmarks of AD include neuronal loss, abundant accumulations of abnormal, hyperphosphorylated cytoskeletal proteins in neuronal perikarya and dystrophic fibers, and increased expression and abnormal processing of amyloid-beta precursor protein (AβPP), leading to AβPP-Aβ peptide deposition in neurons, plaques, and vessels. A definitive diagnosis of AD requires more-than-normal aging densities of neurofibrillary tangles, neuritic plaques, and AβPP-Aβ deposits in the brain but particularly in corticolimbic structures (**Figs. 3–5**). The pathognomonic molecular abnormalities that correspond with these dementia-associated structural lesions include accumulations of insoluble aggregates of abnormally phosphorylated and ubiquitinated tau, and neurotoxic AβPP-Aβ as oligomers, fibrillar aggregates, or plaques. Secreted neurotoxic AβPP-Aβ oligomers inhibit synaptic plasticity, learning, and memory via impairments in hippocampal long-term potentiation.[32]

AD is a Metabolic Disease with Brain Insulin/IGF Resistance

For the better part of the last 3 decades, AD research was largely focused on the pathogenic roles of hyperphosphorylated tau and AβPP-Aβ, despite hints that insulin resistance and metabolic dysfunction were important factors.[33,34] With the wealth of data collected over the past 8 to10 years, it is fair to state that AD should be regarded as a metabolic disease that is mediated by brain insulin and IGF resistance.[35,36] This concept is supported by the findings that AD shares many features in common with systemic insulin-resistance diseases. For example, reduced insulin-stimulated growth and survival signaling, increased oxidative stress, proinflammatory cytokine activation, mitochondrial dysfunction, and impaired energy metabolism all occur in peripheral insulin-resistance diseases as well as in AD (**Table 1**).[20,37,38] In the early stages of disease, AD is marked by reductions in cerebral glucose utilization[39–41]; as AD progresses, brain metabolic derangements,[42,43] including impairments in insulin

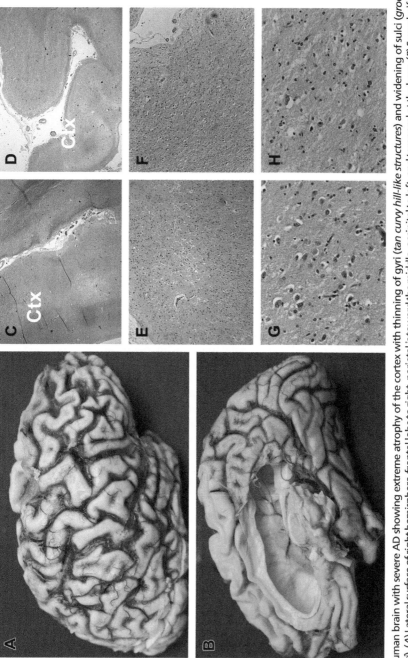

Fig. 3. Human brain with severe AD showing extreme atrophy of the cortex with thinning of gyri (*tan curvy hill-like structures*) and widening of sulci (*grooves between gyri*). (*A*) Lateral surface of right hemisphere–frontal lobe to right, parietal is toward the middle, occipital to left, and temporal at the base. (*B*) Same half-brain as in (*A*) showing medial surface with frontal pole to the left, occipital on the right. Frontal, parietal, and temporal lobes are markedly atrophic. (*C, E, G*) Represent histologic images of the left temporal lobe and (*D, F, H*) represent the right temporal lobe shown at low (*C, D*), medium (*E, F*) and high (*G, H*) magnifications to illustrate more severe atrophy of the cortex (Ctx) with extensive replacement of neurons in the right compared with left temporal lobe. Note absence (loss) of large neuronal cell bodies in (*H*) compared with (*G*). Both sides are severely damaged; but asymmetry is not uncommon, meaning that neurodegeneration does not arise in all brain regions or progress in both hemispheres at the same time ([*C–H*] Luxol fast blue, hematoxylin-eosin, original magnifications: *C, D* = ×20; *E, F* = ×100; *G, H* = ×400).

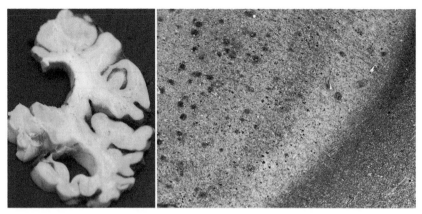

Fig. 4. Left: Coronal section through the right cerebral hemisphere showing extreme atrophy of the hippocampus, thalamus, and white matter, with compensatory enlargement of the ventricles. Right: Histologic section through the hippocampus stained to illustrate abundant senile plaques and neurofibrillary tangles replacing the normal architecture (Bielschowsky silver impregnation) (original magnification ×100).

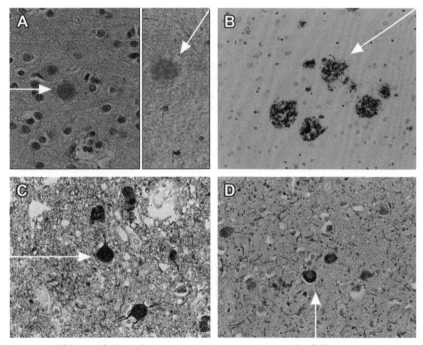

Fig. 5. Typical histopathologic lesions in AD. Arrows point to the following: (A) dense core plaques in cerebral cortex (*Congo red*); (B) amyloid precursor protein-amyloid beta (AβPP-Aβ) immunoreactivity in cortical plaques; (C) phospho-tau immunoreactive neurofibrillary tangles accumulated in cortical neurons; and (D) ubiquitin immunostained neurofibrillary tangles in neurons. Fine dotlike and linear structures in the background neutrophil of (C, D) represent dystrophic neuritis. Immunoreactivity was detected with biotinylated secondary antibody, horseradish peroxidase conjugated streptavidin, and diaminobenzidine (brown precipitate). Background structures were stained with hematoxylin (original magnifications: A, C, D = ×200; B = ×100).

Table 1
Mechanisms and consequences of cellular injury and degeneration in insulin-resistance diseases

Mediator of Injury	Mechanisms and Consequences of Injury
Inflammation	Activation of proinflammatory cytokines
Stress	ER, oxidative, and nitrosative stress; DNA, RNA, protein damage and adduct formation
Cell injury/death	Activation of proapoptosis pathways
Metabolic deficiencies	Dysregulated lipid metabolism, lipid peroxidation
Mitochondrial dysfunction	Reduced ATP production, increased reactive oxygen species
Vascular	Stress and mechanical injuy, ischemic tissue damage, end-organ hypertensive injury with microhemorrhages and toxin exposure

signaling, insulin-responsive gene expression, glucose utilization, and energy production, and stress worsen.[35,36,44]

Brain Insulin and IGF Resistance and Deficiency in AD-Human Studies

Human postmortem studies have convincingly shown that brain insulin resistance with reduced activation of receptors and downstream neuronal survival and plasticity mechanisms are consistent and fundamental abnormalities in AD.[35,36,44] Importantly, IGF-1 and IGF-2 networks were also found to be impaired,[35,36] meaning that their crosstalk functions were also deficient. Deficits in brain insulin and IGF signaling worsen as AD progresses,[35] along with declines in brain energy production, gene expression, and plasticity.[33] One of the most important realizations from these studies was that nearly all of the critical features of AD, including the activation of the kinases responsible for aberrant phosphorylation of tau and formation of neurofibrillary tangles, dystrophic neuritic plaques and neutrophil threads, AβPP and accumulation and toxicity, oxidative and endoplasmic reticulum stress, mitochondrial dysfunction, and cholinergic dyshomeostasis, can be explained by brain insulin/IGF resistance.

Does AD = Type 3 Diabetes?

Although the term type 3 diabetes is controversial, it serves to inform that the fundamental abnormalities in AD are quite similar to those present in type 1 and type 2 diabetes, except the primary target is the brain.[35,36] Like type 1 diabetes (T1DM) in which insulin deficiency is the underlying problem, in AD, neuronal expression of insulin polypeptide gene and insulin levels in brain and cerebrospinal fluid (CSF) are reduced.[34–36] As in T2DM, which has insulin resistance at its core, early AD is marked by insulin resistance and desensitization of insulin receptors in the brain; as AD progresses, these deficits worsen. In essence, AD can be regarded as a brain form of diabetes that has elements of both insulin resistance (T2DM) and insulin deficiency (T1DM). Although T1DM and T2DM can be associated with cognitive impairment and drive the onset or worsen the clinical course of AD, it is important to know that AD often occurs in people who do not have diabetes mellitus (**Table 2**). The notion that AD is a diabetes-type metabolic disease that is mediated by brain insulin and IGF resistance is further supported by human and experimental studies showing neuroprotective effects of glucagonlike peptide-1,[45] IGF-1,[46] and caloric restriction[47] with respect to brain aging and insulin resistance.

Table 2
Comparison of T1DM, T2DM, and type 3 diabetes

Target Effects	T1DM	T2DM	Type 3 Diabetes
Insulin ligand	Reduced	Increased	Reduced
Insulin receptor	Unaffected or increased	Reduced activation	Reduced activation and expression
Glucose utilization	Decreased	Decreased	Decreased
Primary targets	Pancreas, (brain)	Skeletal muscle, adipose tissue, vessels	Brain: neurons, white matter
Secondary targets	Brain, retina, blood vessels, kidneys, skin, peripheral and autonomic nerves	Brain, blood vessels, kidneys, peripheral and autonomic nerves, retina, skin	Brain satiety centers with increased proneness to obesity

The inclusion of AD within the spectrum of insulin-resistance diseases opens doors for endocrinologists and specifically diabetologists to detect disease earlier in patients with overlapping organ-system involvement and also helps design and monitor the effects of treatment. The wealth of clinical, translational, and basic science data accrued by experts in the field could be extended to AD to accelerate the development of programs to better control and possibly cure AD. Similarly, the clustering of other insulin-resistance diseases, such as metabolic syndrome, NAFLD, and polycystic ovarian disease, under one analytical roof could lead to better management of these diseases and also increase the likelihood that their causes could be found.

Experimental Evidence that Type 3 Diabetes = Sporadic AD

Experimental intracerebroventricular injections of streptozotocin, a prodiabetes drug, produce deficits in brain energy metabolism,[48] impairments in spatial learning and memory, brain insulin resistance, brain insulin deficiency, and AD-type neurodegeneration but not diabetes mellitus.[48,49] In contrast, intraperitoneal or intravenous administration of streptozotocin causes diabetes mellitus with mild hepatic steatosis and modest degrees of neurodegeneration.[50,51] Therefore, these experiments unequivocally demonstrate that brain diabetes (type 3) can occur independent of T1DM and T2DM and vice versa (**Fig. 6**).

Because streptozotocin is a nitrosamine-related toxin, which may be highly relevant to its overall effects, the specific consequences of brain insulin and IGF resistance are not tested by models generated with this and related compounds. To address this point, further studies were performed using small interfering RNA (siRNA) duplex molecules to silence insulin or IGF receptor expression in the brain.[52] This approach avoided the genotoxic and nitrosative damage produced by streptozotocin.[50] The inhibition of brain insulin and IGF receptor expression with siRNA molecules was found to be sufficient to cause cognitive impairment and hippocampal degeneration with AD-type impairments in protein and gene expression.[52] However, the phenotype was mild compared with the effects of streptozotocin. Therefore, oxidative and nitrosative damage may also be needed to produce a model that is entirely reflective of sporadic AD in humans.

Metabolic Deficits in AD: the Starving Brain

Insulin and IGF signaling regulate glucose utilization and ATP production in the brain. In AD, deficits in cerebral glucose utilization and metabolism occur early and before

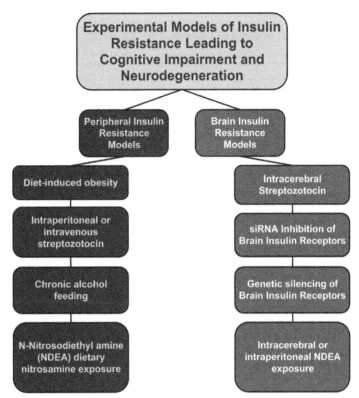

Fig. 6. Experimental models of peripheral and brain insulin resistance that lead to neurode-generation. siRNA, small interfering RNA.

cognitive decline.[53] Therefore, impairments in brain insulin signaling are probably pivotal to AD pathogenesis.[36] Oxidative stress stemming from insulin resistance or other superimposed diseases can damage mitochondria, further impairing electron transport and ATP production. In addition, oxidative stress activates proinflammatory networks that cause organelle dysfunction; disinhibits proapoptosis mechanisms; stimulates AβPP expression[54] and cleavage to neurotoxic fibrils[55]; and activates GSK-3β, which promotes tau phosphorylation (**Table 3**).[15,35,56]

The glucose transporter 4 (GLUT4) mediates glucose uptake in the brain,[57] which is abundantly expressed along with insulin receptors in the medial temporal lobe and other targets of AD.[15,20] Insulin stimulates GLUT4 mRNA expression and GLUT4 protein trafficking from the Golgi to the plasma membrane where it engages in glucose uptake. In AD, because GLUT4 expression is preserved,[36] deficits in brain glucose utilization and energy metabolism vis-à-vis brain insulin/IGF resistance could be mediated in part by functional impairments in GLUT4 (ie, posttranslational mechanisms responsible for GLUT4 trafficking to the plasma membrane).

Chronic Ischemic Cerebral Microvascular Disease

Cerebral microvascular disease is a consistent feature of AD, and recognized mediator of cognitive impairment (**Fig. 7**). Postmortem studies demonstrated similar degrees of dementia in people with severe classical AD and those with moderate AD plus chronic ischemic encephalopathy. The ischemic injury mainly consists of

Table 3
Role of insulin resistance or insulin deficiency in the molecular and pathologic features of AD

Alzheimer Pathology	Role of Insulin Resistance/Deficiency
Phospho-tau neuronal cytoskeletal lesions	Increased activation of GSK-3β caused by inhibition of insulin signaling and increased oxidative stress
Amyloid pathology	Formation of toxic amyloid-beta soluble oligomeric fibrils
Cell injury/death	Activation of proapoptosis pathways; inhibition of prosurvival mechanisms; increased endoplasmic reticulum, oxidative, and nitrosative stress; macromolecular adducts
Impaired glucose utilization	Reduced glucose uptake, impaired GLUT4 function, reduced signaling downstream of the insulin receptor through IRS, PI3K, and Akt
Impaired learning and memory	Inhibition of growth pathways needed for synapse formation and remodeling, reduced cholinergic and other neurotransmitter functions, impaired neurogenesis
Microvascular disease	Hyperinsulinemia in T2DM, possibly local insulin resistance
White matter atrophy	Cerebral microvascular disease, inhibition of myelin maintenance by oligodendrocytes
Cholinergic functional deficits	Inhibition of choline acetyltransferase expression, which is regulated by insulin/IGF-1
Mitochondrial dysfunction	Oxidative stress-induced DNA damage leading to reduced ATP production and increased levels of reactive oxygen species
Neuroinflammation	Activation of proinflammatory cytokines

multifocal small infarcts and leukoaraiosis (ie, extensive white matter fiber attrition with pallor of myelin staining) and prominent cerebral microvascular disease (see **Fig. 7**; **Fig. 8**).[58] T2DM and hypertension cause microvascular disease throughout the body, including the brain. Evidence that microvascular disease contributes to neurodegeneration was suggested by the finding that the medial temporal lobe, which houses the hippocampus, undergoes progressive atrophy with advancing stages of T2DM.[59] Perhaps the regular finding of chronic ischemic leukoencephalopathy (white matter atrophy and fiber degeneration) with microvascular disease in AD is just another manifestation of brain diabetes. It is noteworthy that besides the impairments in brain glucose metabolism, white matter atrophy is one of the earliest abnormalities in AD.[60]

Hyperinsulinemia causes progressive injury to microvessels. Chronic microvascular injury is characterized by reactive proliferation of endothelial cells, thickening of the intima, fibrosis of the media, and narrowing of the lumens. Mural scarring reduces vascular compliance and compromises blood flow and nutrient delivery, particularly in periods of high metabolic demand. Moreover, weakened and damaged blood vessels are leaky and permeable to toxins,[61,62] which together could contribute to increased frequencies of microhemorrhage and perivascular white matter tissue loss in T2DM and AD. Therefore, hyperinsulinemia ultimately produces a state of chronic hypoperfusion with toxic/metabolic/ischemic tissue degeneration in the brain. These pathologic processes have not received adequate attention, and their mechanistic links to cognitive impairment in diabetes and AD are only in the rudimentary stages of investigation.

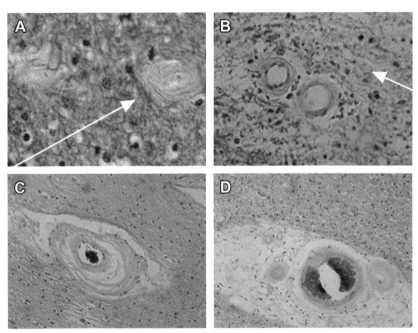

Fig. 7. Microvascular disease contributes to cognitive impairment and neurodegeneration in AD. (*A*) Arteriolosclerosis and capillary sclerosis are associated with fibrotic thickening of vessel walls and extreme narrowing of the lumens (*arrow*). (*B*) Arteriosclerosis results in chronic ischemic injury with rarefaction of white matter fibers (loss of dense Luxol fast blue myelin staining in vicinity of blood vessels [*arrow*]). Note fibrosis of vessel walls and perivascular microhemorrhages in center. These abnormalities reflect increased stiffness and reduce vascular compliance, together with weakness and leakiness of vascular walls. (*C*) Marked fibrotic thickening and damage to vessel wall caused by destruction (clearing) of the media. Tissue surrounding vessel in center is lost. Adjacent myelin is stained blue (Luxol fast blue). (*D*) Large area of perivascular tissue loss and further pallor adjacent to lacunar infarct. Note small vessels with tiny lumens and rigid fibrotic vessels in the middle of the perivascular lacunar infarct ([*A–D*] Luxol fast blue, hematoxylin-eosin).

BRAIN METABOLIC DERANGEMENTS IN OTHER NEURODEGENERATIVE DISEASES

Advances in neuroimaging, including positron emission tomography, magnetic resonance imaging (MRI), functional MRI, and magnetic spectroscopy, together with molecular and biochemical biomarkers have helped demonstrate the common themes surrounding disease mechanisms among clinically and pathologically diverse sets of neurodegenerative diseases.[63–65] For example, like AD, other major neurodegenerative diseases are associated with deficits in brain metabolism. Parkinson-dementia with Lewy bodies (DLB), frontotemporal lobar dementia, motor neuron disease, and multiple systems atrophy are all associated with brain accumulations of misfolded ubiquitinated proteins (often cytoskeletal) and increased levels of oxidative stress, neuroinflammation, autophagy, mitochondrial dysfunction, apoptosis, and necrosis.[66–70] Parkinson disease (PD) has epidemiologic links to diabetes mellitus,[45] and experimental PD is associated with insulin resistance in the basal ganglia.[71] Finally, impairments in insulin and IGF signaling exist in human brains with PD or DLB, although the nature and distribution of abnormalities differ from those in AD.[72] Therefore, many sporadic human neurodegenerative diseases could potentially be

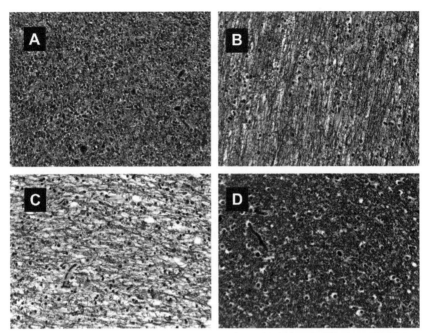

Fig. 8. White matter fiber loss in AD. Myelin is produced by oligodendrocytes, which are insulin and IGF-1 responsive. Insulin resistance impairs oligodendrocyte function. In AD, brain insulin/IGF-1 resistance develop early in the course of neurodegeneration, and the earliest abnormalities include impairments in glucose metabolism and white matter atrophy. White matter from the (A) anterior frontal, (B) posterior frontal, (C) parietal, and (D) occipital lobes (Luxol fast blue). The normal appearance of staining is depicted in (D), an area least affected by AD. The pink coloration in (A, B) reflect loss of myelin and myelinated fibers. The extreme pallor of myelin staining in (C) corresponds to the severity of neurodegeneration and extensive fiber loss.

approached from diagnostic and therapeutic perspectives through knowledge gained in endocrinology and specifically diabetology.

UNDERLYING CAUSES OF BRAIN INSULIN RESISTANCE IN AD
Aging

Insulin and IGF resistance increase with aging, whereas longevity is associated with the preservation of insulin/IGF responsiveness.[73–75] Furthermore, evidence suggests that chronic stress over a lifespan damages cells because of excessive signaling through insulin/IGF-1 receptors.[76] Correspondingly, neuronal overexpression of IRS2 leads to increased fat mass, insulin resistance, and glucose intolerance with aging.[77] These findings suggest that chronic overuse of insulin/IGF signaling networks, which occurs with hyperinsulinemia and insulin resistance, accelerates aging.

Declines in growth hormone levels and metabolism also promote aging because of the anabolic deficiencies that accelerate metabolic dysfunction.[78] Because growth hormone deficiency promotes obesity[79] and obesity promotes insulin resistance and hyperinsulinemia, aging-associated declines in growth hormone could be a cause of insulin resistance.[80] Because this concept is broadly applicable to insulin resistance–related degenerative diseases, efforts should be made to improve our understanding of cellular aging, with the goal of preventing or delaying the onset of neurodegeneration.

Arguments could be made that insulin resistance, cognitive impairment, and AD are inevitable consequences of aging[81] because aging-associated chronic low-grade inflammation[82,83] causes insulin resistance.[83,84] Because inflammation and insulin resistance increase oxidative stress, over time, reactive oxygen species and advanced glycation end-products accumulate, driving mitochondrial dysfunction, DNA damage, and cell death cascades,[80] which are pivotal to aging-associated cognitive impairment and brain atrophy.

On the other hand, opposing arguments offer an alternative perspective and suggest that other intrinsic host factors, lifetime exposures, and lifestyle choices dictate the quality of aging and propensity to develop insulin-resistance diseases. An excellent example of this phenomenon exists with respect to postpolio syndrome, in which people who recovered from childhood poliomyelitis exhibit high rates of motor neuron disease as middle-aged adults.[85,86] During childhood, recovery from poliomyelitis was enabled by the vigorous regenerative and reparative activities of the youthful plastic central nervous system (CNS). However, with aging, the regenerative capacity of the CNS declines. Individuals develop postpolio motor neuron disease because the underlying previously damaged motor neuron system gets exposed, resulting in significant weakness caused by denervation myopathy.[87,88] In contrast, aging of the previously undamaged CNS results in mild weakness and reduced mobility; this suggests that chronic enrichment and protection of neuronal circuitry may be required to maintain excellent brain function throughout the normal human lifespan.

Lifestyle Choices and Aging

Obesity, T2DM, NAFLD/nonalcoholic steatohepatitis (NASH), metabolic syndrome, and AD have grown in prevalence to epidemic proportions in many societies.[29,89,90] In recent years, countries throughout the world have witnessed rapid increases in the prevalence rates of insulin-resistance diseases and their consequences in non-aged individuals, including adolescents and children.[81] These trends have been linked to obesity and sedentary lifestyles. Because the spectra of insulin resistance–related diseases are nearly identical across different age groups, it could be argued that certain lifestyles, habits, and behaviors cause disease by accelerating aging. By the same token, lifestyle modifications could potentially retard aging and defer or prevent aging-associated insulin-resistance diseases, including neurodegeneration.

Obesity and Cognitive Impairment

Obesity significantly increases the risk for cognitive impairment and leads to brain insulin resistance because of the disruption of homeostatic mechanisms.[11,91–93] Concerns about obesity's effects on the brain arose from studies showing an increased risk for mild cognitive impairment (MCI) or AD-type dementia in individuals with glucose intolerance, deficits in insulin secretion, T2DM, obesity/dyslipidemic disorders, or NASH.[20,94–96] Other studies correlated obesity with deficits in executive function[96,97] and eventual development of AD.[98] These concepts were confirmed in experimental animal models of diet-induced obesity with T2DM.[47,91,99,100] Perhaps the most convincing evidence that obesity contributes to cognitive impairment was provided by studies showing that weight-loss reversal of insulin resistance improves cognitive performance[101,102] and neuropsychiatric function[103] and that adherence to Mediterranean diets reduces metabolic risk for AD.[104]

T2DM

The molecular and biochemical abnormalities in AD mimic the effects of T2DM on skeletal muscle and NASH on liver. Epidemiologic and longitudinal studies demonstrated increased risks for MCI or AD in people with glucose intolerance, T2DM, obesity/dyslipidemic disorders, or deficits in insulin secretion.[105–107] More recently, investigators linked increased rates of cognitive impairment to chronic hyperglycemia,[108] which precedes the diagnosis of T2DM. Similarly, postmortem studies revealed that peripheral insulin resistance contributes to cognitive impairment and AD progression,[109,110] whereas experimental studies showed that diet-induced obesity with T2DM leads to deficits in spatial learning and memory,[99] brain atrophy with brain insulin resistance, neuroinflammation, oxidative stress, and deficits in cholinergic function.[91,111]

NAFLD/NASH

Several studies have shown that cognitive impairment and neuropsychiatric dysfunction occur with steatohepatitis caused by obesity, alcohol abuse, chronic hepatitis C virus infection, Reyes syndrome, or nitrosamine exposure.[111–114] Mechanistically, steatohepatitis (ie, inflammation with fatty liver disease) increases ER stress, oxidative damage, mitochondrial dysfunction, and lipid peroxidation, which together drive hepatic insulin resistance.[93] Hepatic insulin resistance dysregulates lipid metabolism and promotes lipolysis,[115] which increases the production of toxic lipids, including ceramides, which further impair insulin signaling, mitochondrial function, and cell viability.[93,116,117] Liver disease worsens as ER stress and mitochondrial dysfunction exacerbate insulin resistance,[11] lipolysis, and ceramide accumulation.[118–120]

Experimental models of NAFLD with T2DM and visceral obesity are associated with brain atrophy, neurodegeneration, and cognitive impairment.[56,91,100,111,114] In humans with NASH, the rates of neuropsychiatric disease, including depression and anxiety,[121] and the risks for developing cognitive impairment[122] are increased. In fact, cognitive impairment and neuropsychiatric dysfunction correlate more with steatohepatitis and insulin resistance than obesity or T2DM.[123,124] Therefore, the potential roles of steatohepatitis and hepatic insulin resistance in relation to neurodegeneration must be considered. To this end, the author and colleagues hypothesized that increased levels of cytotoxic ceramides generated in liver (or visceral adipose tissue) could cause neurodegeneration.[56,100,111,114] In humans and experimental models with steatohepatitis, ceramide gene expression and ceramide levels are increased regardless of the cause.[19,20,91,125–128] Correspondingly, CNS exposures to cytotoxic ceramides cause AD-type molecular and biochemical abnormalities in vitro[129,130] and cognitive-motor deficits, brain insulin resistance, oxidative stress, metabolic dysfunction, and neurodegeneration with features similar to AD in vivo.[128] Ex vivo treatment of frontal lobe slice cultures with long-chain ceramide-containing plasma from obese rats with steatohepatitis produces neurotoxic responses with impairments in viability and mitochondrial function.[125] This concept illustrates how peripheral insulin-resistance diseases might cause or contribute to cognitive impairment and neurodegeneration.

Metabolic Syndrome

Metabolic syndrome is a cluster of disease processes that pivots around insulin resistance, visceral obesity, hypertension, and dyslipidemia.[131] Metabolic syndrome increases the risk for coronary artery disease, atherosclerosis, and T2DM and is frequently associated with NAFLD/NASH, proinflammatory and prothrombotic states, and sleep apnea.[131] Studies have linked peripheral insulin resistance,[132] visceral obesity,[133] and metabolic syndrome[134–136] to brain atrophy, cognitive impairment, and declines in executive function. These associations sound an alarm in light of the recent increases in the prevalence of metabolic syndrome among adults and children.[137] If T2DM, obesity, metabolic syndrome, and NAFLD/NASH could actually be demonstrated to serve as cofactors in the pathogenesis and progression of neurodegeneration, then aggressive efforts would be needed to treat and prevent the full spectrum of systemic insulin-resistance diseases. Accordingly, antihyperglycemic or insulin sensitizer agents have already been shown to reduce AD clinical manifestations and pathology.[56,138–143]

SUMMARY

Brain insulin/IGF resistance initiates a cascade of progressive oxidative stress, neuro-inflammation, impaired cell survival, mitochondrial dysfunction, dysregulated lipid metabolism, and ER stress. Continued compromise of neuronal and glial functions causes cognitive impairment and the eventual development of neurodegeneration. Because many of the molecular and cellular abnormalities in AD exist in systemic/peripheral insulin resistance, such as in obesity, T2DM, and NAFLD/NASH, common mechanisms of insulin and IGF resistance should be investigated. By regarding these clinically diverse diseases as fundamentally related on molecular, biochemical, and perhaps etiologic bases, their clustering beneath an umbrella term of *insulin resistance spectrum disorders* could accelerate the discovery of new treatments and improve the understanding of disease pathogenesis and progression.

REFERENCES

1. Best CH, Scott DA. The preparation of insulin. J Biol Chem 1923;57:709–23.
2. Roth J, Qureshi S, Whitford I, et al. Insulin's discovery: new insights on its ninetieth birthday. Diabetes Metab Res Rev 2012;28(4):293–304.
3. Gilchrist JA, Best CH, Banting FG. Observations with insulin on Department of Soldiers' Civil Re-Establishment Diabetics. Can Med Assoc J 1923;13(8):565–72.
4. Gualandi-Signorini AM, Giorgi G. Insulin formulations–a review. Eur Rev Med Pharmacol Sci 2001;5(3):73–83.
5. Heinemann L, Richter B. Clinical pharmacology of human insulin. Diabetes Care 1993;16(Suppl 3):90–100.
6. Dave N, Hazra P, Khedkar A, et al. Process and purification for manufacture of a modified insulin intended for oral delivery. J Chromatogr A 2008;1177(2):282–6.
7. Freiherr J, Hallschmid M, Frey WH 2nd, et al. Intranasal insulin as a treatment for Alzheimer's disease: a review of basic research and clinical evidence. CNS Drugs 2013;27(7):505–14.
8. Ott V, Benedict C, Schultes B, et al. Intranasal administration of insulin to the brain impacts cognitive function and peripheral metabolism. Diabetes Obes Metab 2012;14(3):214–21.
9. Plum MB, Sicat BL, Brokaw DK. Newer insulin therapies for management of type 1 and type 2 diabetes mellitus. Consult Pharm 2003;18(5):454–65.
10. Zeyda M, Stulnig TM. Obesity, inflammation, and insulin resistance–a mini-review. Gerontology 2009;55(4):379–86.
11. Capeau J. Insulin resistance and steatosis in humans. Diabetes Metab 2008;34(6 Pt 2):649–57.

12. Dai Z, Wu F, Yeung EW, et al. IGF-IEc expression, regulation and biological function in different tissues. Growth Horm IGF Res 2010;20(4):275–81.
13. Matheny RW Jr, Nindl BC, Adamo ML. Minireview: mechano-growth factor: a putative product of IGF-I gene expression involved in tissue repair and regeneration. Endocrinology 2010;151(3):865–75.
14. Kuemmerle JF. Insulin-like growth factors in the gastrointestinal tract and liver. Endocrinol Metab Clin North Am 2012;41(2):409–23, vii.
15. de la Monte SM, Wands JR. Review of insulin and insulin-like growth factor expression, signaling, and malfunction in the central nervous system: relevance to Alzheimer's disease. J Alzheimers Dis 2005;7(1):45–61.
16. D'Ercole AJ, Ye P. Expanding the mind: insulin-like growth factor I and brain development. Endocrinology 2008;149(12):5958–62.
17. Freude S, Schilbach K, Schubert M. The role of IGF-1 receptor and insulin receptor signaling for the pathogenesis of Alzheimer's disease: from model organisms to human disease. Curr Alzheimer Res 2009;6(3):213–23.
18. Zeger M, Popken G, Zhang J, et al. Insulin-like growth factor type 1 receptor signaling in the cells of oligodendrocyte lineage is required for normal in vivo oligodendrocyte development and myelination. Glia 2007;55(4):400–11.
19. de la Monte SM, Longato L, Tong M, et al. The liver-brain axis of alcohol-mediated neurodegeneration: role of toxic lipids. Int J Environ Res Public Health 2009;6(7):2055–75.
20. de la Monte SM, Longato L, Tong M, et al. Insulin resistance and neurodegeneration: roles of obesity, type 2 diabetes mellitus and non-alcoholic steatohepatitis. Curr Opin Investig Drugs 2009;10(10):1049–60.
21. Gronke S, Clarke DF, Broughton S, et al. Molecular evolution and functional characterization of Drosophila insulin-like peptides. PLoS Genet 2010;6(2): e1000857.
22. Shanik MH, Xu Y, Skrha J, et al. Insulin resistance and hyperinsulinemia: is hyperinsulinemia the cart or the horse? Diabetes Care 2008;31(Suppl 2):S262–8.
23. Dankner R, Chetrit A, Shanik MH, et al. Basal-state hyperinsulinemia in healthy normoglycemic adults is predictive of type 2 diabetes over a 24-year follow-up: a preliminary report. Diabetes Care 2009;32(8):1464–6.
24. Garcia RG, Rincon MY, Arenas WD, et al. Hyperinsulinemia is a predictor of new cardiovascular events in Colombian patients with a first myocardial infarction. Int J Cardiol 2011;148(1):85–90.
25. Kasai T, Miyauchi K, Kajimoto K, et al. The adverse prognostic significance of the metabolic syndrome with and without hypertension in patients who underwent complete coronary revascularization. J Hypertens 2009;27(5): 1017–24.
26. Agnoli C, Berrino F, Abagnato CA, et al. Metabolic syndrome and postmenopausal breast cancer in the ORDET cohort: a nested case-control study. Nutr Metab Cardiovasc Dis 2010;20(1):41–8.
27. Faulds MH, Dahlman-Wright K. Metabolic diseases and cancer risk. Curr Opin Oncol 2012;24(1):58–61.
28. Colonna SV, Douglas Case L, Lawrence JA. A retrospective review of the metabolic syndrome in women diagnosed with breast cancer and correlation with estrogen receptor. Breast Cancer Res Treat 2012;131(1):325–31.
29. de la Monte SM, Neusner A, Chu J, et al. Epidemiological trends strongly suggest exposures as etiologic agents in the pathogenesis of sporadic Alzheimer's disease, diabetes mellitus, and non-alcoholic steatohepatitis. J Alzheimers Dis 2009;17(3):519–29.

30. Cummings JL. Definitions and diagnostic criteria. 3rd edition. London: Informa UK Limited; 2007.
31. Gustaw-Rothenberg K, Lerner A, Bonda DJ, et al. Biomarkers in Alzheimer's disease: past, present and future. Biomark Med 2010;4(1):15–26.
32. Walsh DM, Klyubin I, Fadeeva JV, et al. Naturally secreted oligomers of amyloid beta protein potently inhibit hippocampal long-term potentiation in vivo. Nature 2002;416(6880):535–9.
33. Frolich L, Blum-Degen D, Bernstein HG, et al. Brain insulin and insulin receptors in aging and sporadic Alzheimer's disease. J Neural Transm 1998;105(4–5): 423–38.
34. Hoyer S. Glucose metabolism and insulin receptor signal transduction in Alzheimer disease. Eur J Pharmacol 2004;490(1–3):115–25.
35. Rivera EJ, Goldin A, Fulmer N, et al. Insulin and insulin-like growth factor expression and function deteriorate with progression of Alzheimer's disease: link to brain reductions in acetylcholine. J Alzheimers Dis 2005;8(3):247–68.
36. Steen E, Terry BM, Rivera EJ, et al. Impaired insulin and insulin-like growth factor expression and signaling mechanisms in Alzheimer's disease–is this type 3 diabetes? J Alzheimers Dis 2005;7(1):63–80.
37. de la Monte SM. Therapeutic targets of brain insulin resistance in sporadic Alzheimer's disease. Front Biosci (Elite Ed) 2012;E4:1582–605.
38. de la Monte SM, Re E, Longato L, et al. Dysfunctional pro-ceramide, ER stress, and insulin/IGF signaling networks with progression of Alzheimer's disease. J Alzheimers Dis 2012;30(0):S217–29.
39. Caselli RJ, Chen K, Lee W, et al. Correlating cerebral hypometabolism with future memory decline in subsequent converters to amnestic pre-mild cognitive impairment. Arch Neurol 2008;65(9):1231–6.
40. Mosconi L, Pupi A, De Leon MJ. Brain glucose hypometabolism and oxidative stress in preclinical Alzheimer's disease. Ann N Y Acad Sci 2008;1147:180–95.
41. Langbaum JB, Chen K, Caselli RJ, et al. Hypometabolism in Alzheimer-affected brain regions in cognitively healthy Latino individuals carrying the apolipoprotein E epsilon4 allele. Arch Neurol 2010;67(4):462–8.
42. Hoyer S, Nitsch R. Cerebral excess release of neurotransmitter amino acids subsequent to reduced cerebral glucose metabolism in early-onset dementia of Alzheimer type. J Neural Transm 1989;75(3):227–32.
43. Hoyer S, Nitsch R, Oesterreich K. Predominant abnormality in cerebral glucose utilization in late-onset dementia of the Alzheimer type: a cross-sectional comparison against advanced late-onset and incipient early-onset cases. J Neural Transm Park Dis Dement Sect 1991;3(1):1–14.
44. Talbot K, Wang HY, Kazi H, et al. Demonstrated brain insulin resistance in Alzheimer's disease patients is associated with IGF-1 resistance, IRS-1 dysregulation, and cognitive decline. J Clin Invest 2012;122(4):1316–38.
45. Salcedo I, Tweedie D, Li Y, et al. Neuroprotective and neurotrophic actions of glucagon-like peptide-1: an emerging opportunity to treat neurodegenerative and cerebrovascular disorders. Br J Pharmacol 2012;166(5):1586–99.
46. Piriz J, Muller A, Trejo JL, et al. IGF-I and the aging mammalian brain. Exp Gerontol 2011;46(2–3):96–9.
47. Mattson MP. The impact of dietary energy intake on cognitive aging. Front Aging Neurosci 2010;2:5.
48. Weinstock M, Shoham S. Rat models of dementia based on reductions in regional glucose metabolism, cerebral blood flow and cytochrome oxidase activity. J Neural Transm 2004;111(3):347–66.

49. Lester-Coll N, Rivera EJ, Soscia SJ, et al. Intracerebral streptozotocin model of type 3 diabetes: relevance to sporadic Alzheimer's disease. J Alzheimers Dis 2006;9(1):13–33.
50. Bolzan AD, Bianchi MS. Genotoxicity of streptozotocin. Mutat Res 2002; 512(2–3):121–34.
51. Koulmanda M, Qipo A, Chebrolu S, et al. The effect of low versus high dose of streptozotocin in cynomolgus monkeys (Macaca fascilularis). Am J Transplant 2003;3(3):267–72.
52. de la Monte SM, Tong M, Bowling N, et al. si-RNA inhibition of brain insulin or insulin-like growth factor receptors causes developmental cerebellar abnormalities: relevance to fetal alcohol spectrum disorder. Mol Brain 2011;4:13.
53. Hoyer S. Causes and consequences of disturbances of cerebral glucose metabolism in sporadic Alzheimer disease: therapeutic implications. Adv Exp Med Biol 2004;541:135–52.
54. Chen GJ, Xu J, Lahousse SA, et al. Transient hypoxia causes Alzheimer-type molecular and biochemical abnormalities in cortical neurons: potential strategies for neuroprotection. J Alzheimers Dis 2003;5(3):209–28.
55. Tsukamoto E, Hashimoto Y, Kanekura K, et al. Characterization of the toxic mechanism triggered by Alzheimer's amyloid-beta peptides via p75 neurotrophin receptor in neuronal hybrid cells. J Neurosci Res 2003;73(5):627–36.
56. de la Monte SM, Tong M, Lester-Coll N, et al. Therapeutic rescue of neurodegeneration in experimental type 3 diabetes: relevance to Alzheimer's disease. J Alzheimers Dis 2006;10(1):89–109.
57. Gonzalez-Sanchez JL, Serrano-Rios M. Molecular basis of insulin action. Drug News Perspect 2007;20(8):527–31.
58. Etiene D, Kraft J, Ganju N, et al. Cerebrovascular pathology contributes to the heterogeneity of Alzheimer's disease. J Alzheimers Dis 1998;1(2):119–34.
59. Korf ES, White LR, Scheltens P, et al. Brain aging in very old men with type 2 diabetes: the Honolulu-Asia Aging Study. Diabetes Care 2006;29(10):2268–74.
60. de la Monte SM. Quantitation of cerebral atrophy in preclinical and end-stage Alzheimer's disease. Ann Neurol 1989;25(5):450–9.
61. Kincaid-Smith P. Hypothesis: obesity and the insulin resistance syndrome play a major role in end-stage renal failure attributed to hypertension and labelled 'hypertensive nephrosclerosis'. J Hypertens 2004;22(6):1051–5.
62. Matsumoto H, Nakao T, Okada T, et al. Insulin resistance contributes to obesity-related proteinuria. Intern Med 2005;44(6):548–53.
63. O'Brien JT. Role of imaging techniques in the diagnosis of dementia. Br J Radiol 2007;80(Spec No 2):S71–7.
64. Poljansky S, Ibach B, Hirschberger B, et al. A visual [18F]FDG-PET rating scale for the differential diagnosis of frontotemporal lobar degeneration. Eur Arch Psychiatry Clin Neurosci 2011;261(6):433–46.
65. Teune LK, Bartels AL, de Jong BM, et al. Typical cerebral metabolic patterns in neurodegenerative brain diseases. Mov Disord 2010;25(14):2395–404.
66. Nijholt DA, De Kimpe L, Elfrink HL, et al. Removing protein aggregates: the role of proteolysis in neurodegeneration. Curr Med Chem 2011;18(16):2459–76.
67. Uehara T. Accumulation of misfolded protein through nitrosative stress linked to neurodegenerative disorders. Antioxid Redox Signal 2007;9(5): 597–601.
68. Hol EM, Fischer DF, Ovaa H, et al. Ubiquitin proteasome system as a pharmacological target in neurodegeneration. Expert Rev Neurother 2006;6(9): 1337–47.

69. Kahle PJ, Haass C. How does parkin ligate ubiquitin to Parkinson's disease? EMBO Rep 2004;5(7):681–5.
70. Turner BJ, Atkin JD. ER stress and UPR in familial amyotrophic lateral sclerosis. Curr Mol Med 2006;6(1):79–86.
71. Morris JK, Seim NB, Bomhoff GL, et al. Effects of unilateral nigrostriatal dopamine depletion on peripheral glucose tolerance and insulin signaling in middle aged rats. Neurosci Lett 2011;504(3):219–22.
72. Tong M, Dong M, de la Monte SM. Brain insulin-like growth factor and neurotrophin resistance in Parkinson's disease and dementia with Lewy bodies: potential role of manganese neurotoxicity. J Alzheimers Dis 2009;16(3):585–99.
73. Sato N, Takeda S, Uchio-Yamada K, et al. Role of insulin signaling in the interaction between Alzheimer disease and diabetes mellitus: a missing link to therapeutic potential. Curr Aging Sci 2011;4(2):118–27.
74. Holzenberger M. Igf-I signaling and effects on longevity. Nestle Nutr Workshop Ser Pediatr Program 2011;68:237–45 [discussion: 246–9].
75. Schuh AF, Rieder CM, Rizzi L, et al. Mechanisms of brain aging regulation by insulin: implications for neurodegeneration in late-onset Alzheimer's disease. ISRN Neurol 2011;2011:306905.
76. Valentini S, Cabreiro F, Ackerman D, et al. Manipulation of in vivo iron levels can alter resistance to oxidative stress without affecting ageing in the nematode C. elegans. Mech Ageing Dev 2012;133(5):282–90.
77. Zemva J, Udelhoven M, Moll L, et al. Neuronal overexpression of insulin receptor substrate 2 leads to increased fat mass, insulin resistance, and glucose intolerance during aging. Age (Dordr) 2012;35(5):1881–97.
78. Castilla-Cortazar I, Garcia-Fernandez M, Delgado G, et al. Hepatoprotection and neuroprotection induced by low doses of IGF-II in aging rats. J Transl Med 2011;9:103.
79. Luque RM, Lin Q, Cordoba-Chacon J, et al. Metabolic impact of adult-onset, isolated, growth hormone deficiency (AOiGHD) due to destruction of pituitary somatotropes. PloS One 2011;6(1):e15767.
80. Srikanth V, Westcott B, Forbes J, et al. Methylglyoxal, cognitive function and cerebral atrophy in older people. J Gerontol A Biol Sci Med Sci 2012;68(1):68–73.
81. Williamson R, McNeilly A, Sutherland C. Insulin resistance in the brain: an old-age or new-age problem? Biochem Pharmacol 2012;84(6):737–45.
82. Oxenkrug G. Interferon-gamma - inducible inflammation: contribution to aging and aging-associated psychiatric disorders. Aging Dis 2011;2(6):474–86.
83. Horrillo D, Sierra J, Arribas C, et al. Age-associated development of inflammation in Wistar rats: effects of caloric restriction. Arch Physiol Biochem 2011; 117(3):140–50.
84. Cai D, Liu T. Inflammatory cause of metabolic syndrome via brain stress and NF-kappaB. Aging (Albany NY) 2012;4(2):98–115.
85. Birk TJ. Poliomyelitis and the post-polio syndrome: exercise capacities and adaptation–current research, future directions, and widespread applicability. Med Sci Sports Exerc 1993;25(4):466–72.
86. Jubelt B, Cashman NR. Neurological manifestations of the post-polio syndrome. Crit Rev Neurobiol 1987;3(3):199–220.
87. Gordon T, Hegedus J, Tam SL. Adaptive and maladaptive motor axonal sprouting in aging and motoneuron disease. Neurol Res 2004;26(2):174–85.
88. Dalakas MC. Pathogenetic mechanisms of post-polio syndrome: morphological, electrophysiological, virological, and immunological correlations. Ann N Y Acad Sci 1995;753:167–85.

89. Chiang DJ, Pritchard MT, Nagy LE. Obesity, diabetes mellitus, and liver fibrosis. Am J Physiol Gastrointest Liver Physiol 2011;300(5):G697–702.

90. Vernon G, Baranova A, Younossi ZM. Systematic review: the epidemiology and natural history of non-alcoholic fatty liver disease and non-alcoholic steatohepatitis in adults. Aliment Pharmacol Ther 2011;34(3):274–85.

91. Lyn-Cook LE Jr, Lawton M, Tong M, et al. Hepatic ceramide may mediate brain insulin resistance and neurodegeneration in type 2 diabetes and non-alcoholic steatohepatitis. J Alzheimers Dis 2009;16(4):715–29.

92. de la Monte SM, Wands JR. Alzheimer's disease is type 3 diabetes: evidence reviewed. J Diabetes Sci Technol 2008;2(6):1101–13.

93. Kraegen EW, Cooney GJ. Free fatty acids and skeletal muscle insulin resistance. Curr Opin Lipidol 2008;19(3):235–41.

94. Luchsinger JA, Reitz C, Patel B, et al. Relation of diabetes to mild cognitive impairment. Arch Neurol 2007;64(4):570–5.

95. Craft S. Insulin resistance and Alzheimer's disease pathogenesis: potential mechanisms and implications for treatment. Curr Alzheimer Res 2007;4(2):147–52.

96. Lokken KL, Boeka AG, Austin HM, et al. Evidence of executive dysfunction in extremely obese adolescents: a pilot study. Surg Obes Relat Dis 2009;5(5):547–52.

97. Gunstad J, Paul RH, Cohen RA, et al. Elevated body mass index is associated with executive dysfunction in otherwise healthy adults. Compr Psychiatry 2007;48(1):57–61.

98. Yaffe K. Metabolic syndrome and cognitive decline. Curr Alzheimer Res 2007;4(2):123–6.

99. Winocur G, Greenwood CE. Studies of the effects of high fat diets on cognitive function in a rat model. Neurobiol Aging 2005;26(Suppl 1):46–9.

100. Moroz N, Tong M, Longato L, et al. Limited Alzheimer-type neurodegeneration in experimental obesity and Type 2 diabetes mellitus. J Alzheimers Dis 2008;15(1):29–44.

101. Baker LD, Frank LL, Foster-Schubert K, et al. Aerobic exercise improves cognition for older adults with glucose intolerance, a risk factor for Alzheimer's disease. J Alzheimers Dis 2010;22(2):569–79.

102. Baker LD, Frank LL, Foster-Schubert K, et al. Effects of aerobic exercise on mild cognitive impairment: a controlled trial. Arch Neurol 2010;67(1):71–9.

103. Bryan J, Tiggemann M. The effect of weight-loss dieting on cognitive performance and psychological well-being in overweight women. Appetite 2001;36(2):147–56.

104. Gu Y, Luchsinger JA, Stern Y, et al. Mediterranean diet, inflammatory and metabolic biomarkers, and risk of Alzheimer's disease. J Alzheimers Dis 2010;22(2):483–92.

105. Martins IJ, Hone E, Foster JK, et al. Apolipoprotein E, cholesterol metabolism, diabetes, and the convergence of risk factors for Alzheimer's disease and cardiovascular disease. Mol Psychiatry 2006;11(8):721–36.

106. Pasquier F, Boulogne A, Leys D, et al. Diabetes mellitus and dementia. Diabetes Metab 2006;32(5 Pt 1):403–14.

107. Whitmer RA. Type 2 diabetes and risk of cognitive impairment and dementia. Curr Neurol Neurosci Rep 2007;7(5):373–80.

108. Crane PK, Walker R, Hubbard RA, et al. Glucose levels and risk of dementia. N Engl J Med 2013;369(6):540–8.

109. Nelson PT, Smith CD, Abner EA, et al. Human cerebral neuropathology of type 2 diabetes mellitus. Biochim Biophys Acta 2008;1792(5):454–69.

110. Janson J, Laedtke T, Parisi JE, et al. Increased risk of type 2 diabetes in Alzheimer disease. Diabetes 2004;53(2):474–81.

111. Tong M, Longato L, de la Monte SM. Early limited nitrosamine exposures exacerbate high fat diet-mediated type2 diabetes and neurodegeneration. BMC Endocr Disord 2010;10(1):4.

112. Perry W, Hilsabeck RC, Hassanein TI. Cognitive dysfunction in chronic hepatitis C: a review. Dig Dis Sci 2008;53(2):307–21.

113. Weiss JJ, Gorman JM. Psychiatric behavioral aspects of comanagement of hepatitis C virus and HIV. Curr HIV/AIDS Rep 2006;3(4):176–81.

114. Tong M, Neusner A, Longato L, et al. Nitrosamine exposure causes insulin resistance diseases: relevance to type 2 diabetes mellitus, non-alcoholic steatohepatitis, and Alzheimer's disease. J Alzheimers Dis 2009;17(4):827–44.

115. Kao Y, Youson JH, Holmes JA, et al. Effects of insulin on lipid metabolism of larvae and metamorphosing landlocked sea lamprey, Petromyzon marinus. Gen Comp Endocrinol 1999;114(3):405–14.

116. Holland WL, Summers SA. Sphingolipids, insulin resistance, and metabolic disease: new insights from in vivo manipulation of sphingolipid metabolism. Endocr Rev 2008;29(4):381–402.

117. Langeveld M, Aerts JM. Glycosphingolipids and insulin resistance. Prog Lipid Res 2009;48(3–4):196–205.

118. Kaplowitz N, Than TA, Shinohara M, et al. Endoplasmic reticulum stress and liver injury. Semin Liver Dis 2007;27(4):367–77.

119. Malhi H, Gores GJ. Molecular mechanisms of lipotoxicity in nonalcoholic fatty liver disease. Semin Liver Dis 2008;28(4):360–9.

120. Sundar-Rajan S, Srinivasan V, Balasubramanyam M, et al. Endoplasmic reticulum (ER) stress & diabetes. Indian J Med Res 2007;125(3):411–24.

121. Elwing JE, Lustman PJ, Wang HL, et al. Depression, anxiety, and nonalcoholic steatohepatitis. Psychosom Med 2006;68(4):563–9.

122. Felipo V, Urios A, Montesinos E, et al. Contribution of hyperammonemia and inflammatory factors to cognitive impairment in minimal hepatic encephalopathy. Metab Brain Dis 2011;27(1):51–8.

123. Schmidt KS, Gallo JL, Ferri C, et al. The neuropsychological profile of alcohol-related dementia suggests cortical and subcortical pathology. Dement Geriatr Cogn Disord 2005;20(5):286–91.

124. Kopelman MD, Thomson AD, Guerrini I, et al. The Korsakoff syndrome: clinical aspects, psychology and treatment. Alcohol Alcohol 2009;44(2):148–54.

125. de la Monte SM. Triangulated mal-signaling in Alzheimer's disease: roles of neurotoxic ceramides, ER stress, and insulin resistance reviewed. J Alzheimers Dis 2012;30:S231–49.

126. de la Monte SM, Tong M, Lawton M, et al. Nitrosamine exposure exacerbates high fat diet-mediated type 2 diabetes mellitus, non-alcoholic steatohepatitis, and neurodegeneration with cognitive impairment. Mol Neurodegener 2009;4:54.

127. de la Monte SM, Tong M, Nguyen V, et al. Ceramide-mediated insulin resistance and impairment of cognitive-motor functions. J Alzheimers Dis 2010;21(3): 967–84.

128. Tong M, de la Monte SM. Mechanisms of ceramide-mediated neurodegeneration. J Alzheimers Dis 2009;16(4):705–14.

129. Alessenko AV, Bugrova AE, Dudnik LB. Connection of lipid peroxide oxidation with the sphingomyelin pathway in the development of Alzheimer's disease. Biochem Soc Trans 2004;32(Pt 1):144–6.

130. Adibhatla RM, Hatcher JF. Altered lipid metabolism in brain injury and disorders. Subcell Biochem 2008;49:241–68.
131. Kassi E, Pervanidou P, Kaltsas G, et al. Metabolic syndrome: definitions and controversies. BMC Med 2011;9:48.
132. Tan ZS, Beiser AS, Fox CS, et al. Association of metabolic dysregulation with volumetric brain magnetic resonance imaging and cognitive markers of subclinical brain aging in middle-aged adults: the Framingham Offspring Study. Diabetes Care 2011;34(8):1766–70.
133. Debette S, Beiser A, Hoffmann U, et al. Visceral fat is associated with lower brain volume in healthy middle-aged adults. Ann Neurol 2010;68(2):136–44.
134. Hassenstab JJ, Sweat V, Bruehl H, et al. Metabolic syndrome is associated with learning and recall impairment in middle age. Dement Geriatr Cogn Disord 2010;29(4):356–62.
135. Frisardi V, Solfrizzi V, Capurso C, et al. Is insulin resistant brain state a central feature of the metabolic-cognitive syndrome? J Alzheimers Dis 2010;21(1):57–63.
136. Yates KF, Sweat V, Yau PL, et al. Impact of metabolic syndrome on cognition and brain: a selected review of the literature. Arterioscler Thromb Vasc Biol 2012;32(9):2060–7.
137. Burns JM, Honea RA, Vidoni ED, et al. Insulin is differentially related to cognitive decline and atrophy in Alzheimer's disease and aging. Biochim Biophys Acta 2012;1822(3):333–9.
138. Benedict C, Hallschmid M, Schmitz K, et al. Intranasal insulin improves memory in humans: superiority of insulin aspart. Neuropsychopharmacology 2007;32(1):239–43.
139. Craft S, Baker LD, Montine TJ, et al. Intranasal insulin therapy for Alzheimer disease and amnestic mild cognitive impairment: a pilot clinical trial. Arch Neurol 2011;69(1):29–38.
140. Holscher C. Incretin analogues that have been developed to treat type 2 diabetes hold promise as a novel treatment strategy for Alzheimer's disease. Recent Pat CNS Drug Discov 2010;5(2):109–17.
141. Krikorian R, Eliassen JC, Boespflug EL, et al. Improved cognitive-cerebral function in older adults with chromium supplementation. Nutr Neurosci 2010;13(3):116–22.
142. Reger MA, Watson GS, Green PS, et al. Intranasal insulin improves cognition and modulates {beta}-amyloid in early AD. Neurology 2008;70(6):440–8.
143. Luchsinger JA. Type 2 diabetes, related conditions, in relation and dementia: an opportunity for prevention? J Alzheimers Dis 2010;20(3):723–36.

Interactions Between Diabetes and Anxiety and Depression
Implications for Treatment

Alexander Bystritsky, MD, PhD[a],*, Jessica Danial, MA[b],
David Kronemyer, MA[a]

KEYWORDS

- Anxiety • Cognitive behavioral therapy • Cognitive restructuring • Depression
- Diabetes

KEY POINTS

- A bidirectional relationship exists between anxiety and depression and diabetes.
- A person with a general medical condition such as diabetes is likely to experience anxiety and depression.
- Persons with anxiety and depression may engage in coping strategies such as overeating, causing weight gain and exacerbating conditions such as metabolic syndrome, which is a precursor to diabetes.
- Clinicians must use caution when using pharmacologic interventions to treat anxiety and depression, because they might be counterproductive.
- Cognitive behavior therapy is the most effective therapeutic intervention for diabetes-related anxiety and depression. It can be conceptualized using the alarms-beliefs-coping (A-B-C) model.

According to statistics developed by the World Health Organization, more than 350 million persons worldwide will be diagnosed with diabetes by 2030.[1] Age of onset is trending younger, magnifying the adverse effects of the disease.[2,3] It entails a significant social cost burden, including not only direct health care expenses but also expenses associated with increased mortality and lost productivity.[4] Not surprisingly, epidemiologic studies have shown that persons with diabetes are more depressed (a worldwide prevalence

Funding Support: Gerald J. and Dorothy R. Friedman New York Foundation for Medical Research.
Financial Disclosures: A. Bystritsky is founder and stockholder of Brainsonix Corporation.
[a] Department of Psychiatry and Biobehavioral Sciences, Semel Institute for Neuroscience and Human Behavior, David Geffen School of Medicine, University of California, Los Angeles, 300 UCLA Medical Plaza, Room 2330, Los Angeles, CA 90095-6968, USA; [b] California School of Professional Psychology, Alliant International University, Los Angeles, CA 91803, USA
* Corresponding author.
E-mail address: abystritsky@mednet.ucla.edu

Endocrinol Metab Clin N Am 43 (2014) 269–283
http://dx.doi.org/10.1016/j.ecl.2013.10.001
0889-8529/14/$ – see front matter © 2014 Elsevier Inc. All rights reserved.

rate of 10%–15%) and anxious (a worldwide prevalence rate of approximately 40%)[5] compared with the normal population (depression, 1.6%[6]; anxiety, 7.3%[7]).

However, this is only half of the story. From a biopsychosocial perspective, persons who are depressed or anxious may tend to engage in diabetes-risk behavior, such as overeating, in an attempt to relieve their symptoms. An extensive body of literature has examined the relationship between obesity and diabetes.[8] The American Medical Association recently recognized obesity as a disease.[9] It is also now a recognized psychopathology, explicitly linking it with diabetes.

This article reviews some of the complex associations between diabetes and anxiety and depression, and also pharmaceutical and cognitive behavioral strategies to address these issues from a psychiatric and psychological perspective.

SUBTYPES OF DIABETES AND THEIR RELATIONSHIP TO ANXIETY AND DEPRESSION

The well-recognized subtypes of diabetes each relate differentially to anxiety and depression. Type I diabetes mellitus (T1DM) usually has an early onset and progresses slowly over the lifetime.[10] T1DM is treated with insulin; additional treatment is usually for symptomatic management of various complications, which may be numerous. This need for lifelong treatment presents a challenge for people who live with chronic illness, because it interferes significantly with their quality life. Not surprisingly, many persons with T1DM develop clinically significant depression and anxiety. Type 2 diabetes mellitus (T2DM), however, usually develops later in life and is associated with an unhealthy lifestyle or metabolic problems, both of which may be sequelae of depression or its treatment.[11] Recent studies indicate a more complex relationship between T2DM and depression, suggesting that onset of diabetes frequently follows depression, complicating the course of treatment and interfering with treatment compliance.[12]

COMPLEX RELATIONSHIPS BETWEEN ANXIETY AND DEPRESSION AND DIABETES

Many complex relationships exist between medical illnesses and psychiatric syndromes such as anxiety and depression.[13] Both acute and chronic illnesses produce stress that could lead to anxiety and depression. The underlying disease could induce biological changes affecting the brain and inducing or enhancing psychopathology. The psychiatric syndrome, in turn, could result in behaviors that produce, exacerbate, or alter the course of medical illness. Treatment of the illness could produce psychiatric side effects. Side effects of psychiatric medications, in turn, are capable of causing medical problems or worsening their course. Clinicians must be keenly aware of these reciprocal, mutually interactive relationships in order to treat patients effectively.

DIABETES ASSOCIATION WITH DEPRESSION AND ANXIETY

A well-established relationship exists between diabetes and anxiety/depression. Adverse medical diagnoses are one of the leading triggers for anxious/depressive episodes.[14] In a recent meta-analysis, Smith and colleagues[15] analyzed 12 studies including 12,626 persons with diabetes. They found a pooled odds ratio (OR) of 1.20 (95% confidence interval [CI], 1.10–1.31) for anxiety disorders and an even higher pooled OR of 1.48 (95% CI, 1.02–1.93) for elevated anxiety symptoms. Park and colleagues[16] conducted a similar meta-analysis for persons with diabetes and comorbid depression. They analyzed 10 studies including 42,363 persons and found a pooled OR of 1.50 (95% CI, 1.35–1.66).

Sullivan and colleagues[17] recently studied 3000 middle-aged participants with T2DM who were at risk for cardiovascular events. They assessed both cognitive capacity and extent of depression over a 40-month period. They found that participants who were more depressed showed greater cognitive decline. Typical demographic and clinical covariates did not significantly change the outcome. Although the authors did not discuss possible interventions, their findings are highly significant in tracing the cause of depression in persons with T2DM. These patients are initially somewhat depressed, and then become increasingly depressed as their illness progresses, which creates a cognitive environment predisposing them to even further depression.

The authors conducted only 3 assessments: at baseline, 20 months, and 40 months. Had they conducted more, they may have found a dynamic, nonlinear process. The progression of depression is first influenced by physiologic variables; that is, the patient's perception of symptoms associated with illness. The patient may be triggered to ruminate over her/his symptoms by alarm-related sensations akin to panic, arising out of conditions such as hypoglycemia, metabolic syndrome, and the need to comply with a rigorous treatment regimen. Second, this progression is influenced by cognitive/affective variables, including the patient's perception of increased depression and accompanying cognitive decline.

To a large extent the relationships between these 2 stages can be understood by using simple conditioning models. Symptoms are the unconditioned stimulus and perception of these symptoms results in depression, the unconditioned response. The patient, however, then extrapolates contextual elements from the unconditioned stimulus. For example, the environment in which symptoms are experienced (conditioned stimulus) can become paired or associated with their perception, further exacerbating depression (conditioned response). Another way of looking at it is that the patient experiences symptoms as aversive. The patient attempts to avert them (and their associated cognitive/affective effects) through treatment, such as using insulin to maintain blood glucose levels. This symptom-reducing behavior should be a negative reinforcer, reducing the patient's predilection toward depressing thoughts. If treatment, however, is unsuccessful in remediating or forestalling symptoms, or the patient experiences further cognitive decline, then the patient becomes even more depressed. Instead of reducing depression, unsuccessful treatment exacerbates it. The patient becomes aware of this cognitive decline when behavioral experiments are unsuccessful in altering the environmental contingencies.

The *Diagnostic and Statistical Manual of Mental Disorders* (Fifth Edition) (DSM-5), recently published by the American Psychiatric Association,[18] recognizes these connections. Disruptive mood dysregulation disorder (§296.99), major depressive disorder (§296.xx), persistent depressive disorder (dysthymia) (§300.4), premenstrual dysphoric disorder (§625.4), and unspecified depressive disorders (§311) all may be triggered by diabetes-related concerns. Persons with diabetes have a litany of feared outcomes. These include physical impairment caused by diabetes or obesity; financial cost, logistics, and side effects of treatment; loss of employment; impact of disease on family and friends; and, in extreme cases, loss of body parts and premature demise. The same analysis applies to anxiety. Acute stress disorder (§308.3), adjustment disorder (§309.24), agoraphobia (§300.22), body dysmorphic disorder (§300.7), generalized anxiety disorder (§300.02), obsessive-compulsive disorder (§300.3), panic disorder (§300.01), and social anxiety disorder (§300.23) all follow a similar template.

DEPRESSION AND ANXIETY ASSOCIATION WITH DIABETES

Depression or anxiety also could be a contributing factor to the development of diabetes. This type of psychogenic "reverse causal" or "mental causation" model has been hypothesized between depression and anxiety and primary care diagnoses such as cardiovascular disease[19,20] and cancer.[21,22] Research is now focusing on it in connection with diabetes. An example of how it might work is as follows: anxiety is associated with poor glycemic control.[23] Depression is associated with insulin resistance.[24] Both also are associated with sleep disturbance. The combination of these factors increases vulnerability to obesity and associated cardiometabolic disease.[25] Other contributing factors are physical inactivity, a sedentary lifestyle, appetite dysregulation, and poor dietary habits, all of which may result in overeating, which also may result in obesity. Obesity in turn may trigger more anxiety. To contend with anxiety-depression symptoms, patients engage in coping strategies that place them at further risk for diabetes, such as more overeating. In persons genetically prone to diabetes, this combination of circumstances might produce its actual occurrence. **Fig. 1** depicts some of these interactions.

The clinician also should be sensitive to cultural concepts of psychological distress. Diabetes prevalence has been associated with persons of ethnic minority descent, particularly persons of Hispanic origin.[26] Their experience of the relationship between a psychological diagnosis and a primary care medical diagnosis may be completely different from that of the dominant culture in their respective areas of influence.

METABOLIC SYNDROME

Obesity and overweight also may activate metabolic syndrome, a diabetes precursor.[27] Metabolic syndrome is a cluster of risk factors for cardiovascular disease and diabetes that occur together more often than by chance alone.[28] Although some studies suggest evidence to the contrary,[29] recent research suggests that metabolic syndrome can be caused by psychiatric conditions, just as by any other primary care medical diagnoses.[30,31] This finding may be because of considerations such as dysregulation of the hypothalamic-pituitary-adrenal axis and sympathetic nervous system, precipitated by stress, which increases production of cortisol and, in turn,

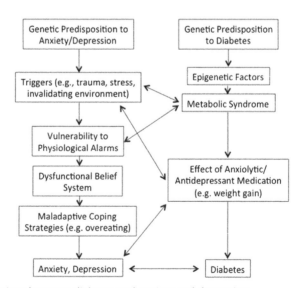

Fig. 1. Interactions between diabetes and anxiety and depression.

raises glucose and insulin levels.[32] Estimates of worldwide prevalence of metabolic syndrome range from 8% to 43%, depending on gender, age, and environment (urban vs rural).[33]

EPIGENETIC RISK

Genome-wide association studies have identified at least 40 genes associated with T1DM[34] and at least 30 genes associated with T2DM.[35,36] The genetics of depression[37–39] and anxiety[40,41] also are increasingly well understood.

Another factor that must be considered is epigenetic risk. Diseases such as diabetes are influenced not only by genes but also by epigenetic, nonhereditary environmental variation.[42,43] In the case of a phenotypical characteristic such as obesity, parental genetic contribution actually may be less important than epigenetic variation.[44] Epigenetic factors also influence the genetic profile of depression[45,46] and anxiety.[47,48] For these reasons, recent research has identified epigenetic factors as the most important determinant of diabetes susceptibility.[43] In psychiatry, this relationship is also known as diathesis-stress, wherein environmental conditions interact with genetic predisposition to express a phenotypical trait characteristic of a psychiatric disorder.[49,50]

TREATMENT OF DEPRESSION: EFFECT OF MEDICATION

The problem presented by psychiatric diagnoses is exacerbated when a psychiatrist prescribes anxiolytics, antidepressants, or neuroleptics, which frequently have direct side effects such as weight gain.[51] Although the mediating-moderating mechanisms have yet to be clarified, use of antidepressant medications also may be sufficient in and of itself to initiate new-onset diabetes.[52] These complex relationships might result in clinical confusion and misdiagnosis. Illustrating the pernicious interaction between psychiatric medication and weight gain. Obesity and overweight in turn are leading risk factors for diabetes (a recent meta-analysis estimated the adjusted relative risk [RR] to be 7.28).[53]

Serotonin reuptake inhibitors (eg, fluoxetine, sertraline, paroxetine) and atypical neuroleptic medications (eg, risperidone, olanzapine, ziprasidone) increasingly are used alone or in combination to treat anxiety and depression.[54,55] All of these medications are capable of producing weight gain and metabolic abnormalities. Some data directly link these medications with the development of diabetes. Also, both classes of medication are associated with insulin resistance,[56–59] which raises an important clinical point. Although treatment of depression and anxiety in the diabetic population is important, it is not risk-free. The clinician must consider the risk/benefit ratio and clearly inform the patient of the complicating factors that have been discussed. Physicians and patients must collaborate in the development of an appropriate treatment plan, which the patient is capable of implementing.

ANTIDEPRESSANTS AND ANTIPSYCHOTICS: FURTHER ANALYSIS OF RISK/BENEFIT

Tricyclic antidepressants (TCAs) and monoamine oxidase inhibitors (MAOIs) that are less frequently used in clinical practice seem to be effective therapy for depression in patients with diabetes. However, evidence shows that these agents may destabilize glycemic control.[60,61] One study showed that selective serotonin reuptake inhibitor (SSRI) antidepressants may help improve glycemic control in some patients with comorbid diabetes and depression.[62] This study and others suggest that SSRIs are the preferred pharmacologic intervention for patients with comorbid depression and diabetes.[63,64] Within this group, Lexapro (escitalopram) and Zoloft (sertraline) are preferable because they have minimal inhibitory effect on the cytochrome P-450 2D6 and 3A4 iso-enzymes that are responsible for the metabolism of many drugs used to treat diabetes.[65]

On the other hand, all SSRI antidepressants typically cause weight gain, especially with prolonged use, thereby increasing risk of diabetes for some patients.[66] A large meta-analysis involving 2934 screened articles on the use of TCAs, SSRIs, serotonin and norepinephrine reuptake inhibitors (SNRIs), and other antidepressants, and the associated risk of diabetes, agreed with this assessment.[67] The authors concluded that use of antidepressants was significantly associated with an increased risk of diabetes in a random effects model (RR, 1.49; 95% confidence interval [CI], 1.29–1.71). In subgroup analyses, the risk of diabetes increased among users of SSRIs (RR, 1.35; 95% CI, 1.15–1.58) and TCAs (RR, 1.57; 95% CI, 1.26–1.96). The subgroup analyses were consistent with overall results regardless of study type, information source, country, duration of medication, or study quality. The subgroup results considering body weight, depression severity, and physical activity also showed a positive association (RR, 1.14; 95% CI, 1.01–1.28).

Overall, these results suggest that the use of antidepressants is associated with an increased risk of diabetes. However, other meta-analyses suggest beneficial effects on glucose homeostasis of hydrazine-type MAOIs and SSRIs in patients with diabetes or those with comorbid depression and diabetes. Noradrenergic substances (and also dual-acting antidepressants) seem to impair glucose tolerance.[68] Whether favorable effects on mood regulation outweigh adverse metabolic effects is unknown; mood regulation could be at the expense of worsening glycemic control.[69] Effective treatment with antidepressants likely improves glucose homeostasis in patients with depression but not diabetes in the short run, whereas long-term effects are unclear. Treatment with SSRIs may improve glycemic control for some patients with depression and diabetes, whereas noradrenergic antidepressants, dual-action antidepressants and TCAs may cause the metabolic situation to deteriorate. The effects of other antidepressants that do not cause weight gain, such as bupropion or newer agents, require further investigation before reliable conclusions can be drawn.[70]

Antipsychotics as a group have been associated with metabolic syndrome, weight gain, and diabetes.[71] A recent meta-analysis[72] analyzed 88,467 cases; 6109 persons with diabetes were matched to 61,090 controls. The risk of diabetes was not statistically different across the atypical antipsychotics. On the other hand, longer exposure to any antipsychotic (odds ratio [OR], 1.009; 95% CI, 1.006–1.011 for each 30-day period) and current use of antipsychotics (OR, 1.26; 95% CI, 1.17–1.36) were associated with diabetes. One study reviewing 60 reports[73] affirmed diabetic ketoacidosis as a rare but serious risk associated with almost all atypical antipsychotics. Liability varied between agents, at least partially mirroring the risk of weight gain. More than one-third of cases had no weight gain or loss; 61% of those required ongoing treatment for glycemic control. Death occurred in 7.25% of cases. Although rare, clinicians must remain vigilant of this complication given its acute onset and potential lethality. Older adults without schizophrenia or bipolar disorder seem to be more at risk of new-onset treatment-dependent diabetes and hyperlipidemia associated with atypical antipsychotic use.[74] Overall, studies seem to agree that the antipsychotic medications that are widely used in clinical practice for nonpsychotic anxiety and depression have the potential to increase the risk of diabetes and its complications.[75,76] The metabolic parameters associated with diabetes should be monitored more carefully with prolonged use of both antidepressant and antipsychotic medications.

TREATMENT OF DIABETES AS RISK FACTOR OF DEPRESSION AND ANXIETY

Few data are available on the interaction among depression, antidepressant treatment, and medications used in the treatment of T2DM. Insulin excess could lead to hypoglycemic seizures and subsequent anxiety and depression.[77] Poor control of diabetes, however, can lead to fatigue and deteriorating mood, which mimics depression. Although no studies have been published, metformin and sulfourea drugs have been anecdotally associated with improvement in depression; however, both have anxiety and depression as potential side effects.

OTHER BIOLOGIC TREATMENT MODALITIES FOR DEPRESSION

Several studies conclude that some other antidepressants recently approved on the market with low drug-drug interaction (eg, milnacipran) may improve management of depression in the diabetic population.[78] However, this medication has a strong norepinephrine component to its mechanism of action that was implicated in the deregulation of glycemic control.

Some time has passed since significant scientific advances have been made in anxiolytics or antidepressants. The authors believe that brain stimulation has significant potential to bridge the gap between cognitive behavioral therapy and psychotropic medication. Other treatments include repetitive transcranial magnetic stimulation (rTMS), recently approved by the U.S. Food and Drug Association for unipolar depression,[79] and daily left prefrontal rTMS (DrTMS). A recent study[80] showed that the odds of attaining remission with DrTMS were 4.2 times greater than with an inactive control.

Other new minimally or noninvasive neuromodulation technologies include magnetic resonance–guided rTMS, cranial electrotherapy stimulation, transcranial direct-current stimulation, and low-intensity focused-ultrasound pulse. Surgical technologies nearing market include vagus nerve stimulation; deep brain stimulation; implanted electrocortical stimulation; epidural cortical stimulation; and high-intensity focused-ultrasound.[81] The efficacy of these third-wave therapies in treating anxiety or depression associated with diabetes has not yet been studied.

COGNITIVE BEHAVIORAL THERAPY INTERVENTIONS

One also should consider the use of cognitive behavior therapy (CBT). CBT is widely regarded as the paradigm of an empirically supported therapy,[82] and numerous studies validate its efficacy in a variety of treatment contexts.[83] In most instances, it is more effective than other forms of psychotherapy[84] and a useful adjunct to pharmacotherapy for most types of treatment-resistant psychopathology, primarily depressive/anxiety disorders.[85] CBT theorizes that adverse psychological, affective, and behavioral outcomes do not result from facts or states of affairs in a person's real or imaginal world. Rather, events or situations engender thoughts or beliefs (CBT frequently uses these terms interchangeably), which then cause subjective personal distress or maladaptive social behavior.[86,87] Epigenetic risk, which now has been identified as an important diabetes precursor, primarily arises from environmental factors. It follows that it should be more manageable than purely genetic risk using CBT techniques.

Within the CBT framework, the best way to regard the depression/anxiety complex from a case conceptualization standpoint is by using an alarm-belief-coping (A-B-C) model. Alarms are activated by triggers, which are events or situations that occur in the real world. These triggers also can be an intrusive recollection of a past event, which creates tension, pressure, or stress. Beliefs are the thoughts that alarms provoke. Coping strategies are the way one contends with the anxiety-producing complex created by the mutually reinforcing network of alarms and beliefs.[14,88] **Fig. 2** diagrams this process.

CBT has been successfully used in the medical setting for a variety of lifestyle changes, such as reducing obesity.[89] Specific programs have been developed for the management of diabetes-related depression.[90] A collaborative care approach is producing favorable results in managing anxiety in a primary care setting.[91] Other important components of a comprehensive program of psychological interventions include family and group treatment. Organizations and support groups also have shown efficacy in medical and psychiatric settings.[92]

HOW TO IMPROVE CARE FOR DIABETES AND ANXIETY AND DEPRESSION

Better clinical models are needed to treat people with combined medical-psychiatric illness. Instead of resorting to static diagnostic criteria, clinicians should use more of a dimensional criteria-set for comorbid primary care conditions such as diabetes. This approach is more suitable because it incorporates epidemiologic, etiologic, and idiographic factors that situate patients on a diagnostic spectrum.[93] It is disappointing that instead of recognizing this, the authors of DSM-5 largely retained an obsolete categorical approach.[94] A categorical approach requires a person to meet a set of specified criteria to qualify for a diagnosis. A dimensional approach, on the other hand, evaluates the patient along a continuum of different symptoms, syndromes, and cognitive phenotypes.[95] Symptoms are particular features of a disorder, which can be ascertained from subjective self-reports and clinical judgments of behavior. Symptoms tend to co-occur in clusters, which are called *syndromes*. Symptoms and syndromes are components of higher-order constructs, such as mood disorders, which are called *cognitive phenotypes*. If anxiety is the syndrome, then the physiologic sensations characteristic of panic disorder (eg, hypoglycemia) are a symptom, and a dysfunctional belief hierarchy (eg, "I'll always be ill" or "There's nothing I can do about it") is a cognitive phenotype.[96] Using this approach, a patient's concern over a medical

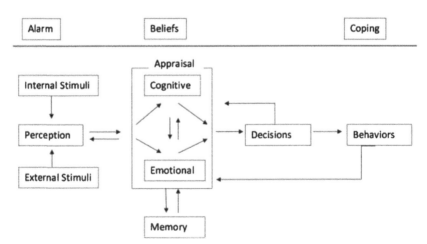

Fig. 2. The alarms-beliefs-coping (A-B-C) model of anxiety and depression. (*From* Bystritsky A, Nierenberg AA, Feusner JD, et al. Computational non-linear dynamical psychiatry: a new methodological paradigm for diagnosis and course of illness. J Psychiatr Res 2012;6(4):428–35; with permission.)

condition such as diabetes could be situated along an anxiety-depression scale ranging from no causal relationship/no patient concern to demonstrated causal relationship/high patient concern.

This form of case conceptualization also has implications for the delivery of health care services. The processes of anxiety and depression is nonlinear, dynamic, and interactive.[88] As a result, a patient's clinical presentation may become accentuated or pathologized at any point within the dimensional cycle. For example, compulsive behavior may be a consequence of beliefs associated with illness rather than obsessional thinking. Negative thought patterns characteristic of persons with diabetes in fact may be a form of conditioned problem-solving coping behavior in response to dysfunctional beliefs, not a precipitating cause of them.

This model is more plausible for understanding the relationship among depression, anxiety, and primary care diagnoses such as diabetes. It also requires keen understanding of how different treatments of diabetes and anxiety/depression interact. Case conceptualization using this type of transdiagnostic approach, and treatment of these diagnoses using a unified protocol, should be standard procedure, not the exception.[97–99] The National Institute of Mental Health[100] recently announced that it no longer will use DSM criteria in awarding research grants. It recognizes that syndromes such as anxiety and depression are ataxonic and multidimensional.[101] Instead, funding will be directed toward projects using multiple data sources, ranging from behavioral symptoms to neuroimaging results. A transdiagnostic approach in turn implicates what might be characterized as a trans-treatment response, addressing all symptoms at once regardless of their provenance or origin. This approach will become increasingly important as expanding mental health care needs collide with the Patient Protection and Affordable Care Act,[102] prompting physicians and therapists to collaborate to improve outcomes and control costs.[103]

At the same time, each person's psychological response to a medical condition such as diabetes is unique, and therefore clinical interventions must be sensitive to individual differences. Even though these responses are conceptualized nomothetically, they require an idiographic treatment strategy.[104] The National Institute of Mental Health's recent vision statement[105] emphasizes this mandate:

> In general, traditional intervention research has focused on comparing how groups of individuals receiving an experimental intervention fare against a comparison group that does not receive that intervention. This approach has given us information about treatments for selected groups of people but not necessarily about how to choose the best treatment for a specific individual. We need personalized medicine: tailoring pharmacologic, behavioral, and other forms of treatment to the needs of each individual. A new generation of clinical trials is needed to gather a wider array of data and examine the kinds of questions that can be used for personalized decision-making in medicine.

An important component of this model will be the use of computer-assisted technology to empower patients and enable them to collaborate proactively in every phase of their treatment.[106–108]

SUMMARY

Anxiety and depression are among the most common forms of psychopathology, affecting millions of persons worldwide. They result in an insidious, mutually reinforcing hierarchy of enhanced alarm sensitivity, dysfunctional beliefs, and maladaptive coping behaviors. This template is exacerbated when overlaid with a serious primary care diagnosis, such as diabetes. Any serious primary care diagnosis has the potential to cause anxiety and depression. Conversely, anxiety and depression increase epigenetic risk, which intensify the danger from hybrid biologic/environmental factors, such as metabolic syndrome. CBT is highly useful for addressing factors contributing to metabolic syndrome, such as obesity. Psychotropic medication is a useful adjunct to psychotherapy. Medications used to treat anxiety and depression, however, create their own diathesis-stress type of risk. The result is a confusing and potentially destabilizing clinical presentation; all of these variables must be considered when treating patients.

REFERENCES

1. Wild S, Roglic G, Green A, et al. Global prevalence of diabetes: estimates for the year 2000 and projections for 2030. Diabetes Care 2004;27:1047–53.
2. Pinhas-Hamiel O, Zeitler P. The global spread of type 2 diabetes mellitus in children and adolescents. J Pediatr 2005;146(5):693–700.
3. Hannon TS, Rao G, Arslanian SA. Childhood obesity and type 2 diabetes mellitus. Pediatrics 2005;116(2):473–80.
4. Hogan P, Dall T, Nikolov P, et al. Economic costs of diabetes in the US in 2002. Diabetes Care 2003;26(3):917–32.
5. Lin EH, Korff MV, Alonso J, et al. Mental disorders among persons with diabetes–results from the World Mental Health Surveys. J Psychosom Res 2008; 65(6):571–80.
6. Richards D. Prevalence and clinical course of depression: a review. Clin Psychol Rev 2011;31(7):1117–25.
7. Baxter AJ, Scott KM, Vos T, et al. Global prevalence of anxiety disorders: a systematic review and meta-regression. Psychol Med 2013;43(5):897–910.
8. Willett WC, Hu FB, Thun M. Overweight, obesity, and all-cause mortality. J Am Med Assoc 2013;309(16):1681.
9. Pollack A. A.M.A. recognizes obesity as a disease. New York Times 2013. Available at: http://www.nytimes.com/2013/06/19/business/ama-recognizes-obesity-as-a-disease.html?_r=0. Accessed August 15, 2013.
10. Atkinson MA, Eisenbarth GS. Type 1 diabetes: new perspectives on disease pathogenesis and treatment. Lancet 2001;358(9277):221–9.
11. Casey DE. Metabolic issues and cardiovascular disease in patients with psychiatric disorders. Am J Med 2005;118(2):15–22.
12. Bogner HR, Morales KH, deVries HF, et al. Diabetes mellitus and depression treatment to improve medication adherence: a randomized controlled trial. Ann Fam Med 2012;10(1):15–22.
13. North CS, Hong BA, Alpers DH. Relationship of functional gastrointestinal disorders and psychiatric disorders: implications for treatment. World J Gastroenterol 2007;13(14):2020–7.
14. Bystritsky A, Khalsa SS, Cameron ME, et al. Current diagnosis and treatment of anxiety disorders. P T 2013;38(1):30–57.
15. Smith KJ, Béland M, Clyde M, et al. Association of diabetes with anxiety: a systematic review and meta-analysis. J Psychosom Res 2013;74(2):89–99.
16. Park M, Katon WJ, Wolf FM. Depression and risk of mortality in individuals with diabetes: a meta-analysis and systematic review. Gen Hosp Psychiatry 2013; 35(3):217–25.
17. Sullivan MD, Katon WJ, Lovato LC, et al. Association of depression with accelerated cognitive decline among patients with type 2 diabetes in the ACCORD-MIND trial. JAMA Psychiatry 2013;70(10):1041–7.

18. American Psychiatric Association. Diagnostic and statistical manual of mental disorders (DSM-5). 5th edition. Washington, DC: American Psychiatric Publishing; 2013.
19. Chavez CA, Ski CF, Thompson DR. Depression and coronary heart disease: apprehending the elusive black dog. Int J Cardiol 2012;158(3):335–6.
20. Leung YW, Flora DB, Gravely S, et al. The impact of premorbid and postmorbid depression onset on mortality and cardiac morbidity among patients with coronary heart disease: meta-analysis. Psychosom Med 2012;74(8):786–801.
21. Pössel P, Adams E, Valentine JC. Depression as a risk factor for breast cancer: investigating methodological limitations in the literature. Cancer Causes Control 2012;23(8):1223–9.
22. Whitley E, Batty GD, Mulheran PA, et al. Psychiatric disorder as a risk factor for cancer: different analytic strategies produce different findings. Epidemiology 2012;23(4):543–50.
23. Anderson RJ, Grigsby AB, Freedland KE, et al. Anxiety and poor glycemic control: a meta-analytic review of the literature. Int J Psychiatry Med 2002;32(3):235–47.
24. Kan C, Silva N, Golden SH, et al. A systematic review and meta-analysis of the association between depression and insulin resistance. Diabetes Care 2013; 36(2):480–9.
25. Knutson KL. Does inadequate sleep play a role in vulnerability to obesity? Am J Human Biol 2012;24(3):361–71.
26. Casagrande SS, Fradkin JE, Saydah SH, et al. The prevalence of meeting A1C, blood pressure, and LDL goals among people with diabetes, 1988-2010. Diabetes Care 2013;36(8):2271–9.
27. Dunkley AJ, Charles K, Gray LJ, et al. Effectiveness of interventions for reducing diabetes and cardiovascular disease risk in people with metabolic syndrome: systematic review and mixed treatment comparison meta-analysis. Diabetes Obes Metab 2012;14(7):616–25.
28. Alberti KG, Eckel RH, Grundy SM, et al. Joint scientific statement harmonizing the metabolic syndrome: a joint interim statement of the International Diabetes Federation Task Force on Epidemiology and Prevention; National Heart, Lung, and Blood Institute; American Heart Association; World Heart Federation; International Atherosclerosis Society; and International Association for the Study of Obesity. Circulation 2009;120:1640–5.
29. Hildrum B, Mykletun A, Midthjell K, et al. No association of depression and anxiety with the metabolic syndrome: the Norwegian HUNT study. Acta Psychiatr Scand 2009;120(1):14–22.
30. Ohaeri JU, Akanji AO. Metabolic syndrome in severe mental disorders. Metab Syndr Relat Disord 2011;9(2):91–8.
31. Pan A, Keum NN, Okereke OI, et al. Bidirectional association between depression and metabolic syndrome: a systematic review and meta-analysis of epidemiological studies. Diabetes Care 2012;35(5):1171–80.
32. Champaneri S, Wand GS, Malhotra SS, et al. Biological basis of depression in adults with diabetes. Curr Diab Rep 2010;10(6):396–405.
33. Eckel RH, Grundy SM, Zimmet PZ. The metabolic syndrome. Lancet 2005; 365(9468):1415–28.
34. Barrett JC, Clayton DG, Concannon P, et al. Genome-wide association study and meta-analysis find that over 40 loci affect risk of type 1 diabetes. Nat Genet 2009;41:703–7.
35. Newgard CB, Attie AD. Getting biological about the genetics of diabetes. Nat Med 2010;16:388–91.

36. Voight BF, Scott LJ, Steinthorsdottir V, et al. Twelve type 2 diabetes susceptibility loci identified through large-scale association analysis. Nat Genet 2010;42: 579–89.
37. Cohen-Woods S, Craig IW, McGuffin P. The current state of play on the molecular genetics of depression. Psychol Med 2013;43(4):673–87.
38. Lohoff FW. Overview of the genetics of major depressive disorder. Curr Psychiatry Rep 2010;12(6):539–46.
39. Wray NR, Pergadia ML, Blackwood DH, et al. Genome-wide association study of major depressive disorder: new results, meta-analysis, and lessons learned. Mol Psychiatry 2012;17:36–48.
40. Webb BT, Guo AY, Maher BS, et al. Meta-analyses of genome-wide linkage scans of anxiety-related phenotypes. Eur J Hum Genet 2012;20:1078–84.
41. Smoller JW, Block SR, Young MM. Genetics of anxiety disorders: the complex road from DSM to DNA. Depress Anxiety 2009;26(11):965–75.
42. Drong AW, Lindgren CM, McCarthy MI. The genetic and epigenetic basis of type 2 diabetes and obesity. Clin Pharmacol Ther 2012;92(6):707–15.
43. Ling C, Groop L. Epigenetics: a molecular link between environmental factors and type 2 diabetes. Diabetes 2009;58(12):2718–25.
44. Moore GE, Stanier P. Fat dads must not be blamed for their children's health problems. BMC Med 2013;11:30.
45. Krishnan V, Nestler EJ. The molecular neurobiology of depression. Nature 2008; 455:894–902.
46. Labonté B, Turecki G. The epigenetics of depression and suicide. In: Petronis A, Mill J, editors. Brain, behavior and epigenetics. New York: Springer Science+''' Business Media; 2011. p. 49–70.
47. Dias BG, Banerjee SB, Goodman JV, et al. Towards new approaches to disorders of fear and anxiety. Curr Opin Neurobiol 2013;23(3):346–52.
48. Hamilton SP. Linkage and association studies of anxiety disorders. Depress Anxiety 2009;26(11):976–83.
49. Belsky J, Pluess M. Beyond diathesis stress: differential susceptibility to environmental influences. Psychol Bull 2009;135(6):885–908.
50. Belsky J, Jonassaint C, Pluess M, et al. Vulnerability genes or plasticity genes? Mol Psychiatry 2009;14:746–54.
51. Kivimäki M, Hamer M, Batty GD, et al. Antidepressant medication use, weight gain, and risk of type 2 diabetes: a population-based study. Diabetes Care 2010;33(12):2611–6.
52. Bhattacharjee S, Bhattacharya R, Kelley GA, et al. Antidepressant use and new-onset diabetes: a systematic review and meta-analysis. Diabetes Metab Res Rev 2013;29(4):273–84.
53. Abdullah A, Peeters A, Courten MD, et al. The magnitude of association between overweight and obesity and the risk of diabetes: a meta-analysis of prospective cohort studies. Diabetes Res Clin Pract 2010;89(3):309–19.
54. Bschor T. Therapy-resistant depression. Expert Rev Neurother 2010;10(1): 77–86.
55. Philip NS, Carpenter LL, Tyrka AR, et al. Pharmacologic approaches to treatment resistant depression: a re-examination for the modern era. Expert Opin Pharmacother 2010;11(5):709–22.
56. Citrome LL, Jaffe AB. Relationship of atypical antipsychotics with development of diabetes mellitus. Ann Pharmacother 2003;37(12):1849–57.
57. Malone M. Medications associated with weight gain. Ann Pharmacother 2005; 39(12):2046–55.

58. Nguyen HT, Arcury TA, Grzywacz JG, et al. The association of mental conditions with blood glucose levels in older adults with diabetes. Aging Ment Health 2012; 16(8):950–7.

59. Penckofer S, Quinn L, Byrn M, et al. Does glycemic variability impact mood and quality of life? Diabetes Technol Ther 2012;14(4):303–10.

60. Goodnick PJ, Henry JH, Buki VM. Treatment of depression in patients with diabetes mellitus. J Clin Psychiatry 1995;56(4):128–36.

61. Lustman PJ, Griffith LS, Clouse RE, et al. Effects of nortriptyline on depression and glycemic control in diabetes: results of a double-blind, placebo-controlled trial. Psychosom Med 1997;59(3):241–50.

62. Ghaeli P, Shahsavand E, Mesbahi M, et al. Comparing the effects of 8-week treatment with fluoxetine and imipramine on fasting blood glucose of patients with major depressive disorder. J Clin Psychopharmacol 2004;24(4): 386–8.

63. Katon WJ, Young BA, Russo J, et al. Association of depression with increased risk of severe hypoglycemic episodes in patients with diabetes. Ann Fam Med 2013;11(3):245–50.

64. Gehlawat P, Gupta R, Rajput R, et al. Diabetes with comorbid depression: role of SSRI in better glycemic control. Asian J Psychiatr 2013;6(5):364–8.

65. Greenblatt DJ, von Moltke LL, Harmatz JS, et al. Human cytochromes and some newer antidepressants: kinetics, metabolism, and drug interactions. J Clin Psychopharmacol 1999;19(Suppl 5):23S–35S.

66. Papakostas GI. Managing partial response or nonresponse: switching, augmentation, and combination strategies for major depressive disorder. J Clin Psychiatry 2009;70(Suppl 6):16–25.

67. Allemann S, Houriet C, Diem P, et al. Self-monitoring of blood glucose in non-insulin treated patients with type 2 diabetes: a systematic review and meta-analysis. Curr Med Res Opin 2009;25(1):2903–13.

68. Hennings JM, Schaaf L, Fulda S. Glucose metabolism and antidepressant medication. Curr Pharm Des 2012;18(36):5900–19.

69. Isaac R, Boura-Halfon S, Gurevitch D, et al. Selective serotonin reuptake inhibitors (SSRIs) inhibit insulin secretion and action in pancreatic cells. J Biol Chem 2013;288(8):5682–93.

70. Deuschle M. Effects of antidepressants on glucose metabolism and diabetes mellitus type 2 in adults. Curr Opin Psychiatry 2013;26(1):60–5.

71. Mitchell AJ, Vancampfort D, Sweers K, et al. Prevalence of metabolic syndrome and metabolic abnormalities in schizophrenia and related disorders–a systematic review and meta-analysis. Schizophr Bull 2013;39(2):306–18.

72. Moisan J, Turgeon M, Desjardins O, et al. Comparative safety of antipsychotics: another look at the risk of diabetes. Can J Psychiatry 2013;58(4):218–24.

73. Guenette MD, Hahn M, Cohn TA, et al. Atypical antipsychotics and diabetic ketoacidosis: a review. Psychopharmacology (Berl) 2013;226(1):1–12.

74. Thakurathi N, Henderson DC. Atypical antipsychotics are associated with incident diabetes in older adults without schizophrenia or bipolar disorder. Evid Based Ment Health 2012;15(3):61.

75. McIntyre RS, Soczynska JK, Konarski JZ, et al. The effect of antidepressants on glucose homeostasis and insulin sensitivity: synthesis and mechanisms. Expert Opin Drug Saf 2006;5(1):157–68.

76. Meltzer HY. Putting metabolic side effects into perspective: risks versus benefits of atypical antipsychotics. J Clin Psychiatry 2001;62(Suppl 27):35–9 [discussion: 40–1].

77. MacLeod KM, Hepburn DA, Frier BM. Frequency and morbidity of severe hypo-glycaemia in insulin-treated diabetic patients. Diabet Med 1993;10(3):238–45.

78. Hofman P. Treatment of patients with comorbid depression and diabetes with metformin and milnacipran. Neuropsychiatr Dis Treat 2010;6(Suppl I):9–15.

79. Daskalakis ZJ. Repetitive transcranial magnetic stimulation for the treatment of depression: to stimulate or not to stimulate? J Psychiatry Neurosci 2005; 30(2):81–2.

80. George MS, Lisanby SH, Avery D, et al. Daily left prefrontal transcranial mag-netic stimulation therapy for major depressive disorder: a sham-controlled ran-domized trial. Arch Gen Psychiatry 2010;67(5):507–16.

81. Bystritsky A, Korb AS, Douglas PK, et al. A review of low-intensity focused ultra-sound pulsation. Brain Stimul 2011;4(3):125–36.

82. Butler AC, Chapman JE, Forman EM, et al. The empirical status of cognitive-behavioral therapy: a review of meta-analyses. Clin Psychol Rev 2006;26(1): 17–31.

83. Hofman SG, Asnaani A, Vonk IJ, et al. The efficacy of cognitive behavioral ther-apy: a review of meta-analyses. Cognit Ther Res 2012;36(5):427–40.

84. Tolin DF. Is cognitive-behavioral therapy more effective than other therapies? Clin Psychol Rev 2010;30(6):710–20.

85. Wiles N, Thomas L, Abel A, et al. Cognitive behavioural therapy as an adjunct to pharmacotherapy for primary care based patients with treatment resistant depression: results of the CoBalT randomised controlled trial. Lancet 2013; 381(9864):375–84.

86. Friedman ES, Thase ME. Cognitive and behavioral therapies. In: Fatemi SH, Clayton PJ, editors. The medical basis of psychiatry. 3rd edition. Totowa (NJ): Humana Press; 2008. p. 635–49.

87. González-Prendes AA, Resko SM. Cognitive-behavioral theory. In: Ringel S, Brandell JR, editors. Trauma: contemporary directions in theory, practice, and research. Thousand Oaks (CA): SAGE Publications, Inc; 2012. p. 14–40.

88. Bystritsky A, Nierenberg AA, Feusner JD, et al. Computational non-linear dynamical psychiatry: a new methodological paradigm for diagnosis and course of illness. J Psychiatr Res 2012;46(4):428–35.

89. Fabricatore AN. Behavior therapy and cognitive-behavioral therapy of obesity: is there a difference? J Am Diet Assoc 2007;107(1):92–9.

90. Anderson RJ, Freedland KE, Clouse RE, et al. The prevalence of comorbid depression in adults with diabetes: a meta-analysis. Diabetes Care 2001; 24(6):1069–78.

91. Roy-Byrne P, Katon W, Cowley DS, et al. A randomized trail of collaborative care for patients with panic disorder in primary care. Arch Gen Psychiatry 2001; 58(9):869–76.

92. Due-Christensen M, Zoffman V, Hommel E, et al. Can sharing experiences in groups reduce the burden of living with diabetes, regardless of glycaemic con-trol? Diabet Med 2012;29(2):251–6.

93. DeFife JA, Peart J, Bradley B, et al. Validity of prototype diagnosis for mood and anxiety disorders. JAMA Psychiatry 2013;70(2):140–8.

94. Gros DF, Simms LJ, Antony MM. A hybrid model of social phobia: an analysis of so-cial anxiety and related symptoms of anxiety. J Clin Psychol 2011;67(3):293–307.

95. Helzer JE, Kraemer HC, Krueger RF. The feasibility and need for dimensional psychiatric diagnoses. Psychol Med 2006;36:1671–80.

96. Bilder RM, Howe A, Novak N, et al. The genetics of cognitive impairment in schizophrenia: a phenomic perspective. Trends Cogn Sci 2011;15(9):428–35.

97. Clark DA. Cognitive behavioral therapy for anxiety and depression: possibilities and limitations of a transdiagnostic perspective. Cogn Behav Ther 2009; 38(Suppl 1):29–34.

98. Dudley R, Kuyken W, Padesky CA. Disorder specific and trans-diagnostic case conceptualization. Clin Psychol Rev 2011;31(2):213–24.

99. Norton PJ, Barrera TL. Transdiagnostic versus diagnosis-specific CBT for anxiety disorders: a preliminary randomized controlled noninferiority trial. Depress Anxiety 2012;29(10):874–82.

100. National Institute of Mental Health. NIMH Research Domain Criteria (RDoC). Available at: http://www.nimh.nih.gov/research-funding/rdoc/nimh-research-domain-criteria-rdoc.shtml. Accessed August 15, 2013.

101. Bernstein A, Stickle TR, Zvolensky MJ, et al. Dimensional, categorical, or dimensional-categories: testing the latent structure of anxiety sensitivity among adults using factor-mixture modeling. Behav Ther 2010;41(4):515–29.

102. Patient Protection and Affordable Care Act, Pub L No 111–148, 124 Stat 119, 42 USC §18001 (2010).

103. Gorman A. Seeing the whole patient–Health care law prompts physicians and therapists to collaborate. Los Angeles Times 2013. Available at: http://www.latimes.com/news/local/la-me-clinic-mental-health-20130610,0, 1529192.story. Accessed August 15, 2013.

104. Persons JB, Roberts NA, Zalecki CA, et al. Naturalistic outcome of case formulation-driven cognitive-behavior therapy for anxious depressed outpatients. Behav Res Ther 2006;44(7):1041–51.

105. National Institute of Mental Health. The National Institute of Mental Health Strategic Plan. Available at: http://www.nimh.nih.gov/about/strategic-planning-reports/index.shtml. Accessed August 15, 2013.

106. Sullivan G, Craske MG, Sherbourne C, et al. Design of the coordinated anxiety learning and management (CALM) study: innovations in collaborative care for anxiety disorders. Gen Hosp Psychiatry 2007;29(5):379–87.

107. Roy-Byrne P, Craske MG, Sullivan G, et al. Delivery of evidence-based treatment for multiple anxiety disorders in primary care: a randomized controlled trial. J Am Med Assoc 2010;303(19):1921–8.

108. Craske MG, Stein MB, Sullivan G, et al. Disorder-specific impact of coordinated anxiety learning and management treatment for anxiety disorders in primary care. Arch Gen Psychiatry 2011;68(4):378–88.

Index

Note: Page numbers of article titles are in **boldface** type.

A

Abdominal obesity, in metabolic syndrome, 11β-HSD1 role in, 86
    prevention strategies for, 13–14
    waist circumference in, 2–4
        suggested cutoffs for, 3, 5
  polycystic ovary syndrome associated with, 7
ABPI (ankle brachial pressure index), in PAD diagnosis, 157–158
ACCORD trial, of diabetes, effect on cardiovascular outcomes, 28–30, 32–33, 49–50
    fracture risk and, 238
    hypertension and, 109
Acetylsalicylic acid (ASA). See *Aspirin.*
Acute coronary syndromes, 67
  non–ST elevation, 67
AD. See *Alzheimer disease (AD).*
Adenosine monophosphate–activated kinase (AMPK), in glucocorticoid-induced insulin resistance, 84–85
Adenosine-stress radionuclide myocardial perfusion imaging, for CHD in asymptomatic patients, 34
Adhesion molecules, in atherosclerosis, vascular cell, 151–152
    with PAD, 154
Adipocytes, in adipogenesis, 80
  in OSA, 195
Adipogenesis, GCs regulation of, 79–80
  in PCOS, 135
Adipokines, in diabetes, atherosclerosis and, 27
    cancer and, 178–179
  in metabolic syndrome, 12
  in OSA, 195
  white adipose secretion of, GCs regulation of, 80–81
Adiponectin, in cancer and diabetes, 178–179
  white adipose secretion of, GCs regulation of, 80–81
    OSA and, 195
Adipose tissue, GCs regulation of functionality, mass, and distribution, 76–85
    11β-HSD1 as gatekeeper of, 81–82, 85–86
    adipogenesis, 79–80
    brown adipose, 81–82
    Cushing syndrome, 78–80
    white adipose de novo lipogenesis, 78
    white adipose insulin sensitivity, 78–79, 88
    white adipose lipolysis, 76–78
    white adipose mass and distribution, 79–80
    white adipose secretory profile, 80–81

Endocrinol Metab Clin N Am 43 (2014) 285–329
http://dx.doi.org/10.1016/S0889-8529(13)00131-X
0889-8529/14/$ – see front matter © 2014 Elsevier Inc. All rights reserved.

endo.theclinics.com

Adipose (*continued*)
  in metabolic syndrome, pathophysiology of, 10–11, 76
    secretory products of, 12
  in PCOS, 135–136
  inflammation of, hypoxia and, 195
  remodeling of, in adipogenesis, 80
  visceral, hypertension and, in diabetes, 106
    OSA and, 195
  vitamin D and insulin metabolism in, 208–210
Adolescent age group, hypertension in, with diabetes, 105
  metabolic syndrome in, 3, 7
  PCOS in, 128, 131–132
Adult criteria, for metabolic syndrome, 2–3
ADVANCE trial, of diabetes effect on cardiovascular outcomes, 28–30, 32
Advanced glycation end products (AGEs), in diabetes, bone and, 234–235
    CAD and, 60
    cardiomyopathy and, 48
    PAD and, 153–154
    vasculature and, 43–44
  receptors of. See *RAGE (receptor of advanced glycation end products)*.
Age/aging, as PAD risk factor, 150
  brain insulin resistance in AD associated with, 257–258
  diabetes and, hypertension in, 105
    osteoporosis-associated fracture in, 237, 239
Age-specific criteria, for metabolic syndrome, 2–3
Age-specific prevalence, of metabolic syndrome, 6–7
  of PCOS, 128, 131–132
Alarm-belief-coping (A-B-C) model, of anxiety/depression connection to diabetes, 275–276
Albuminuria, in diabetes, cardiovascular disease and, 42
    RAAS blockade effect on, 111–112
Alcohol restriction, for hypertension, 110
Aldosterone, hypertension and, in diabetes, 106–107
Alendronate, for osteoporosis, 239
Alzheimer disease (AD), in diabetes, 246
    as metabolic with brain insulin/IGF resistance, 249, 252
      human studies of, 252
    as T3DM, 252–253
      experimental evidence for sporadic AD, 253–254
    chronic ischemic cerebral microvascular disease and, 254–257
    clinical diagnosis of, 248–249
    insulin resistance and, 248, 252, 257
      sporadic, 253–254
    metabolic deficits in, 253–255
    neuropathology of, 249–251
    occurrence of, 246, 248
    underlying causes of, 257–260
      aging as, 257–258
      lifestyle choices as, 258
      metabolic syndrome as, 259–260
      NAFLD/NASH as, 259

obesity as, 258–259
T2DM as, 259
Amenorrhea, in PCOS, 125–126
American Association of Clinical Endocrinologists (AACE), metabolic syndrome definition
  of, 2, 4–5
American College of Cardiology (ACC), revascularization guidelines of, 63, 66
American Diabetes Association (ADA), on ABPI screening for PAD, 158
  on dyslipidemia treatment, 49–50
  on hypertension treatment, 32, 108–109
  on metabolic syndrome, concerns expressed by, 15–16
    definition of, 2–5
American Heart Association (AHA), metabolic syndrome definition of, 2–5
  preventive aspirin recommendations of 33, 2–5
Amlodipine, for hypertension, 111–112, 114
Amyloid-beta precursor protein (AbPP), in AD, 246, 249, 251–252
    insulin resistance/deficiency and, 254–255
Anabolic agents, for osteoporosis, 239
  insulin as, 236
Androgen Excess Society (AES) criteria, for PCOS, 124–125
Androgens. See also *Testosterone.*
  excess of. See *Hyperandrogenism.*
  prenatal exposure to, in PCOS, 129, 134
Angiogenesis, in cancer and diabetes, 176–177
  in PAD, 153, 163
Angiography, in PAD diagnosis, 159–160
Angioplasty, with/without stents, for PAD, 162
Angiotensin II (Ang II), in hypertension, with diabetes, 106–107, 111
Angiotensin II receptor, in cardiomyopathy, with diabetes, 47
Angiotensin receptor blockers (ARBs), for hypertension, in diabetes, 33, 68, 111
    in metabolic syndrome, 15
Angiotensin-converting enzyme, in diabetes, atherosclerosis and, 27
Angiotensin-converting enzyme inhibitors (ACEIs), for hypertension, in diabetes, 33, 111,
  114
    in metabolic syndrome, 15
Angiotensinogen (AGT), in hypertension, 106
Ankle brachial pressure index (ABPI), in PAD diagnosis, 157–158
Anovulation, in PCOS, 124–126, 129
    treatment of, 136–138
Antiandrogenic agents, for PCOS, 138
Antidepressants, diabetes and, effects of, 270, 273
    risk/benefit analysis of, 273–274
Antihypertensive agents, in diabetes, 111–113
    clinical trials on, 108–109
Antilipid agents. See also *specific classification or drug.*
  for CAD prevention in diabetics, 31–32, 49–50, 68
  for metabolic syndrome, 14–15
Antiplatelet agents, for cardiovascular disease, 60, 68
  for PAD, 161
Antipsychotics, diabetes and, effects of, 270, 273
    risk/benefit analysis of, 274
Antiresorptives, for osteoporosis, 239

Antithrombotic agents, with PCI, for CAD, 67
Anxiety, interactions between diabetes and, **269–283**
 association with diabetes, 271–272
 cognitive impairment with, 270–271
 complex relationships in, 270
 depression treatment in, 273–276
  biologic modalities, 275
  cognitive behavioral therapy interventions, 275–276
  improving care, 276–277
  medication effects, 270, 273
  risk/benefit analysis, 273–274
 diabetes association with, 270–271
 diabetes subtypes in, 270
 diabetes treatment in, as risk factor, 275
  improving care, 276–277
 epigenetic risk for, 273, 275
 key points on, 269–270
 metabolic syndrome and, 272–273
Anxiolytics, diabetes and, risk/benefit analysis of, 273, 275
Apnea, during OSA, 191–192
 CPAP considerations of, 200
 severity indices of, 193
Apoptosis. See *Cellular injury/death.*
Appetite, GCs regulation of, 85
 in metabolic syndrome, 13
Arterial disease, cardiovascular. See *Cardiovascular disease (CVD).*
 in lower limbs. See *Peripheral arterial disease (PAD).*
Artery grafts, for CABG, 63–64
Aspirin, for cardiovascular disease, 33, 68
 for PAD, 161
Atherosclerosis, in diabetes, 27–28, 42, 60
 in PAD, 150–154
 OSA impact on, 193–194
 risk of, cardiovascular. See *Cardiovascular disease (CVD).*
 coronary. See *Coronary artery disease (CAD).*
 in diabetes, 27–28, 42
 in metabolic syndrome, 1–3
 in PCOS, 129–130
Autoimmunity, in PCOS, 136
Autonomic nervous system, in OSA, 191
Autonomic neuropathy, cardiac, in diabetic cardiomyopathy, 47–48

B

Bare-metal stents (BMSs), for cardiovascular disease, 60, 68
BARI 2D trial, of diabetes effect on cardiovascular outcomes, 30, 34, 60, 67
Berlin questionnaire, for OSA, 199
β-Blockers, for hypertension, in diabetes, 113
 in metabolic syndrome, 15
β-Cell function, in metabolic syndrome, 13
 adipose tissue and, 10–13

in OSA, 190
   IH impact on, 194
      human studies linking, 195–196
  in PCOS, 135
  in T2DM, 208
   vitamin D impact on, 208–209
Biologic modalities, for depression, 275
Biopsychosocial perspective, of diabetes, 270
Bisphosphonates, for osteoporosis, 239
Bladder cancer, diabetes and, 169–171
Blood glucose level, after meals. See *Postprandial glucose.*
  decreased. See *Hypoglycemia.*
  fasting. See *Fasting glucose (FG).*
  in metabolic syndrome definitions, 2–3, 5
  increased. See *Hyperglycemia.*
Blood pressure (BP), control in diabetes, for cardiovascular disease, 32–33
    hypertension guidelines for, 108–109
  in metabolic syndrome, 1–3, 5, 13
  in PAD, 151, 161
  increased. See *Hypertension (HTN).*
BMD. See *Bone mineral density (BMD).*
Body mass index (BMI), in cancer and diabetes, 179
  in diabetes, bone loss and, 235
    effect on PCI outcomes, 68
  in metabolic syndrome, 3–4, 13
  in obesity definition, 168–169
  in OSA, 189–191
Bone abnormalities, craniofacial, OSA and, 191, 198
Bone formation, glucocorticoids effect on, 239
  in diabetes, 239
  markers of, 236–237
Bone loss, in diabetes, 234
    T1D vs. T2D, 234–237
      differences of, 236–237
      similarities of, 234–235
Bone marrow (BM), vascular progenitor cells in, 45
Bone marrow–derived cells. See also *Macrophages.*
  in metabolic syndrome, 12
Bone mineral density (BMD), in diabetes, fracture risk and, 234, 236
    management applications of, 238–239
    quantification of, 237
Bone resorption, in diabetes, 235, 237, 239
  markers of, 237
Bone turnover, in diabetes, 235, 237, 239
Bone-specific alkaline phosphatase (BSAP), in bone turnover, 237
BP. See *Blood pressure (BP).*
Bradykinin, in diabetes, atherosclerosis and, 27
Brain insulin/IGF resistance, cognitive impairment and, as metabolic AD, 249, 252
    experimental models of, 253–254, 259
    human studies of, 252
    in other neurodegenerative diseases, 256–257

Brain (*continued*)
      systemic insulin-resistance diseases mediation of, 246–247
      underlying causes of, 257–260
          aging as, 257–258
          lifestyle as, 258
          metabolic syndrome as, 259–260
          NAFLD/NASH as, 259
          obesity as, 258–259
          T2DM as, 259
Brain signaling pathways, insulin and IGFs, 248
      with AD, 253–254
   satiety, 13, 85
Brain tissue, chronic ischemic microvascular disease impact on, 254–257
   in glucocorticoid-induced insulin resistance, 84–85
   metabolic derangements of, cognitive impairment with. See *Brain insulin/IGF resistance.*
      in other neurodegenerative diseases, 256–257
Breast cancer, diabetes and, 169–172
      IGF-1 effects on, 173–174
      inflammation in, 178–179
      IR expression in, 176
Breathing, occluded, during OSA, 191–192, 199
Brown adipose tissue, GCs regulation of, 81–82
      11β-HSD1 role in, 81–82, 85
Buerger test, for PAD, 157
Bypass surgery, for CAD. See *Coronary artery bypass graft (CABG).*
   for PAD, 156, 162

C

CABG. See *Coronary artery bypass graft (CABG).*
CAD. See *Coronary artery disease (CAD).*
Calcium channel blockers (CCBs), for hypertension, 111–112, 114
Calcium hemostasis, as PAD risk factor, 151, 154
   in vitamin D and insulin metabolism, 208–210, 217, 225
Calcium intake, for osteoporosis, 238–239
Calcium scores, coronary artery, for CHD in asymptomatic patients, 34
Caloric intake, in hypertension, and diabetes, 110
   in metabolic syndrome, 10–13. See also *Diet.*
   in PCOS, 137
Cancer, diabetes and, **167–185**
      biologic mechanisms linking, 171–177
          hyperglycemia in, 176–177
          hyperinsulinemia in, 175–176
          IGF-1 in, 172–175
          inflammation in, 178
          insulin resistance in, 175–176
          T2DM, obesity, and metabolic syndrome in, 10, 171–172
      epidemiology of, 167–171
          incidence in, 169–170
          mortality in, 170–171
          T2DM, obesity, and metabolic syndrome in, 10, 167–169
      inflammation in, 177–179

        adipokines and, 178–179
        cytokines and, 177–178
     introduction to, 167
     key points on, 167
     summary overview of, 179–180
  endometrial, PCOS and, 131
Cancer mortality, diabetes and, 170–171
Carbenoxolone, potential role in humans, 86–87
Cardiac autonomic neuropathy (CAN), in diabetic cardiomyopathy, 47–48
Cardiomyopathy, in diabetes. See *Diabetic cardiomyopathy (DCM)*.
Cardiovascular disease (CVD), Cushing syndrome and, 79–80
  diabetes mellitus and, cardiomyopathy in, 45–49
        altered substrate metabolism, 46–47
        cardiac autonomic neuropathy, 47–48
        cardiovascular findings, 48
        definition of, 45–46
        diagnosing, 48–49
        mechanisms of, 42, 46–47
        myocardial fibrosis, 47–48
        renin-angiotensin system activation, 47
     clinical implications of, 49–52
        CAD outcomes, 50–52
        CAD risk factors, 49–50
        heart failure, 46, 52
     coronary artery disease with, interventions for, **59–73**. See also *Coronary artery bypass graft (CABG); Percutaneous coronary intervention (PCI)*.
     outcomes of, 50–52
     risk factors of, 49–50
        dyslipidemia as, 49–50
        glycemic control as, 50
        hypertension as, 50
     epidemiology of, 26
     glycemic control for, 28–31
       as risk mitigation, 28–31
       choosing right agent, 29–31
       intensive, 28–29
     heart failure with, 46, 52
     hypertension as risk factor for, 32, 50, 103, 105
       treatment of, 108–109
     introduction to, 25, 41–42
     key points on, 25, 41
     pathogenesis of, **41–57**
     pathophysiology of, 27–28
     risk assessment for events, 26–27
     risk factors and medical therapy, **25–40**
     risk mitigation for, 28–34
       aspirin as, 33
       CHD diagnosis in asymptomatic patients as, 33–34
       glycemic control as, 28–31
       hypertension control as, 32–33
       lipid-lowering therapy as, 31–32

Cardiovascular (*continued*)
    revascularization as, 34
  summary overview of, 34–35, 52–53
  vasculature in, 42–45
    cardiomyopathy findings, 48
    impaired reverse cholesterol transport, 43, 45
    microvasculature dysfunction, 42, 44
    oxidative stress effects on, 42–44
    summary of relationships between, 42–43, 45
    vascular progenitor cell dysfunction, 43–45
  metabolic syndrome and, as risk factor, 1–2, 8–10
    residual, 15
  controversies regarding, 15–16
  pathophysiology of, 11–12
  prevention of, 8, 13–15
  OSA impact on, 187, 193–194
  PCOS and, 129–130
  peripheral. See *Peripheral arterial disease (PAD)*.
Cardiovascular events, major, following revascularization for CAD, 61, 63, 67–68
  risk of. See *Risk entries*.
  with hypertension in diabetes, 104–105
Case conceptualization, of anxiety/depression connection to diabetes, 276–277
Causal model/relationships, in anxiety/depression connection to diabetes, 276–277
  reverse, 271–272
Cellular injury/death, in insulin-resistance diseases, 249, 252
  AD pathology of, 246, 254–255
  chronic ischemic cerebral microvascular disease and, 254–257
Ceramides, in brain insulin/IGF resistance, 246–247, 259
Cerebral microvascular disease, chronic ischemic, in AD, 254–257
Cervical cancer, diabetes and, 172
CHD (coronary heart disease). See *Coronary artery disease (CAD)*.
Cholecalciferol (vitamin D3), physiology of, 206
  supplementation influence on T2DM, 217, 225
    randomized controlled trials of, 217–224
Cholesterol absorption inhibitors, for atherosclerosis, 14
Cholesterol disorders. See *Dyslipidemia*.
Cholesterol transport, GCs regulation of, 83
  impaired reverse, in diabetes, 43, 45
Cholinergic functional deficits, in AD, 252, 255
Chronic ischemic cerebral microvascular disease, in AD, 254–257
Chronic ischemic encephalopathy, in AD, 254
Cigarette smoking, PAD related to, 150
  lifestyle modifications for, 159–160
Cilostazol, for PAD, 161
Claudication, in PAD. See *Intermittent claudication (IC)*.
Clopidrogrel, for PAD, 161
Coagulation cascade, in atherosclerosis, 153
  PAD and, 154
Cognitive behavioral therapy (CBT), for depression, diabetes and, 275–276
Cognitive impairment, in diabetes, **245–267**
  Alzheimer disease as, 246

    as metabolic with brain insulin/IGF resistance, 249, 252
        human studies of, 252
    as T3DM, 252–253
        experimental evidence for sporadic AD, 253–254
    chronic ischemic cerebral microvascular disease and, 254–257
    clinical diagnosis of, 248–249
    insulin resistance and, 248, 252, 257
        sporadic, 253–254
    metabolic deficits in, 253–255
    neuropathology of, 249–251
    occurrence of, 246, 248
    underlying causes of, 257–260
        aging as, 257–258
        lifestyle choices as, 258
        metabolic syndrome as, 259–260
        NAFLD/NASH as, 259
        obesity as, 258–259
        T2DM as, 259
  anxiety/depression with, 270–271
  brain insulin/IGF resistance and, as metabolic AD, 249, 252
        human studies of, 252
        underlying causes of, 257–260
    in other neurodegenerative diseases, 256–257
    systemic insulin-resistance diseases mediation of, 246–247
  insulin resistance in, 248–249
    AD and, 249, 252, 257
  insulin signaling in, 246–248
  introduction to, 245–246
  key points on, 245
  neurodegeneration as, 248–257
  summary overview of, 260
Cognitive phenotypes, in anxiety/depression connection to diabetes, 276–277
  in experimental sporadic AD, 253
Collagen-matrix remodeling, in diabetes, atherosclerosis and, 28, 60
    vascular pathogenesis and, 44, 153–154
Colorectal cancer, diabetes and, 169–172, 174
Comorbidities, of diabetes, cardiovascular risk assessment and, 27, 32
    fracture risk and, 235
    mental health. See *Anxiety; Depression.*
  of OSA, treatment considerations for, 200
Computer-assisted technology, for hypertension management, 114–115
  for patient empowerment in mental health treatment, 277
Conditioning models, simple, of anxiety/depression connection to diabetes, 271
Congestive heart failure (CHF), in diabetes, 46, 52
Continuous positive airway pressure (CPAP), for OSA, 200
    HbA1c changes with, 197
    impact on metabolic syndrome, 197–198
    insulin sensitivity changes with, 196–197
    observational studies of, 190
Coronary artery bypass graft (CABG), for CAD, in diabetes, 34, 50, 52
    as better than PCI, 61, 65–66

Coronary (*continued*)
  comparative outcome findings, 60–63
  conduit choice, 63–64
  guidelines and other issues, 63
  risk scoring, 64–65
  with PCI, 63–64
Coronary artery calcium scores (CACS), for CHD in asymptomatic patients, 34
Coronary artery disease (CAD), diabetes and, 42
  diagnosis in asymptomatic patients, 33–34
  interventions for, **59–73**
    atherosclerosis and, 60
    CABG as, as better than PCI, 65–66
      comparative outcome findings, 60–63
      conduit choice, 63–64
      glucose control perioperatively, 66–67
      guidelines and other issues, 63
      risk scoring, 64–65
      with PCI, 63–64
    introduction to, 59–60
    key points on, 59
    PCI as, CABG as better than, 65–66
      comparative outcome findings, 61–63
      current role for, 67–68
      with CABG, 63–64
    PTCA as, 60–61
    revascularization options in, 60–63
    stents as, 34, 50, 52
      comparative outcome findings, 60–65, 68
      with PCI, 67–68
    summary overview of, 68
  metabolic syndrome and, 2
  outcomes of, 50–52
  risk factors of, 26–27, 49–50
    dyslipidemia as, 49–50
    glycemic control as, 2, 50
    hypertension as, 50
  glucose control perioperatively, and diabetes, interventions for, CABG as, 66–67
  PCOS and, 130
Cortex atrophy, in AD, 249–250, 255
Cortisol, glucocorticoid excess and, 76, 83
  11β-HSD1 expression and, 86
  common obesity and, 87
  in Cushing syndrome, 79
Country-specific criteria, for obesity, in metabolic syndrome, 3, 6
Country-specific prevalence, of diabetes, vitamin D impact on, 211, 225
  with cancer, 170
  with hypertension, 105
  of metabolic syndrome, 3, 6
CPAP. See *Continuous positive airway pressure (CPAP)*.
Craniofacial skeletal structure, OSA and, 191, 198
C-Reactive protein (CRP), in Cushing syndrome, 79

in diabetes, cancer and, 177
    hypertension and, 107, 110
in metabolic syndrome, 11–12
in PAD, 151, 155
Critical limb ischemia (CLI), in PAD, 155–156
    surgical interventions for, 162
Cross-sectional studies, of vitamin D status association with T2DM, 210–211
Cushing syndrome, GCs regulation of adipose tissue and, 76, 78–80
    11β-HSD1 role in, 86
    adipokine secretion in, 80–81
    circulating lipids in, 83–84
    hepatic steatosis in, 83
    obesity development and, 87
    paradoxical actions of, 88
Cytokines, in AD, 249, 254–255
    in atherosclerosis, 152
    in diabetes, cancer and, 177–178
        hypertension and, 106–107
        vitamin D impact on, 209–210
    in metabolic syndrome, 11–12
    OSA impact on, 193–194
        adipose tissue and, 195
    white adipose secretion of, GCs regulation of, 81, 88
Cytoskeletal protein accumulations, in AD, 249–251

D

Dairy intake, for osteoporosis, 238
DASH diet, for hypertension, 110
    for metabolic syndrome, 14
DCCT trial, of diabetes effect on cardiovascular outcomes, 30
DCCT-EDIC trial, of diabetes effect on cardiovascular outcomes, 29–30
D-dimer, as PAD progression predictor, 155
De novo lipogenesis, in white adipose, GCs regulation of, 78
Dementia, brain metabolic derangements in other, 256–257
    degrees in AD, 248, 254–255
Denervation, renal, for hypertension, 115
Depression, interactions between diabetes and, **269–283**
    association with diabetes, 271–272
    cognitive impairment with, 270–271
    complex relationships in, 270
    depression treatment in, 273–276
        biologic modalities, 275
        cognitive behavioral therapy interventions, 275–276
        improving care, 276–277
        medication effects, 270, 273
        risk/benefit analysis, 273–274
    diabetes association with, 270–271
    diabetes subtypes in, 270
    diabetes treatment in, as risk factor, 275
        improving care, 276–277

Depression (*continued*)
  epigenetic risk for, 273, 275
  key points on, 269–270
  metabolic syndrome and, 272–273
Diabetes mellitus (DM), anxiety and depression interactions between, **269–283**
  complex relationships in, 270
  depression/anxiety association with diabetes, 271–272
  depression/anxiety treatment in, 273–276
    biologic modalities, 275
    cognitive behavioral therapy interventions, 275–276
    improving care, 276–277
    medication effects, 270, 273
    risk/benefit analysis, 273–274
  diabetes association with anxiety/depression, 270–271
  diabetes subtypes in, 270
  diabetes treatment in, as risk factor, 275
    improving care, 276–277
  epigenetic risk for, 273, 275
  key points on, 269–270
  metabolic syndrome and, 272–273
  cancer and, **167–185**. See also *Cancer; Type 2 diabetes mellitus (T2DM).*
  cardiovascular disease and, cardiomyopathy in, 45–49
      altered substrate metabolism, 46–47
      cardiac autonomic neuropathy, 47–48
      cardiovascular findings, 48
      definition of, 45–46
      diagnosing, 48–49
      mechanisms of, 42, 46–47
      myocardial fibrosis, 47–48
      renin-angiotensin system activation, 47
    clinical implications of, 49–52
      CAD outcomes, 50–52
      CAD risk factors, 49–50
      heart failure, 46, 52
    coronary artery disease with, interventions for, **59–73**. See also *Coronary artery bypass graft (CABG); Percutaneous coronary intervention (PCI).*
    outcomes of, 50–52
    risk factors of, 49–50
        dyslipidemia as, 49–50
        glycemic control as, 50
        hypertension as, 50
    epidemiology of, 26
    glycemic control for, 28–31
      as risk mitigation, 28–31
      choosing right agent, 29–31
      intensive, 28–29
    heart failure with, 46, 52
    introduction to, 25, 41–42
    key points on, 25, 41
    pathogenesis of, **41–57**
    pathophysiology of, 27–28

   risk assessment of events, 26–27
   risk factors and medical therapy, **25–40**
   risk mitigation for, 28–34
      aspirin as, 33
      CHD diagnosis in asymptomatic patients as, 33–34
      glycemic control as, 28–31
      hypertension control as, 32–33
      lipid-lowering therapy as, 31–32
      revascularization as, 34
   summary overview of, 34–35, 52–53
   vasculature in, 42–45
      cardiomyopathy findings, 48
      impaired reverse cholesterol transport, 43, 45
      microvasculature dysfunction, 42, 44
      oxidative stress effects on, 42–44
      summary of relationships between, 42–43, 45
      vascular progenitor cell dysfunction, 43–45
cognitive impairment and, **245–267**
   Alzheimer disease as, as metabolic with brain insulin/IGF resistance, 249, 252
         human studies of, 252
      as T3DM, 252–253
         experimental evidence for sporadic AD, 253–254
      chronic ischemic cerebral microvascular disease and, 254–257
      clinical diagnosis of, 248–249
      insulin resistance and, 248, 252, 257
         sporadic, 253–254
      metabolic deficits in, 253–255
      neuropathology of, 249–251
      occurrence of, 246, 248
      underlying causes of, 257–260
   anxiety/depression with, 270–271
   brain insulin/IGF resistance and, as metabolic AD, 249, 252
         human studies of, 252
         underlying causes of, 257–260
      in other neurodegenerative diseases, 256–257
      systemic insulin-resistance diseases mediation of, 246–247
   insulin resistance in, AD and, 249, 252, 257
   insulin signaling in, 246–248
   introduction to, 245–246
   key points on, 245
   neurodegeneration as, 248–257
   summary overview of, 260
hypertension in, 42, 50. See also *Hypertension (HTN)*.
   cardiovascular disease risk mitigation, 32–33, 108–109
   type 2, **103–122**. See also *Type 2 diabetes mellitus (T2DM)*.
metabolic syndrome and, as risk factor, 1–2, 9–10
   pathophysiology of, 11–12
   prevention of, 8
non–insulin dependent, in PCOS, 134, 137
obstructive sleep apnea and, **187–204**. See also *Obstructive sleep apnea (OSA)*.
osteoporosis-associated fracture and, **233–243**

Diabetes (*continued*)
    introduction to, 233–234
    key points on, 233
    management of, 238–239
    quantifying risk of, 237
    T1D vs. T2D and bone, 234–237
      differences of, 236–237
      similarities of, 234–235
    treatment of, 239
  PAD and, 153
    as risk factor, 150–151
    hypercoagulability with, 154
    hyperglycemia with, 153–154
    impaired lipid metabolism with, 154
    pathogenesis of, 153–154
    platelet dysfunction with, 153–154
  PCOS and, 126, 129–130
  prevalence of, 25–26, 41–42, 59, 233
  social costs of, 269–270
  type 1. See *Type 1 diabetes mellitus (T1DM)*.
  type 2. See *Type 2 diabetes mellitus (T2DM)*.
  type 3, AD as, 252–253
    experimental evidence for sporadic, 253–254
  types of, comparison of, 252–253
  vitamin D and, **205–232**
    association with T1DM, 225–226
    association with T2DM, biologic plausibility of, 208–210
      cross-sectional studies of status influence on, 210–211
      insulin secretion and, 208–209
      insulin sensitivity and, 208–210
      longitudinal studies of status influence on, 211–217
      supplementation influence on, 217–225
      systemic inflammation and, 209–210
    for osteoporosis, 238–239
    intake requirements for, 207–208
    introduction to, 205–206
    key points on, 205
    physiology review of, 206
    status classification of, 206–207
    summary overview of, 226–227
Diabetic cardiomyopathy (DCM), 45–49
  altered substrate metabolism in, 46–47
  cardiac autonomic neuropathy in, 47–48
  cardiovascular findings in, 48
  definition of, 45–46
  diagnosing of, 48–49
  mechanisms of, 42, 46–47
  myocardial fibrosis in, 47–48
  renin-angiotensin system activation in, 47
Diabetic ketoacidosis, caused by antidepressants, 274
Diabetic nephropathy. See *Renal disease*.

Diabetic neuropathy, 42
    autonomic, in cardiomyopathy, 47–48
Diacylglycerol (DAC), in diabetes, with PAD, 154
Diagnostic and Statistical Manual of Mental Disorders (Fourth Edition) (DSM-4), AD in, 249
Diagnostic and Statistical Manual of Mental Disorders (Fifth Edition) (DSM-5), anxiety/
    depression connection to diabetes in, 271
        categorical vs. dimensional, 276–277
Diastolic dysfunction, in diabetic cardiomyopathy, 46–49, 52
Diastolic hypertension, in diabetes, combined pharmacologic therapy for, 114
Diet, cancer and diabetes associated with, 170, 174
    metabolic syndrome associated with, 10–13
        prevention strategies for, 13–15
    prenatal, in PCOS, 128–129
Dietary interventions/modifications, for hypertension, 110
    for metabolic syndrome, 13–15
    for osteoporosis, in diabetes, 238–239
Dietary supplements, for cardiovascular disease, in diabetes, 32
    in metabolic syndrome, 13–15
    for osteoporosis, 238–239
Dipeptidyl-peptidase 4 (DPP-4) inhibitors, for diabetes, as hypertension treatment,
    113–114
        cardiovascular disease risk, 31
Disturbed sleep, insulin resistance linked to, 195–196
Diuretics, for hypertension, in diabetes, 112, 114
    in metabolic syndrome, 15
Drug-eluting stents (DES), for cardiovascular disease, in diabetes, 50, 52
        CABG vs., 60–65
DXA scan, in diabetes, for fracture risk, 237–238
        for OSA, 190
Dyslipidemia, GCs regulation of circulating lipids and, 83–84
    in diabetes, as CAD risk factor, 49–50
        cardiovascular disease risk mitigation, 31–32
    in metabolic syndrome, 1–2, 15
        CPAP impact on, 198
        definition comparisons of, 2–4
        pathophysiology of, 10–13
        prevention strategies for, 13–15
            secondary targets of, 15
    in PAD, 154
        as risk factor, 151
        risk modification for, 160–161
    in PCOS, 126, 128, 136
        adolescents and, 131–132
    NCEP/ATPIII on, 2
Dysmetabolic phenotypes, of metabolic syndrome components, 2
    primary diseases associated with, 7–8

E

Echocardiography, for diabetic cardiomyopathy, 48–49
Elastin, in diabetes, vascular pathogenesis and, 44

Electroencephalogram (EEG), for OSA, 191–192, 196, 199
Embolus, in atherosclerosis with PAD, 153
Encephalopathy, chronic ischemic, in AD, 254
Endarterectomy, for PAD, 162
Endometrial cancer, diabetes and, 169–170
    PCOS and, 131
End-organ effects, of diabetes, 42–43
Endothelial cells/endothelium, in AD, 255
    in diabetes, atherosclerosis and, 27, 154
        changes in glomerular, 42–43
        hypertension and, 106–107
            pharmacologic therapy effect on, 112–113
        vascular pathogenesis and, 43–45
    in PAD, atherosclerosis and, 153–154
Endothelial progenitor cells, dysfunction of, in diabetes, 44–45
Endovascular techniques, for PAD, 162
Energy balance, excess, in metabolic syndrome, 10–11
    glucocorticoids function in, 76–77
Energy production, brain, 245–246
        in AD, 249, 252–254
Environment, in diabetes interaction between anxiety/depression, 273, 275
    in metabolic syndrome, pathophysiology of, 12–13
Epidemiology, of AD, with diabetes, 246, 248
    of cancer, in diabetes, 167–171
            incidence, 169–170
            mortality, 170–171
            T2DM, obesity, and metabolic syndrome, 10, 167–169
    of cardiovascular disease, in diabetes, 26
    of diabetes mellitus, 25–26, 41–42, 59, 233
    of hypertension, in T2DM, 105
    of metabolic syndrome, 3, 6–8, 258
    of obesity and overweight, 2
    of OSA, in T2DM, 190
Epigenetic factors, of anxiety/depression risk, in diabetes, 273, 275
    of metabolic syndrome, 13
Epithelial-to-mesenchymal transition (EMT), in cancer and diabetes, hyperglycemia and,
    176
        IGF-1 and, 173–174
        insulin resistance and, 175
Epworth Sleepiness Scale (ESS), 198–199
Ergocalciferol (vitamin D2), physiology of, 206
    supplementation influence on T2DM, 217, 225
        randomized controlled trials of, 217–224
ESHRE/ASRM criteria, for PCOS, 124–125
Esophageal cancer, diabetes and, 170
Estradiol, in PCOS, 137
Ethinylestradiol/cyproterone acetate, for PCOS, 138
Ethnicity, as PAD risk factor, 150
Ethnic-specific criteria, for obesity, in metabolic syndrome, 3, 6
Ethnic-specific prevalence, of diabetes, vitamin D impact on, 211, 225
        with cancer, 170

with hypertension, 105, 109, 114
of metabolic syndrome, 3, 6
OSA and, 191
of PCOS, 128, 130
European Group for the Study of Insulin Resistance (EGIR), on metabolic syndrome,
concerns expressed by, 15–16
definition of, 2, 4–5
Exenatide, for hypertension, 113
Exercise, for hypertension, 110–111
for insulin resistance, in PCOS, 137
for metabolic syndrome, 14–15
for PAD, 161
Exercise stress testing, for CHD in asymptomatic patients, with diabetes, 33
Experimental models, of neurodegeneration, with peripheral and brain insulin resistance,
253–254, 259
Extracellular matrix (ECM), in adipogenesis, 80
in atherosclerosis, with diabetes, 28, 154
with PAD, 152–154
Ezetimibe, for cardiovascular disease, 32

F

Fall risk/prevention, for diabetic patients, 238
Fasting glucose (FG), in diabetes, cardiovascular risk assessment and, 26
in metabolic syndrome, definition comparisons of, 2–4
diabetic outcomes of, 9–10
treatment of, 13–15
in OSA, 189
Fat intake restrictions, for metabolic syndrome, 13–14
Fat mass and distribution, CPAP impact on, 198
white, GCs regulation of, 76, 79–80
11β-HSD1 role in, 81–82, 85
Fat tissue. See *Adipose tissue.*
Fatty acids, free. See *Free fatty acids (FFA).*
in diabetes, atherosclerosis and, 27–28
hyperglycemia and, 176
metabolism of, insulin role in, 246–247
vitamin D impact on, 208–210
Fatty liver disease, as metabolic syndrome outcome, 2, 10
Femoral neck, BMD of, in diabetes, 236–237
fracture of, in diabetes, 239
Ferriman-Gallwey scale, of hirsutism, in PCOS, 126–127
Fetal exposure, to androgens, in PCOS, 129, 134
Fetal undernutrition, in PCOS, 128–129, 131
Fibrates, for cardiovascular disease, 32, 49
Fibrinogen, as PAD progression predictor, 155
Fish oil, for cardiovascular disease, 32
Foot ulceration, in diabetes, with PAD, 151, 156
Fracture risk, in diabetes, 234, 237, 239
osteoporosis-associated, **233–243**. See also *Osteoporosis-associated fracture.*
Fragility fractures, in diabetes, 234–237, 239. See also *Osteoporosis-associated fracture.*

FRAX algorithm, for fracture risk assessment, in diabetes, 237–239
Free fatty acids (FFA), hypoxia impact on, 195
   in diabetic cardiomyopathy, 46–47, 49
   in glucocorticoid-induced insulin resistance, 76, 79
   in metabolic syndrome, 11
   metabolism of, insulin role in, 246–247
FREEDOM trial, of diabetes, effect on cardiovascular outcomes, 34, 51–52
      with revascularization, 59, 62–63, 66

G

GCs. See *Glucocorticoids (GCs).*
Gender, as PAD risk factor, 150
   diabetes and, cardiovascular risk assessment in, 26–27
      hypertension in, 105
      osteoporosis-associated fracture in, 235–237, 239
Genes/genetics, of anxiety/depression connection to diabetes, 273, 275
   of cancer and diabetes, 175–176, 178–179
   of metabolic syndrome, 12–13
   of PCOS, 7, 126, 128–129, 134–135
      severe insulin resistance syndromes and, 135–136
Genetic engineering, for insulin hormone production, 246
Genome-wide association studies (GWAS), of anxiety/depression connection to diabetes, 273
   of metabolic syndrome, 12–13
   of PCOS, 135
Gestational diabetes mellitus (GDM), PCOS and, 126, 131
Glucagon-like peptide 1 (GLP-1) agonists, for diabetes, as hypertension treatment, 113–114
      cardiovascular disease risk, 31
Glucocorticoid-induced insulin resistance, **75–102**
   11β-HSD1 gatekeeper of, 81–82, 85–86
   adipose tissue functionality, mass, and distribution regulation in, 76–85
      adipogenesis, 79–80
      brown adipose, 81–82
      Cushing syndrome, 78–80
      white adipose de novo lipogenesis, 78
      white adipose insulin sensitivity, 78–79, 88
      white adipose lipolysis, 76–78
      white adipose mass and distribution, 79–80
      white adipose secretory profile, 80–81
   brain tissue regulation in, 84–85
   circulating lipids regulation in, 83–84
   future directions for, 89
   hepatic tissue regulation in, 82–83
   intracellular availability regulation in, 81–82, 85–87
   introduction to, 75–76
   key points on, 75
   mechanisms of whole-body, 76–77
   muscle tissue regulation in, 76, 82
   obesity development and, 76, 80, 87
   paradoxical actions, 87–88

summary overview of, 88–89
tissue-specific regulation mechanisms in, 76–83
    adipose tissue, 76–85
    brain, 84–85
    liver, 82–83, 85
    muscle, 76, 82, 85
Glucocorticoid-induced osteoporosis, 239
Glucocorticoids (GCs), 11β-HSD1 expression and, 86
  chronic exposure to, effect on bone, 239
    insulin resistance induced by. See *Glucocorticoid-induced insulin resistance.*
  critical function of, 76–77
  intracellular availability of, 11β-HSD1 as gatekeeper for, 85–87
    in brain, 84–85
    in muscle, 82, 85
    in white vs. brown adipose, 81–82, 85
Gluconeogenesis. See *Hepatic gluconeogenesis.*
Glucose homeostasis/metabolism. See *Glycemic control.*
Glucose insulin potassium (GIK), for diabetes, perioperative with CABG, 66–67
Glucose level. See *Blood glucose level.*
Glucose tolerance, impaired. See *Impaired glucose tolerance (IGT).*
GLUT4, in AD, 247, 254–255
Glycation end products, in diabetes. See *Advanced glycation end products (AGEs).*
Glycemic control, glucocorticoids function in, 76–77
    11β-HSD1 inhibition and, 87
    paradoxical actions of, 87–88
  in AD, 249, 252
    brain insulin signaling deficits and, 253–254
    insulin resistance/deficiency role in, 254–255
  in diabetes, antidepressants effect on, 273–274
    as CAD risk factor, 50
    as PAD risk factor, 154
    bone health and, 235, 238
    cancer and, 174, 176–177
    cardiovascular event risk mitigation, 28–31
      choosing right agent, 29–31
      intensive, 28–29
    perioperative with CABG, 66–67
  in OSA, assessment of, 190
    human studies of, 195–196
    IH impact on, 193
    in T2DM, 188–191
    observational studies of, 188–190
  in PAD, 154, 160
  in PCOS, 133–135
    treatment of, 136–138
  insulin role in, 246–247
    in AD, 254–255
Glycosylated hemoglobin, in diabetes. See *Hemoglobin (HbA1c).*
Grafts, vascular, for CABG, 63–64
    diseased, PCI for, 67–68
    for PAD, 162

Growth factors. See also *Insulin-like growth factors (IGFs).*
    in atherosclerosis, 152–153
        with PAD, 154
    in hyperinsulinemia, cancer and, 175–176
Growth hormone (GH), IGF-1 stimulation by, cancer and, 173–174
Growth hormone deficiency (GHD), brain insulin resistance in AD associated with, 257–258
    metabolic syndrome phenotypes associated with, 8
Growth restriction, intrauterine, in PCOS, 128–129, 131
Gut-derived hormone analogues, for hypertension, 113–114

H

Harmonized criteria, for metabolic syndrome, 3–5
HbA1C. See *Hemoglobin (HbA1c).*
Head and neck cancer, diabetes and, 174
Heart 2D 2009 trial, of diabetes effect on cardiovascular outcomes, 30
Heart disease, valvular, in diabetes, 42
    vascular. See *Cardiovascular disease (CVD).*
Heart failure, in diabetes, 42
        congestive, 46, 52
Heart pump, for CABG, 64
Heart structure and function, altered, in diabetic cardiomyopathy, 46–49, 52
Hemodynamic dysfunction, in diabetic cardiomyopathy, 46–49, 52
Hemoglobin (HbA1c), in diabetes, bone health and, 235, 238
        cardiovascular disease risk, 28–29, 50
        cardiovascular risk assessment and, 26–27
        effect on PCI outcomes, 68
        hypertension and, 110
    in OSA, 191
        CPAP impact on, 197
Hepatic disease, as metabolic syndrome outcome, 2, 10
    brain insulin resistance in AD associated with, 253, 258–260
Hepatic gluconeogenesis, cancer and, 174
    OSA and, 193, 195
    PCOS and, 126
Hepatic steatosis, GCs regulation of, 83, 86
        11β-HSD1 inhibition effect on, 86
    streptozotocin and, 253
Hepatic tissue, IGF-1 production by, 172–174
    in glucocorticoid-induced insulin resistance, 82–83
        11β-HSD1 role in, 81–82, 85
    insulin role in, 247
    lipogenesis in, GCs regulation of, 82–83, 85–86
Hepatitis C infection, cognitive impairment associated with, 259
    hepatocellular cancer associated with, 169
Hepatocellular cancer, diabetes and, 169–170, 174
Hip fracture, in diabetes, 234, 236–237, 239
Hippocampus atrophy, in AD, 249, 251, 255
Hirsutism, in PCOS, 126–127, 129–130
Histopathology, of AD, 249, 251
History taking, for PAD, 157

Home sleep testing (HST), for OSA, 199
Homeostasis model assessment as insulin resistance marker (HOMA-IR), in OSA, 189–190
    CPAP impact on, 196–197
    vitamin D supplementation impact on, 217, 225
HOT trial, on hypertension, in diabetes, 108–109
11β-HSD-1. See *11β-Hydroxysteroid dehydrogenase 1 (11β-HSD1).*
Human chorionic gonadotropin (hCG), in PCOS, 128–129
Human immunodeficiency virus (HIV) infection, metabolic syndrome phenotypes
    associated with, 7–8
Human studies, of brain insulin/IGF resistance, in cognitive impairment, 252
    of intermittent hypoxia impact on OSA, and b-cell function, 195–196
11β-Hydroxysteroid dehydrogenase 1 (11β-HSD1), as intracellular GCs gatekeeper, 85–87
    in brain, 84–85
    in muscle, 82, 85
    in white vs. brown adipose, 81–82, 85
    inhibition of, potential role in humans, 86–87
25-Hydroxyvitamin D (25OHD), in vitamin D, insulin secretion and, 208–209
    insulin sensitivity and, 208–210
    physiology of, 206
    status classification of, 206–207
Hyperandrogenism, in PCOS, 124–126, 128
    in vitro models of, 133–134
    severe insulin resistance syndromes and, 135–136
    treatment of, 129, 136–138
Hypercholesterolemia, in PAD, risk mitigation for, 160–161
Hypercoagulability, in diabetes, with PAD, 154
Hyperglycemia, in diabetes, bone health and, 234, 236, 238
    cancer and, 174, 176–177
    cardiomyopathy and, 46–48
    cardiovascular disease pathophysiology of, 27–28, 60
    cardiovascular risk assessment and, 26–27
    vascular pathogenesis and, 43
    with PAD, 153–154, 160
    in metabolic syndrome, cardiovascular outcomes of, 9
        definition comparisons of, 2–3, 5
        pathophysiology of, 10–13
        prevention strategies for, 13–14
Hyperhomocysteinemia, in PAD, 151, 155
Hyperinsulinemia, in AD, 255
    in diabetes, cancer and, 175–176
        hypertension and, 107
    in PCOS, 133–134, 136
        pregnancy and, 131
Hyperlipidemia. See *Dyslipidemia.*
Hyperphosphorylated tau, in AD, 246, 249, 251–252
    insulin resistance/deficiency and, 254–255
Hypertension (HTN), diabetes and, 42
        as CVD risk factor, 50, 103, 105
        cardiovascular disease risk, 32–33
        T2DM, **103–122**
    metabolic syndrome and, 1–2

Hypertension (*continued*)
    11β-HSD1 inhibition and, 87
    definition comparisons of, 3, 5
    pathophysiology of, 11–12
    prevention strategies for, 13–14
    treatment of, 15
  PAD and, risk mitigation for, 161
  T2DM and, **103–122**
    burden of, 105
    epidemiology of, 105
    hyperinsulinemia in, 107
    insulin resistance in, 107
    introduction to, 103–104
    key points on, 103
    oxidative stress in, 106–107
    pathophysiology of, 105–106
    pharmacologic therapy for, 111–114
      β-blockers as, 113
      calcium channel blockers as, 112
      clinical trials on, 108–109
      combined, 111, 114
      diuretics as, 112
      incretin-based, 113–114
      RAAS blockade as, 111–112
    treatment of, 108–115
      BP targets for, 108–109
      impact of BP control, 108
      lifestyle interventions in, 109–111
      nonpharmacologic therapy in, 109–111
      pharmacologic therapy in, 111–114
      rationale, strategies, and challenges in, 107–109
      renal denervation in, 115
      telehealth in, 114–115
Hyperviscosity state, as PAD risk factor, 151
Hypoglycemia, insulin-related, fracture risk and, 235
    seizures caused by, 275
Hypopituitarism, metabolic syndrome phenotypes associated with, 8
Hypothalamic-pituitary-adrenal (HPA) axis, glucocorticoid excess and, 76, 87
Hypoxemia, nocturnal, 189
Hypoxia, in OSA, adipose tissue, 194–195
    intermittent. See *Intermittent hypoxia (IH)*.

I

IGF. See *Insulin-like growth factor entries*.
IH. See *Intermittent hypoxia (IH)*.
Illness(es), anxiety/depression related to, 270–271, 276–277
  diabetes associated with, cardiovascular risk assessment and, 27, 32
    fracture risk and, 235
  metabolic syndrome phenotypes associated with, 7
  stress syndromes caused by, 270–271, 276–277

Imaging, myocardial, adenosine-stress radionuclide perfusion, for CHD in asymptomatic
    diabetic patients, 34
        for diabetic cardiomyopathy, 48–49
Immune response, in diabetes, hypertension and, 106
Impaired glucose tolerance (IGT). See also *Diabetes mellitus (DM).*
    in PCOS, 125–126, 130
        adolescents and, 132
Incidence, of diabetes, with AD, 246, 248
        with cancer, 169–170
Incretin-based therapy, for hypertension, 113–114
Infections, brain insulin resistance in AD associated with, 258–259
    chronic, in cancer and diabetes, 169, 178
    metabolic syndrome phenotypes associated with, 7–8
    wound. See *Wound entries.*
Infertility, in PCOS, 124–126
        treatment of, 136–138
Inflammation, in diabetes, atherosclerosis and, 27–28, 43, 60
        cancer and, 177–179
        cardiomyopathy and, 46–48
        hypertension and, 106–107
        insulin resistance and, 81
            11β-HSD1 inhibition effect on, 87
        vascular pathogenesis and, 43–44
        vitamin D influence on, 206–210
    in PAD, atherosclerosis progression and, 154–155
    neural, in AD, 254–255, 258
    of adipose tissue, in OSA, 195
    systemic, in insulin-resistance diseases, 249, 252
        in OSA, 192–194
            adipose tissue hypoxia and, 194–195
        in vitamin D and diabetes, 209–210
Inositol nicotinate, for PAD, 162
Insulin homeostasis/metabolism, in OSA, assessment of, 190
    β-cell function in, 194
    human studies of, 195–196
    IH impact on, 193
    in T2DM, 188–190
    observational studies of, 188–190
Insulin hormone, 11β-HSD1 expression and, 86
    as anabolic, 236
    glycemic control role of, 246–247, 254
    in diabetes, cognitive impairment and, 246–247
        hypertension and, 107
        vascular pathogenesis and, 43
    secretion/stimulation of, in vitamin D and diabetes, 208–209
        main targets of, 246–247
        markers of, 175
Insulin receptors (IRs), cancer and, expression in resistance, 175–176
        IGF-1 in, 173–174
    in brain insulin/IGF signaling, 248, 253
    PCOS and, gene mutations of, 134–135

Insulin (*continued*)
    in ovaries, 132
    in severe genetic syndromes, 135–136
    in skin, 132–133
  vitamin D impact on, 208–210
Insulin resistance, AD and, 248, 252, 257
    experimental evidence of sporadic, 253–254, 259
    underlying causes of, 257–260
      aging as, 257–258
      lifestyle as, 258
      metabolic syndrome as, 259–260
      NAFLD/NASH as, 259
      obesity as, 258–259
      T2DM as, 259
  cognitive impairment and, 248–249. See also *Brain insulin/IGF resistance.*
    AD as, 246, 249, 252
      underlying causes of, 257–260
    experimental models of, 253–254, 259
  definition of, 76
  diabetes and, anxiety/depression and, 272–274
    atherosclerosis and, 27–28, 43
    bone and, 236
    cancer and, 175–176
    cardiomyopathy and, 46–47
    hypertension and, 107
  glucocorticoid-induced, **75–102**
    adipose tissue functionality, mass, and distribution regulation in, 76–85
      adipogenesis, 79–80
      brown adipose, 81–82
      Cushing syndrome, 78–80
      white adipose de novo lipogenesis, 78
      white adipose insulin sensitivity, 78–79, 88
      white adipose lipolysis, 76–78
      white adipose mass and distribution, 79–80
      white adipose secretory profile, 80–81
    brain tissue regulation in, 84–85
    circulating lipids regulation in, 83–84
    future directions for, 89
    hepatic tissue regulation in, 82–83
    intracellular availability regulation in, 81–82, 85–87
    introduction to, 75–76
    key points on, 75
    mechanisms of whole-body, 76–77
    muscle tissue regulation in, 76, 82
    obesity development and, 76, 80, 87
    paradoxical actions in, 87–88
    summary overview of, 88–89
    tissue-specific regulation mechanisms in, 76–83
      adipose tissue, 76–85
      brain, 84–85
      liver, 82–83

muscle, 76, 82
long-term consequences of, 129–130, 248–249. See also *specific disease.*
metabolic syndrome and, 1–2
    adipose tissue and, 10–12, 76
    definition comparisons of, 3–4
    European Group for the Study of, 2, 5
    glucocorticoids and. See *Glucocorticoid-induced insulin resistance.*
    pathophysiology of, 10–13
neurodegeneration and, experimental models of, 253–254, 259
OSA and. See also *Obstructive sleep apnea (OSA).*
    assessment of, 190
    IH and, 192–193, 195
    obesity and, 195
    observational studies of, 188–190
    potential pathophysiology link to, 191–192
PCOS and, 132–136
    as long-term consequence, 129–130
    genetics of, 134–135
    in vitro models of, 132–134
    in vivo models of, 134
    mechanism behind association of, 132
    pregnancy and, 131
    prevalence of, 126
    syndromes of severe, 135–136
    treatment of, 129, 131, 136–138
syndromes of severe, in PCOS, 134–136
vitamin D impact on, 209
Insulin sensitivity, in metabolic syndrome, 11–12
in OSA, CPAP therapy impact on, 196–197
in vitamin D and diabetes, 208–210
in white adipose, 11β-HSD1 expression and, 86–87
    GCs regulation of, 78–79
    paradoxical GCs actions in, 87–88
Insulin sensitizers, for diabetes, cardiovascular disease risk mitigation, 29
for PCOS, 129, 131, 137–138
Insulin signaling pathways, in brain, IGFs and, 248
      with AD, 253–254
      with other neurodegenerative diseases, 256–257
in diabetes, cognitive impairment and, 246–248
    with cancer, IGF-1 and, 172–175
      inflammation effect on, 177–179
      IR expression and, 175–176
in metabolic syndrome, 11
in PCOS, 132–133
    gene mutations of, 134–135
    severe insulin resistance syndromes and, 135–136
Insulin therapy, for diabetes, as depression and anxiety risk, 275
    cardiovascular disease risk mitigation, 31
    fracture risk and, 235
    large scale production technologies for, 246
    perioperative with CABG, 66–67

Insulin-like growth factor 1 (IGF-1), in diabetes, cancer and, 172–175
    fracture risk and, 236
Insulin-like growth factor–binding proteins (IGFBP), in cancer and diabetes, 175
   in PCOS, 132–133, 137
   regulation of IGFs, 247
Insulin-like growth factors (IGFs), brain resistance to, cognitive impairment and, 246
    as metabolic AD, 249, 252
    human studies of, 252
    systemic insulin-resistance diseases mediation of, 246–247
    underlying causes of, 257–260
   in PCOS, 132–133
   insulin vs., 247
    signal transduction and, 248
    signaling in brain and, 248, 256–257
Insulin-resistance diseases, systemic, cellular injury and degeneration in, 249, 252
    AD pathology of, 254–255
    mediation of brain insulin/IGF resistance, 246–247
     aging influence on, 257–258
     cognitive impairment and, 246–247
    spectrum of, AD inclusion within, 252–253
      259, experimental evidence for sporadic, 253–254
      molecular and pathologic features of, 254–255
     affecting primary target organs, 248–249
Interleukins (ILs), in cancer and diabetes, 177–178
Intermittent claudication (IC), in PAD, 153, 156
    surgical interventions for, 162
Intermittent hypoxia (IH), in OSA, 192
    chronic, insulin resistance and, 192–193, 195
     oxidative stress and inflammation with, 193–194
    human studies of, 195–196
    impact on β-cell function, 194–195
Intermittent pneumatic compression, for PAD, 163
Internal thoracic artery grafts, for CABG, 63–64
International Diabetes Federation (IDF), metabolic syndrome definition of, 2–5
Intracellular availability, of GCs, in glucocorticoid-induced insulin resistance, 81–82, 85–87
IRs. See Insulin receptors (IRs).
Ischemia, coronary. See Coronary artery disease (CAD).
   in PAD, 155–156
    surgical interventions for, 162
Ischemic cerebral microvascular disease, chronic, in AD, 254–257
Ischemic encephalopathy, chronic, in AD, 254

K

Ketoacidosis, diabetic, caused by antidepressants, 274
Kidney disease. See Renal entries.

L

Learning, impaired, diabetes and, 245, 255
Leptin, in cancer and diabetes, 178–179

white adipose secretion of, 11β-HSD1 expression and, 86
   GCs regulation of, 80, 85
   OSA and, 195
Leukemia, diabetes and, 170
Lifestyle, brain insulin resistance in AD associated with, 258
  metabolic syndrome associated with, 10–12
   aging and, 258
   prevention strategies for, 13–15
Lifestyle interventions, for hypertension, 109–111
  for insulin resistance, in PCOS, 137
  for metabolic syndrome, 13–15
  for PAD, 159–161
Limb ischemia. See *Critical limb ischemia (CLI)*.
Lipid disorders. See *Dyslipidemia.*
Lipids/lipoproteins, circulating, in glucocorticoid-induced insulin resistance, 83–84
    11β-HSD1 inhibition effect on, 86–87
  impaired metabolism of. See *Dyslipidemia.*
  in atherosclerosis, 151–153
  in diabetes, as CAD risk factor, 49–50, 68
   cardiomyopathy and, 46–47
   cardiovascular disease and, 31–32, 45
  in metabolic syndrome, 1–2
   controversies regarding, 16
   CPAP impact on, 198
   definition comparisons of, 2–4
   pathophysiology of, 10–11, 13
   treatment of, 13–15
    secondary targets for, 15
  in PAD, 151, 154, 160–161
   as disease progression predictor, 155
  metabolism of, insulin role in, 247
Lipogenesis, de novo, in white adipose, GCs regulation of, 78
  in hepatic tissue, GCs regulation of, 82–83, 85–86
Lipolysis, in hepatic tissue, GCs regulation of, 82–83, 85–86
  in white adipose, GCs regulation of, 76–78
Lipoprotein (a), as PAD progression predictor, 155
Lipotoxicity, of myocardial cells, 46–47
Liraglutide, for hypertension, 113
Liver cancer, diabetes and, 169–171
Liver disorders, as metabolic syndrome outcome, 2, 10
Liver metabolism. See *Hepatic entries.*
Longitudinal studies, of vitamin D status association with T2DM, 211–217
   random-effects meta-analysis of, 211, 217
   results of, 211–216
LOOK AHEAD trial, of diabetes effect on cardiovascular outcomes, 30
Low birth weight, PCOS and, 128–129, 131
Lower limbs, atherosclerosis in. See *Peripheral arterial disease (PAD).*
Low-salt diet, for hypertension, 110
  for metabolic syndrome, 14
Lung cancer, diabetes and, 171, 174
   MKR mouse model of, 175–176

M

Macrophages, in adipogenesis, 80
    insulin resistance and, 81
    OSA impact on, 195
  in atherosclerosis, diabetes and, 28
    PAD and, 151–153
  in cancer and diabetes, 178
  in metabolic syndrome, 12
Macrovasculature dysfunction, and diabetes, 46
    with hypertension, 108–109
Major adverse cardiovascular and cerebrovascular events (MACCEs), following
  revascularization for CAD, 61, 63, 67–68
Mammary gland, hyperplasia of, diabetes and, 173–175, 178
MAPK pathway activation, in cancer and diabetes, 173–174, 177, 179
Matrix metalloproteinases, in diabetes, atherosclerosis and, 28
Mechanical stretch, in hypertension, 107
Mechano growth factor, 247. See also *Insulin-like growth factors (IGFs)*.
Medical-psychiatric illness, diabetes connection to, 270–271, 276–277
Mediterranean diet, for metabolic syndrome, 14
Memory, impaired, diabetes and, 245, 255
Menopause, diabetes following, cardiovascular risk assessment and, 26
    fracture risk and, 236–237
      management of, 238–239
Menstrual irregularities, in PCOS, 124–126, 128–129
Mental causation model, of anxiety/depression connection to diabetes, 271–272
Mental health, collaborative proactive patient empowerment in treatment of, 277
  connection to diabetes. See *Anxiety; Depression*.
Metabolic control/homeostasis, glucocorticoids function in, 76–77
    in brain, 84–85
    paradoxical actions of, 87–88
  in diabetes, AD and, 253–255
      as metabolic with brain insulin/IGF resistance, 249, 252
    effect on PCI outcomes, 68
  in PCOS, diabetes risk and, 126, 129–130
    phenotypes of, 7, 128, 131, 133
    treatment of, 129, 131
  in systemic insulin-resistance diseases, 249, 252
Metabolic syndrome (MetS), **1–23**
  age-specific criteria for, 3
  anxiety/depression and, 272–274
  brain insulin resistance in AD associated with, 249, 259–260
  consequences of, 8–10
  controversies regarding, 15–16
  definitions for, 2–6
    comparison of, 4–6
    criteria-based, 2–3
  effect on PCI outcomes, 68
  epidemiology of, 3, 6–8
  future considerations of, 16
  genome-wide association studies of, 12–13

in Cushing syndrome, 80
in diabetes, cancer and, biologic mechanisms linking, 10, 171–172, 178
 epidemiology of, 167–169
insulin resistance in, 1–2
 adipose tissue and, 10–12, 76
 definition comparisons of, 3–4
 European Group for the Study of, 2, 5
 glucocorticoid-induced. See *Glucocorticoid-induced insulin resistance.*
 pathophysiology of, 10–13
introduction to, 1–2
key points on, 1
obesity as risk factor marker for, 76, 80
OSA and, CPAP impact on, 197–198
 independent association of, 191
pathophysiology of, 10–13
 portal theory of, 11
primary diseases associated with, 7
summary overview of, 16
treatment of, 13–15
Metformin, for diabetes, 11β-HSD1 inhibition and, 87
 as depression and anxiety risk, 275
 cardiovascular disease risk mitigation, 29
 fracture risk and, 237
for insulin resistance, in PCOS, 129, 131, 137–138
Microenvironment, in diabetes, tumor-growing, 177–179. See also *Cancer.*
Microvascular disease, chronic ischemic cerebral, in AD, 254–257
Microvasculature dysfunction, and diabetes, 28, 42–44, 46
 with hypertension, 108–109
Milnacipran, for depression, diabetes and, 275
Mineralo-corticoid receptor (MR), in hypertension, 106
Mitochondrial dysfunction, in systemic insulin-resistance diseases, 249, 252, 254–255, 259
Mitochondrial respiratory chain, in diabetes, hypertension and, 106
 OSA impact on, 193
Mitogen-activated protein kinase (MAPK), in diabetes, hypertension and, 107
MKR mouse model, of lung cancer, 175–176
Monamine oxidase inhibitors (MAOIs), for depression, diabetes and, 273–274
Muscle tissue, in glucocorticoid-induced insulin resistance, 76, 82, 85
 insulin role in, 246–247
 vitamin D and insulin metabolism in, 208–210
Myocardial cells, lipotoxicity of, 46–47
Myocardial fibrosis, in diabetic cardiomyopathy, 47–48
Myocardial imaging, adenosine-stress radionuclide perfusion, for CHD in asymptomatic diabetic patients, 34
 for diabetic cardiomyopathy, 48–49
Myocardial infarction (MI), in diabetes, 26–27, 33, 42
 hypertension and, 104
 revascularization and, 61, 66
in metabolic syndrome, 2, 8–9

N

NAFLD. See *Nonalcoholic fatty liver disease (NAFLD)*.

Naftidrofuryl oxalate, for PAD, 162

NASH (nonalcoholic steatohepatitis), brain insulin resistance in AD associated with, 258–260

National Cholesterol Education Program (NCEP) Adult Treatment Panel III (ATPIII), metabolic syndrome definition of, definition comparisons of, 2–5
  updated, 3–5
  on dyslipidemia, 2

National Heart Lung and Blood Institute (NHLBI), metabolic syndrome definition of, 2–5

National Institute of Child Health and Human Development (NICHD), PCOS criteria of, 124–125

National Institute of Mental Health, vision statement of, 277

National Osteoporosis Foundation (NOF), diet recommendations for bone health, 238
  on risk quantification for osteoporosis-associated fractures, 237
  pharmacologic recommendations for bone health, 239

Nationality-specific criteria. See *Country-specific criteria*.

Nationality-specific prevalence. See *Country-specific prevalence*.

NCEP/ATPIII. See *National Cholesterol Education Program (NCEP) Adult Treatment Panel III (ATPIII)*.

Nephropathy, diabetic. See *Renal disease*.

Neurodegeneration/neurodegenerative diseases, AD as, 248–257. See also *Alzheimer disease (AD)*.
  brain metabolic derangements in other, 256–257
  chronic ischemic cerebral microvascular disease and, 254–257
  insulin resistance and, 248–249
    experimental models of, 253–254, 259

Neuroleptics, for depression, diabetes and, 273–274

Neuromodulation therapies, for depression, diabetes and, 275

Neuronal loss, in AD, 249–250
    human studies of, 252

Neuropathology, of AD, in diabetes, 249–251

Neuropathy, diabetic, 42
    cardiac autonomic, in cardiomyopathy, 47–48

Neuropeptide Y (NPY), in glucocorticoid-induced insulin resistance, 84

Niacin, for atherosclerosis, 15

Nicotinamide adenine dinucleotide phosphate oxidase (NADPH), in diabetes, hypertension and, 106–107

Nitric oxide (NO), in diabetes, atherosclerosis and, 27
      with PAD, 153–154
    hypertension and, 106–107
    vascular pathogenesis and, 43–44

Nocturnal hypoxemia, 189

Nonalcoholic fatty liver disease (NAFLD), as metabolic syndrome outcome, 10
  brain insulin resistance in AD associated with, 258–260

Nonalcoholic steatohepatitis (NASH), 258–260

Non–insulin dependent diabetes mellitus, in PCOS, 134, 137

Nonpharmacologic therapies, for hypertension, 109–111
  for insulin resistance, in PCOS, 137
  for metabolic syndrome, 13–15

for osteoporosis, in diabetes, 238–239
    for PAD, 159–161
Non–ST elevation acute coronary syndromes, 67
Norepinephrine reuptake inhibitors (NRIs), for depression, diabetes and, 274–275
Novel therapies, for PAD, 162–163
Nuclear transcription factors, in diabetes, cancer and, 177–178
        vitamin D impact on, 210
    redox-sensitive, OSA impact on, 193–195

O

Obesity, abdominal. See *Abdominal obesity.*
    anxiety/depression and, 272–273
    brain insulin resistance in AD associated with, 258–259
    definition of, 168–169
    development of, glucocorticoid-induced insulin resistance and, 76, 80, 87
        11β-HSD1 inhibition effect on, 86–87
    in diabetes, cancer and, biologic mechanisms linking, 10, 171–172, 178
        epidemiology of, 167–169
        hypertension and, 106
    in metabolic syndrome, 1–2, 16
        as risk factor marker, 76, 80
        country-specific criteria for, 3, 6
        definition comparisons of, 3–4
        disease risks and outcomes in, 10
        pathophysiology of, 12–13
        population-specific criteria for, 3, 6
        prevention strategies for, 13–15
    in pediatric age group, 3
    OSA and, 190, 193
        insulin resistance link to, 195
    PCOS and, 126, 130, 137–138
    WHO prevalence statistics on, 2
Observational studies, of OSA, CPAP for, 190
        glycemic control in, 188–190
        T2DM and, 188–190
    of vitamin D association with T1DM, 226
Obstructive sleep apnea (OSA), **187–204**
    adipose tissue hypoxia and, systemic inflammation with, 194–195
    apnea during, 191–192
        clinical score for, 199
        CPAP considerations of, 200
        severity indices of, 193
    BMI and, 189–191
    CPAP for, 200
        HbA1c changes with, 197
        impact on metabolic syndrome, 197–198
        insulin sensitivity changes with, 196–197
        observational studies of, 190
    diagnosis of, 199
    fasting glucose and, observational studies of, 189

Obstructive (*continued*)
    glucose homeostasis/metabolism and, assessment of, 190
        human studies of, 195–196
        IH impact on, 193
        in T2DM, 188–191
        observational studies of, 188–190
    HbA1c and, 191
        CPAP impact on, 197
    inflammation with, systemic, adipose tissue hypoxia and, 194–195
        IH and, 192–194
    insulin homeostasis/metabolism and, assessment of, 190
        β-cell function in, 194
        human studies of, 195–196
        IH impact on, 193
        in T2DM, 188–190
        observational studies of, 188–190
    insulin resistance, assessment of, 190
        IH and, 192–193, 195
        obesity and, 195
        observational studies of, 188–190
        potential pathophysiology link to, 191–192
    insulin sensitivity and, CPAP therapy impact on, 196–197
    intermittent hypoxia in, 192
        chronic, insulin resistance and, 192–193, 195
            oxidative stress and inflammation with, 192–194
        human studies of, 195–196
        impact on β-cell function, 194–195
    introduction to, 187–188
    key points on, 187
    metabolic syndrome and, CPAP impact on, 197–198
        independent association of, 191
    obesity and, 190, 193, 195
    oral glucose tolerance tests and, assessment of, 190
        observational studies of, 188
    oxidative stress with, IH and, 192–194
    pathophysiology of, 191–192
    screening for, in T2DM patients, 198–199
    sympathetic nervous system and, 191
        activation of, 194
    symptoms of, classic, 198
    T2DM and, glycemic control in, 191
        observational studies of, 188–190
        potential pathophysiology link to, 191–192
        prevalence of, 190
        screening for, 198–199
    treatment of, 199–200
Oligomenorrhea, in PCOS, 125–126, 130
        treatment of, 136–138
ONTARGET trial, on hypertension, in diabetes, 109, 111
Oocyte development, in PCOS, 124–126, 129
Oral cavity cancer, diabetes and, 170

Oral contraceptive pills (OCPs), PCOS and, 126, 138
Oral glucose tolerance tests (OGTTs), in OSA, 188, 190
OSA. See *Obstructive sleep apnea (OSA)*.
Osteopenia, of femoral neck, in diabetes, 236
Osteoporosis, description of, 233
    glucocorticoid-induced, 239
    in diabetes, management of, 238–239
        treatment of, 239
    prevention guidelines for, 237
Osteoporosis-associated fracture, diabetes and, **233–243**
        introduction to, 233–234
        key points on, 233
        management of, 238–239
        quantifying risk of, 237
        T1D vs. T2D and bone, 234–237
            differences of, 236–237
            similarities of, 234–235
        treatment of, 239
Ovarian cancer, diabetes and, 171–172
Ovaries, insulin action on growth and function of, 132–133
    polycystic, in adolescence, 128, 131–132
        syndrome of. See *Polycystic ovary syndrome (PCOS)*.
Overweight, anxiety/depression and, 272–273
    WHO prevalence statistics on, 2
Oxidative stress, brain insulin resistance in AD associated with, 254–255, 258
    in diabetes, atherosclerosis and, 27–28
        cardiomyopathy and, 46–47
        hypertension and, 105–106
        vascular pathogenesis and, 42–44
    in metabolic syndrome, 11–12
    in OSA, 192–194
    in systemic insulin-resistance diseases, 249, 252
Oxygen desaturation index (ODI), in nocturnal hypoxemia, 189, 192
Oxygen saturation, in OSA, 189, 192, 199

P

PAD. See *Peripheral arterial disease (PAD)*.
Pain, in PAD, critical, 155–156
        intermittent, 153, 156
Pancreatic beta cells. See *β-Cell function*.
Pancreatic cancer, diabetes and, 169–171
Parasympathetic nervous system, in OSA, 191
Parathyroid hormone (PTH), in diabetes, bone loss and, 235
Parkinson disease (PD), brain metabolic derangements in, 256–257
Parkinson-dementia with Lewy bodies (DLB), 256–257
Pathogenesis/pathophysiology, of atherosclerosis, in diabetes, 60
        in PAD, 151–154
    of cardiovascular disease. See also *Cardiovascular disease (CVD)*.
        with diabetes, **41–57**
    of diabetes, cardiovascular disease and, 27–28

Pathogenesis/pathophysiology (*continued*)
    T2DM, 208
      with PAD, 153–154
  of hypertension, in T2DM, 105–106
  of metabolic syndrome, 10–13, 76
  of OSA, 191–192
  of PAD, atherosclerosis in, 151–154
    diabetes in, 153–154
Patient Protection and Affordable Care Act, 277
PCOS. See *Polycystic ovary syndrome (PCOS).*
Pediatric age group, hypertension in, with diabetes, 105
  metabolic syndrome in, criteria for, 3
    prevalence of, 7
  obesity criteria for, 3
Pentosidine, in diabetes, bone and, 235
Pentoxifylline, for PAD, 161
Percutaneous coronary intervention (PCI), for CAD, in diabetes, 34, 50, 60
    CABG as better than, 61, 65–66
    comparative outcome findings, 61–63
    current role for, 67–68
    with CABG, 63–64
Percutaneous renal sympathetic denervation, for hypertension, 115
Percutaneous transluminal coronary angioplasty (PTCA), for CAD, 60–61
Peripheral arterial disease (PAD), **149–166**
  atherosclerosis in, characteristics of, 150
    pathogenesis of, 151–154
  clinical presentations of, 155–156
    critical limb ischemia as, 156
    intermittent claudication as, 156
  description of, 149
  diabetes complications in, 153
    clinical importance of, 149–150
    hypercoagulability as, 154
    hyperglycemia as, 153–154
    impaired lipid metabolism as, 154
    pathogenesis of, 153–154
    platelet dysfunction as, 154
  diagnosis of, 157–159
    ABPI measurement in, 157–158
    angiography in, 159–160
    clinical examination in, 157
    TcP_{O2} in, 158–159
    treadmill exercise testing in, 158
    ultrasonography in, 158–159
  introduction to, 149–150
  key points on, 149
  management of, 159–163
    angiogenesis for, 153, 163
    drug therapy for, 161–162
      antiplatelet agents, 161
      vasoactive agents, 161–162

future opportunities for, 162–163
    intermittent pneumatic compression for, 163
    lifestyle modifications for, 159–161
        cigarette smoking, 159–160
        exercise, 161
    new therapies for, 162–163
    purpose of, 159
    risk modifications for, 159–161
        hypercholesterolemia, 160–161
        hyperglycemia, 160
        hypertension, 161
    spinal cord stimulation for, 162–163
    surgical intervention for, 156, 162
  predictors of progression of, 154–155
    CRP as, 151, 155
    D-dimer as, 155
    fibrinogen as, 155
    hyperhomocysteinemia as, 151, 155
    lipoprotein (a) as, 155
  risk factors for, 150–151
    age as, 150
    cigarette smoking as, 150
    diabetes as, 150–151
    ethnicity as, 150
    hyperlipidemia as, 151
    hypertension as, 151
    other, 151
    sex as, 150
  summary overview of, 163
Peripheral vascular examination, for PAD, 157
Pharmacologic therapies. See also *specific drug or category.*
  for anxiety/depression, 270, 273–274
  for bone health, in diabetes, 239
  for cardiovascular disease, following PCI, 68
  for dyslipidemia, 31–32, 49–50, 68
  for hypertension, 31, 33, 68, 108–109, 111–114
  for metabolic syndrome, 13–15
  for PAD, 161–162
    antiplatelet agents, 161
    vasoactive agents, 161–162
Pharyngeal cancer, diabetes and, 170
Phenotypes, cognitive, in anxiety/depression connection to diabetes, 276–277
    in experimental sporadic AD, 253
  of metabolic syndrome components, 2
    primary diseases associated with, 7–8
  of PCOS, 7, 126, 128–129, 131, 133–135
Physical activity. See *Exercise.*
Physical examination, for PAD, 157
Pituitary disorders, metabolic syndrome phenotypes associated with, 8
Plaque formation, in AD, 249, 251–252
  in atherosclerosis, with diabetes, 27–28, 45

Plaque (*continued*)
      microvascular, 42–44
    with PAD, 151–154
Plasminogen activator inhibitor (PAI-1), in diabetes, atherosclerosis and, 28
Platelets, in diabetes, activation in atherosclerosis, 28, 60, 154
    dysfunction of, with PAD, 153–154
Pneumatic compression, intermittent, for PAD, 163
Poliomyelitis, CNS recovery from, 258
Polycystic ovary syndrome (PCOS), **123–147**
   clinical features of, 125
      metabolic, 7, 126
      psychological, 128
      reproductive, 125–127
   definitions of, 124–125
   history of, 123–124
   in adolescence, 128, 131–132
   insulin resistance and, 132–136
     as long-term consequence, 129–130
     genetics of, 128–129, 134–135
     in vitro models of, 132–134
     in vivo models of, 134
     mechanism behind association of, 132
     pregnancy and, 131
     prevalence of, 126
     syndromes of severe, 135–136
     treatment of, 129, 131, 136–138
   key points on, 123
   long-term consequences of, 129–131
     cardiovascular disease as, 129–130
     diabetes risk as, 126, 129–130
     endometrial cancer as, 131
     hyperlipidemia as, 128, 130
     insulin resistance as, 129–130
     obesity as, 126, 130
     pregnancy complications as, 131
   metabolic features of, 126
   obesity and, 126, 130, 137–138
   phenotypes associated with, 7, 126, 128–129, 131, 133
   prevalence of, 124
   risk factors for, 128–129
   sonographic depiction of, 124
   summary overview of, 138
   treatment of, 129, 131, 136–138
Polysomnography (PSG), overnight, for OSA, 191–192, 199
P1NP, in bone turnover, diabetes and, 237
Population-specific criteria, for obesity, in metabolic syndrome, 3, 6
Population-specific prevalence, of diabetes, vitamin D impact on, 211, 225
      with cancer, 170
      with hypertension, 105, 109, 114
   of metabolic syndrome, 3, 6
   of OSA, in T2DM, 190

of PCOS, 128, 130
    adolescents and, 128, 131–132
Portal theory, of metabolic syndrome, 11
Postprandial glucose, in diabetes, cardiovascular risk assessment and, 26–27
    in PCOS, 136
Pregnancy, complications of, in PCOS, 131
Prevalence. See also *specific population entries.*
    of cancer, in T2DM, 168
    of diabetes mellitus, 25–26, 41–42, 59, 233
    of metabolic syndrome, 3, 6–8, 258
    of obesity and overweight, 2
    of OSA, in T2DM, 190
Primary diseases, metabolic syndrome phenotypes associated with, 2, 7–8
    stress syndromes caused by, 270, 277
Progenitor cell dysfunction, endothelial, in diabetes, 44–45
    vascular, in diabetes, 43–45
Progesterone, in PCOS, 137
Proinflammatory markers/pathways, in AD, 249, 254–255
    in diabetes, cancer and, 177–179
        hypertension and, 106–107
    of atherosclerosis, 152
    OSA impact on, 192–194
        adipose tissue and, 195
    white adipose secretions in, GCs regulation of, 81, 88
Prostate cancer, diabetes and, 169–170, 172, 174
Protein kinase C (PKC), in diabetes, with PAD, 154
Proteins. See also *specific protein.*
    cytoskeletal accumulations of, in AD, 249–251
Proteinuria, in diabetes, cardiovascular risk assessment and, 27
Psychiatric medications, diabetes and, effects of, 270, 273
        risk/benefit analysis of, 273–274
Psychiatric syndromes, related to stress, 270–271
Psychiatric-medical illness, diabetes connection to, 270–271, 276–277
Psychogenic models, of anxiety/depression connection to diabetes, 271–272
Psychological features, of PCOS, 128
Psychosocial costs, of diabetes, 269–270. See also *Anxiety; Depression.*
    of hypertension, in T2DM, 105
P13K pathway activation, cancer and, 173–175
    in brain insulin/IGF signaling, 248
Pubarche, premature, in PCOS, 128
Pulse examination, for PAD, 157

R

RAAS. See *Renin-angiotensin-aldosterone system (RAAS).*
Radial artery grafts, for CABG, 63–64
RAGE (receptor of advanced glycation end products), in diabetes, bone and, 235
        vasculature and, 43–44, 60
Reactive oxygen species (ROS), in diabetes, cardiomyopathy and, 46–47
        hypertension and, 106
        vascular pathogenesis and, 42–43

Reactive (*continued*)
  in metabolic syndrome, 11–12
  in OSA, 192–194
Redox-sensitive cellular signaling pathways, OSA impact on, 192–195
Renal cancer, diabetes and, 170
Renal denervation (RDN), for hypertension, 115
Renal disease, in diabetes, cardiovascular risk assessment and, 27, 32
    hypertension and, 103–104, 106–107
      incretin-based therapy effect on, 113–114
      RAAS blockade effect on, 111–112
      treatment of, 108–109
    pathogenesis of, 42
Renal insufficiency, chronic, as PAD risk factor, 151
Renin-angiotensin system, activation of, in diabetic cardiomyopathy, 47
Renin-angiotensin-aldosterone system (RAAS), in diabetes, cardiovascular disease risk
  mitigation, 33
    hypertension and, 105–106
      blockade agents for, 111–112
      vitamin D impact on, 209
    in metabolic syndrome, obesity and, 11, 15
Reoxygenation, in OSA, 192–193
Reperfusion techniques, for PAD, 162
Reproductive system, PCOS and, 125–127
    in definition, 124–125
    severe insulin resistance syndromes and, 135–136
Respiratory effort assessment, for OSA, 191, 199
Revascularization, for cardiovascular disease. See *Coronary artery bypass graft (CABG).*
  for PAD, 156, 162
Reverse causal model, of anxiety/depression connection to diabetes, 271–272
Reverse cholesterol transport, impaired, in diabetes, 43, 45
Risk assessment, of cardiovascular events, in diabetes, 26–27
    with CABG, 64–65
    with hypertension, 103–105
Risk factors. See *specific pathology or factor.*
Risk mitigation/modification, for cardiovascular events, in diabetes, 28–34
      aspirin as, 33
      CHD diagnosis in asymptomatic patients as, 33–34
      glycemic control as, 28–31
      hypertension control as, 32–33
      lipid-lowering therapy as, 31–32
      revascularization as, 34
  for PAD, 159–161
    hypercholesterolemia in, 160–161
    hyperglycemia in, 160
    hypertension in, 161
Risk/benefit analysis, of antidepressants and antipsychotics, diabetes and, 273–274
  of revascularization treatment, for CAD, 60–63, 67–68
Rosiglitazone, for diabetes, fracture risk and, 237
  for insulin resistance, in PCOS, 137–138
Rotterdam criteria, for PCOS, 124–125
Rutherford classification, of intermittent claudication, 156

S

Salt-sensitivity, in obesity, 15
Saphenous vein grafts, for CABG, 63–64
Satiety signaling in brain, 13, 85
Sclerostin, in diabetes, bone loss and, 235
Secretory profile, of white adipose. See also *specific hormone.*
    GCs regulation of, 80–81
Sedentary lifestyle, in metabolic syndrome, 10–11
Seizures, from insulin-related hypoglycemia, 275
Selective serotonin reuptake inhibitors (SSRIs), for depression, diabetes and, 273–274
Serotonin and norepinephrine reuptake inhibitors (SNRIs), for depression, diabetes and, 274–275
Sex. See *Gender.*
SHEP trial, on hypertension, in diabetes, 108
Sitagliptin, for hypertension, 113–114
Site-specific prevalence, of cancer, in diabetes, 169–170
Skeletal muscle mass, GCs regulation of, 76, 82
    insulin role in, 246–247
    vitamin D impact on, 208–210
Skeleton. See *Bone entries.*
Sleep apnea, obstructive, **187–204**. See also *Obstructive sleep apnea (OSA).*
Sleep fragmentation, insulin resistance linked to, 195–196
Sleep Heart Health Study (SHHS), 187–188, 190
Small interfering RNA (siRNA), of neurodegeneration, in experimental models of insulin resistance, 253–254
Smooth muscle cells (SMCs), vascular, in atherosclerosis, 151–152
        in diabetes, 43–44
            hypertension and, 106
Snoring, in OSA, 188, 198–199
Social costs, of diabetes, 269–270. See also *Anxiety; Depression.*
    of hypertension, in T2DM, 105
Sodium intake restriction, for hypertension, 110
    low-salt diet, for metabolic syndrome, 14
Sodium metabolism/transport, in diabetes, hypertension and, 106–107
Sodium-glucose cotransporter-2 (SGC-2) inhibitors, for diabetes, cardiovascular disease risk mitigation, 31
Sodium-hydrogen transporter type 3 (NH3), incretin-based therapy effect on, 113–114
Somatomedin C, 247. See also *Insulin-like growth factors (IGFs).*
Spinal cord stimulation, for PAD, 162–163
Spine fractures, in diabetes, 234–236, 239
Spironolactone, for insulin resistance, in PCOS, 137–138
Statins, for cardiovascular disease, in diabetes, 31–32, 49–50
        effect on PCI outcomes, 68
    in metabolic syndrome, 14–15
Steatohepatitis, nonalcoholic, brain insulin resistance in AD associated with, 258–260
Steatosis, hepatic, GCs regulation of, 83, 86
        11β-HSD1 inhibition effect on, 86
    streptozotocin and, 253
Stents, for cardiovascular disease, 34
    bare-metal, 60, 68

Stents (*continued*)
    drug-eluting, 50, 52
        CABG vs., 60–65
      with PCI, 67–68
  for PAD, angioplasty with/without, 162
STOP-Bang questionnaire, for OSA, 198–199
Streptozotocin, in experimental models of T3DM, 253–254
Stress, AD associated with, 257–258
  glucocorticoid excess and, 76
  oxidative. See *Oxidative stress.*
Stress syndromes, leading to anxiety/depression, 270–272
Stress testing. See *Treadmill exercise test.*
Substrate metabolism, altered, in diabetic cardiomyopathy, 46–47
  glucocorticoids function in, 76–77
    insulin resistance and, 76
Sulfonylureas, for diabetes, as depression and anxiety risk, 275
    cardiovascular disease risk mitigation, 29, 31
Surgical intervention/technologies, for CAD. See *Coronary artery bypass graft (CABG)*;
  Percutaneous coronary intervention (PCI).
  for depression, diabetes and, 275
  for PAD, 162
Sympathetic nervous system, in diabetes, hypertension and, 106
    renal denervation of, 115
  in OSA, 191
    activation of, 194
Syndrome X, 1–2. See also *Metabolic syndrome (MetS).*
Syndrome Z, 191
Syndromes vs. symptoms, in anxiety/depression connection to diabetes, 276
SYNTAX study, of diabetes, effect on cardiovascular outcomes, 50, 52
    with revascularization, 61–63, 65–66
Syst-Eur trial, on hypertension, in diabetes, 108
Systolic dysfunction, in diabetic cardiomyopathy, 46–49, 52
Systolic hypertension, in diabetes, combined pharmacologic therapy for, 111, 114

T

T score, in fracture risk assessment, 237–239
T2DM. See *Type 2 diabetes mellitus (T2DM).*
Target vessel revascularization (TVR), 60–62, 66, 68
Tau, hyperphosphorylated, in AD, 246, 249, 251–252
    insulin resistance/deficiency and, 254–255
TcP$_{O2}$ (TRANSCUTANEOUS OXYGEN PRESSURE), IN PAD DIAGNOSIS, 158–159
Telehealth, for hypertension management, 114–115
Teriparatide, for osteoporosis, 239
Testosterone, in PCOS, 129, 137–138
Thalamus atrophy, in AD, 249, 251
Thiazide diuretics, for hypertension, 112
Thiazolidinediones (TZDs), for diabetes, cardiovascular disease risk mitigation, 29
    fracture risk and, 237
  for insulin resistance, in PCOS, 129, 137–138
Thoracic artery grafts, internal, for CABG, 63–64

Thrombospondin-1, in cancer and diabetes, 176–177
Thrombus, in atherosclerosis with PAD, 153–154
    treatment of, 161–162
Tissue-specific regulation mechanisms, in glucocorticoid-induced insulin resistance, 76–83
    adipose tissue, 76–85
    brain, 84–85
    liver, 82–83
    muscle, 76, 82
Toll-like receptors (TLRs), in diabetes, atherosclerosis and, 27
Transcutaneous oxygen pressure (TcP$_{O2}$), IN PAD DIAGNOSIS, 158–159
Transdiagnostic approach, to anxiety/depression connection to diabetes, 277
Treadmill exercise test, for CHD in asymptomatic patients, with diabetes, 33–34
    in PAD diagnosis, 158
Tricyclic antidepressants (TCAs), diabetes and, risk/benefit analysis of, 273–274
Tumor necrosis factor-alpha (TNF-α), in cancer and diabetes, 177–178
Tumor-growing microenvironment, in diabetes, 177–179. See also *Cancer.*
Type 1 diabetes mellitus (T1DM), anxiety/depression relationship to, 270, 273
    comparison to T2DM and T3DM, 252–253
    definition of, 234
    osteoporosis-associated fracture and, T1D vs., 234–237
        differences of, 236–237
        risk quantification of, 237
        similarities of, 234–235
    pathophysiology of, 168
    vitamin D association with, 225–226
Type 2 diabetes mellitus (T2DM), anxiety/depression relationship to, 270, 273, 275
    atherosclerosis acceleration with, 27–28. See also *Cardiovascular disease (CVD).*
    brain insulin resistance in AD associated with, 246, 255, 259
    cancer and, **167–185**
        biologic mechanisms linking, 171–177
            hyperglycemia in, 176–177
            hyperinsulinemia in, 175–176
            IGF-1 in, 172–175
            inflammation in, 178
            insulin resistance in, 175–176
            T2DM, obesity, and metabolic syndrome in, 10, 171–172
        epidemiology of, 167–171
            incidence in, 169–170
            mortality in, 170–171
            T2DM, obesity, and metabolic syndrome in, 10, 167–169
        inflammation in, 177–179
            adipokines and, 178–179
            cytokines and, 177–178
        introduction to, 167
        key points on, 167
        summary overview of, 179–180
    comparison to T1DM and T3DM, 252–253
    definition of, 234
    hypertension and, **103–122**
        burden of, 105
        epidemiology of, 105

Type 2 (*continued*)
    hyperinsulinemia in, 107
    insulin resistance in, 107
    introduction to, 103–104
    key points on, 103
    oxidative stress in, 106–107
    pathophysiology of, 105–106
    pharmacologic therapy for, 111–114
        β-blockers as, 113
        calcium channel blockers as, 112
        clinical trials on, 108–109
        combined, 111, 114
        diuretics as, 112
        incretin-based, 113–114
        RAAS blockade as, 111–112
    treatment of, 108–115
        BP targets for, 108–109
        impact of BP control, 108
        lifestyle interventions in, 109–111
        nonpharmacologic therapy in, 109–111
        pharmacologic therapy in, 111–114
        rationale, strategies, and challenges in, 107–109
        renal denervation in, 115
        telehealth in, 114–115
  metabolic syndrome and, 2
    as risk factor, 9
    cardiovascular outcomes and, 9
    genetic studies of, 12
    prevention of, 13–15
  OSA and, glycemic control in, 191
    observational studies of, 188–190
    potential pathophysiology link to, 191–192
    prevalence of, 190
    screening for, 198–199
  osteoporosis-associated fracture and, T1D vs., 234–237
        differences of, 236–237
        risk quantification of, 237
        similarities of, 234–235
  pathophysiology of, 208
  PCOS and, 126, 132
  prevalence of, 168
  vitamin D association with, biologic plausibility of, 208–210
    cross-sectional studies of status influence on, 210–211
    insulin secretion and, 208–209
    insulin sensitivity and, 208–210
    longitudinal studies of status influence on, 211–217
    supplementation influence on, 217–225
    systemic inflammation and, 209–210
Type 3 diabetes mellitus (T3DM), Alzheimer disease as, 252–253
    experimental evidence for sporadic, 253–254
  comparison to T1DM and T2DM, 252–253

U

UKPDS trial, of diabetes effect on cardiovascular outcomes, 29–30
    hypertension as, 108–109
Ulcers/ulceration, foot, with PAD, 151, 156
Ultrasound probe, Doppler, in PAD diagnosis, 158
Ultrasound scan, duplex, in PAD diagnosis, 159
Undernutrition, fetal, in PCOS, 128–129, 131
Unifying hypothesis, of cardiovascular disease, in diabetes, 43–44
Upper airway occlusion, during OSA, 191, 199
Uterus, in PCOS, 128

V

VADT trial, of diabetes effect on cardiovascular outcomes, 30
Valvular heart disease, in diabetes, 42
Vascular cell adhesion molecules (VCAMs), in atherosclerosis, 151–152
Vascular endothelial growth factor (VEGF), in hyperinsulinemia, cancer and, 175–176
Vascular grafts, for CABG, 63–64
    diseased, PCI for, 67–68
  for PAD, 162
Vascular progenitor cells (VPCs), dysfunction of, in diabetes, 43–45
  in bone marrow, 45
Vascular smooth muscle cells (VSMCs), in atherosclerosis, 151–152
  in diabetes, 43–44
    hypertension and, 106
Vascular wounds, classification of, for PAD, 157
Vasculature, diabetes and, 42–45
    cardiomyopathy findings, 48
    hypertension mechanisms in, 27, 106–107
    impaired reverse cholesterol transport, 43, 45
    microvasculature dysfunction, 44
    oxidative stress effects on, 42–44
    summary of relationships between, 42–43, 45
    vascular progenitor cell dysfunction, 43–45
  in systemic insulin-resistance diseases, 249, 252
  PAD pathophysiology of, 151–154
  PCOS and, 130
Vasoactive agents, for PAD, 161–162
Vasoconstriction, in diabetes, atherosclerosis and, 27
    hypertension and, 107
    with PAD, 154
Vasodilatation, in diabetes, hypertension and, 106–107
Vein grafts, for CABG, 63–64
    diseased, PCI for, 67–68
Ventricular dysfunction, in diabetic cardiomyopathy, 46–49, 52
Vertebral fractures, in diabetes, 234–236, 239
Virilization, in PCOS, 126–127
Vitamin D, and diabetes, **205–232**
    association with T1DM, 225–226
    association with T2DM, biologic plausibility of, 208–210

Vitamin D (*continued*)
        cross-sectional studies of status influence on, 210–211
        insulin secretion and, 208–209
        insulin sensitivity and, 208–210
        longitudinal studies of status influence on, 211–217
        supplementation influence on, 217–225
        systemic inflammation and, 209–210
    for osteoporosis, 238–239
    intake influence on, 207–208
    introduction to, 205–206
    key points on, 205
    physiology influence on, 206
    status classification in, 206–207
    summary overview of, 226–227
  physiology review of, 206
Vitamin D intake, recommendations for, 207–208
Vitamin D receptor, 208–209
Vitamin D status, classification of, 206–207
Vitamin D supplementation, influence on diabetes, 217–225
  recommendations for, 225
von Willebrand factor (vWF), PAD and, 154

W

Waist circumference (WC), in metabolic syndrome, definition comparisons of, 2–4
    prevention strategies based on, 13
    suggested cutoffs for obesity, 3, 5
  in obesity definition, 168
Weight gain, caused by antidepressants, 273–274
Weight loss, for hypertension, 110
  for insulin resistance, in PCOS, 137–138
  for metabolic syndrome, 13–15
White adipose tissue (WAT), GCs regulation of, 11β-HSD1 role in, 81–82, 85
    de novo lipogenesis, 78
    insulin sensitivity, 78–79, 88
    lipolysis, 76–78
    mass and distribution, 79–80
    secretory profile, 80–81
  hypertension and, in diabetes, 106
  hypoxia in, OSA and, 194–195
White matter atrophy, in AD, 249, 251, 255, 257
Wisconsin Sleep Cohort, 189
World Health Organization (WHO), metabolic syndrome definition of, 2, 4–5
  obesity prevalence statistics of, 2
  on diabetes trends, 269
    heart disease and, 42
  on fracture risk assessment, 237
Wound classification, vascular, for PAD, 157
Wound infection, with CABG, deep sternal, 60, 63–64
    prevention of, 66–67

X

Xanthine oxidase (XO), in diabetes, hypertension and, 106

Y

Yeast fermentation, in insulin hormone production, 246

Moving?

Make sure your subscription moves with you!

To notify us of your new address, find your **Clinics Account Number** (located on your mailing label above your name), and contact customer service at:

Email: journalscustomerservice-usa@elsevier.com

800-654-2452 (subscribers in the U.S. & Canada)
314-447-8871 (subscribers outside of the U.S. & Canada)

Fax number: 314-447-8029

Elsevier Health Sciences Division
Subscription Customer Service
3251 Riverport Lane
Maryland Heights, MO 63043

*To ensure uninterrupted delivery of your subscription, please notify us at least 4 weeks in advance of move.